GW00600831

AZAPROPAZONE
20 years of clinical use

AZAPROPAZONE
20 years of clinical use

Edited by

KD Rainsford

Department of Biomedical Sciences
McMaster University Faculty of Health Sciences
Hamilton, Ontario
Canada

KLUWER ACADEMIC PUBLISHERS
DORDRECHT / BOSTON / LONDON

Distributors

for the United States and Canada: Kluwer Academic Publishers, PO Box 358,
Accord Station, Hingham, MA 02018-0358, USA
for all other countries: Kluwer Academic Publishers Group, Distribution Center,
PO Box 322, 3300 AH Dordrecht, The Netherlands

British Library Cataloguing in Publication Data

Azapropazone.
  1. Azapropazone
  I. Rainsford, K.D. (Kim D.), 1941–
615′.7
  ISBN 0-7923-8911-5

Copyright

Published in the United Kingdom by Kluwer Academic Publishers,
PO Box 55, Lancaster, UK.

Kluwer Academic Publishers BV incorporates the publishing programmes of D.
Reidel, Martinus Nijhoff, Dr W. Junk and MTP Press.

Printed in Great Britain by Butler and Tanner Ltd., Frome and London.

CONTENTS

List of contributors

FU Bauer
Siegfried AG
CH-4800 Zofingen
Switzerland

N Bellamy
Department of Rheumatology
Victoria Hospital, Westminster
  Campus
777 Baseline Road East
London, Ontario N6A 4G2
Canada

R Brown
Medical Products Department
E.I. duPont de Nemours and Co.
PO Box 80400, Wilmington
DE 19880
USA

K Brune
Department of Pharmacology
University of Erlangen-Nürnberg
Universitätstr. 22
D-8525 Erlangen
FRG

WW Buchanan
Department of Medicine
McMaster University Faculty of
  Health Sciences
1200 Main St W, Hamilton
Ontario L8N 3Z5
Canada

G Czerniawska-Mysik
Outpatient Allergological Clinic
City Hospital
Skawinska 8
31-066 Krakow
Poland

I ab I Davies
School of Pharmacy
Queen's University of Belfast
Belfast BT9 7BL
Northern Ireland
UK

FM Dean
Department of Chemistry
University of Liverpool
Box 147
Liverpool L69 3BX
UK

D Eggli
Leumberger Medizin Technik AG
CH-8152 Glattbrugg
Switzerland

FC Geerling
Siegfried AG
CH-4800 Zofingen
Switzerland

E Gilleman
Rheuma- und Rehabilitations Klinik
CH-3954 Leukerbad
Switzerland

F Grinlington
Rheumatic Diseases Unit
University of Edinburgh
Northern General Hospital
Edinburgh EH5 2DQ
UK

JL Heidecker
Department of Medical Services
Siegfried AG
CH-4800 Zofingen
Switzerland

A Hemingway
Department of Diagnostic Radiology
Royal Hallamshire Hospital
Sheffield
S10 2JF
UK

JF Hort
A H Robins Co. Ltd.
Sussex Manor Business Park
Gatwick Road
Crawley, W. Sussex RH10 2NH
UK

U Jahn
Department of Biology
Siegfried AG
CH-4800 Zofingen
Switzerland

RM Knabb
Medical Products Department
E.I. duPont de Nemours and Co.
PO Box 80400, Wilmington
DE 19880
USA

O Knüsel
Stv. Chefarzt der Rheumaklinik
 Zurzach
Quellenstrasse
CH-8437 Zurzach
Switzerland

GM Lam
E.I. duPont de Nemours and
 Company (Inc.)
Medical Products Department
Pharmaceuticals Division
Drug Metabolism Section
Stine-Haskell Research Center
Elkton Road
Newark DE 19714
USA

EM Lemmel
Staatliches Rheumakrankenhaus
Baden-Baden
FRG

F Low
X-ray Department
West Middlesex University Hospital
Isleworth TW7 6AF
UK

WM Mackin
Medical Products Department
E.I. duPont de Nemours and Co.
PO Box 80400, Wilmington
DE 19880
USA

KK Maggon
Medical Products Department
Clinical Research
Du Pont de Nemours International
PO Box 50
1218 Le Grand Saconnex
Switzerland

K McCormack
McCormack Ltd.
Church House
Church Square
Leighton Buzzard, Beds LU7 7AE
UK

JC McElnay
School of Pharmacy
Queen's University of Belfast
97 Lisburn Road
Belfast BT9 7BL, Northern Ireland
UK

SA Mousa
Medical Products Department
E.I. duPont de Nemours and Co.
PO Box 80400, Wilmington
DE 19880
USA

FU Niethard
Orthopädische Universitätsklinik
Schlierbacher Landstrasse
D-6900 Heidelberg
FRG

E Nizankowska
Department of Allergy and Clinical
 Immunology
Copernicus Academy of Medicine
Skawinska 8
31-066 Krakow
Poland

G Nuki
Rheumatic Diseases Unit
University of Edinburgh
Northern General Hospital
Edinburgh EH5 2DQ
UK

J Palit
Rheumatic Diseases Unit
University of Edinburgh
Northern General Hospital
Edinburgh EH5 2DQ
UK

JA Pfister
Clinique Rheumatologique
Lavey-les-Bains
Switzerland

KD Rainsford
Dept of Biomedical Sciences
McMaster University Faculty of
  Health Sciences
1200 Main St W, Hamilton
Ontario L8N 3Z5
Canada

S Rashad
Department of Orthopaedic Surgery
West Middlesex University Hospital
Isleworth TW7 6AF
UK

P Revell
Bone and Joint Research Unit
The London Hospital Medical College
London E1 2AD
UK

JG Riddell
School of Pharmacy
Queen's University of Belfast
Belfast BT9 7BL
Northern Ireland
UK

E Schneider
Orthopädische Universitätsklinik
Schlierbacher Landstrasse 200a
D-6900 Heidelberg
FRG

CH Schneider
University of Bern
Institute for Clinical Immunology
Inselspital
CH-3010 Bern
Switzerland

B Simon
Ruprecht-Karls-Universität
  Heidelberg
Medizinische Klinik
Abt. 1.1.4 Gastroenterologie
Bergheimerstrasse 58
D-6900 Heidelberg
FRG

A Szczeklik
Department of Allergy and Clinical
  Immunology
Copernicus Academy of Medicine
Skawinska 8
31-066 Krakow
Poland

MJM Thoolen
Medical Products Department/NEN
E.I. duPont de Nemours and Co.
N. Billerica
Mass.
USA

PBMWM Timmermans
Medical Products Department
E.I. duPont de Nemours and Co.
PO Box 80400, Wilmington
DE 19880
USA

P Turlapaty
Medical Products Department
E.I. duPont de Nemours and Co.
PO Box 80400, Wilmington
DE 19880
USA

M Waldburger
Hôpital cantonal
Fribourg
Switzerland

FS Walker
A H Robins Co. Ltd.
Sussex Manor Business Park
Gatwick Road
Crawley, W. Sussex RH10 2NH
UK

RD Smith
Medical Products Department
E.I. duPont de Nemours and Co.
PO Box 80400, Wilmington
DE 19880
USA

H Spring
Rheuma- und Rehabilitations Klinik
CH-3954 Leukerbad
Switzerland

J Steens
Rumelinbackweg 20
CH-4054 Basel
Switzerland

R Wallace
Rheumatic Diseases Unit
University of Edinburgh
Northern General Hospital
Edinburgh EH5 2DQ
UK

A Wright
School of Pharmacy
Queen's University of Belfast
Belfast BT9 7BL
Northern Ireland
UK

Preface

Azapropazone is a chemically unique non-steroidal anti-inflammatory drug (benzotriazine oxide) which has found successful clinical applications in the therapy of a wide variety of arthritic conditions. This book summarizes the progress and critically reviews the clinical use and experimental studies since its introduction 20 years ago.

Several studies focus on the physiochemical, pharmacological and toxicological properties of this drug. The studies suggest that it has some unique properties compared with other non-steroidal anti-inflammatory drugs. Among these the novel observations are that azapropazone inhibits several non-prostaglandin-related leucocyte functions, especially superoxide anion production. These serve as a basis for investigations which are reviewed showing the potential for the drug to prevent the pathological consequencies of myocardial ischaemia.

The preparation of this book would not have been possible without the cooperation of the four companies who produce, market, or have research involvement with azapropazone, namely Siegfried AG (the manufacturers of the drug), A.H. Robins (U.K.) Co. Ltd., Robapharm AG (Switzerland) and E.I. duPont de Nemours (U.S.A., Switzerland and F.R.G.).

I thank, in particular, Dr J.F. Hort and Mr F.S. Walker of A.H. Robins (U.K.) Co. Ltd., Drs J. Heidecker and A. von Korponay of Siegfried AG and Dr K.K. Maggon of E.I. duPont Europe (Geneva) for their invaluable help in organizing the contributions and their esteemed advice. My thanks also to the Publishing Director at Kluwer Academic Publishers, Lancaster, UK, Dr Peter Clarke, and his Editor, Mr Phil Johnstone, for all their efforts and also those of their colleagues which have enabled smooth publication of this volume. Finally, my sincere thanks to the contributors who had to meet strict deadlines against the inevitable problem of competing professional and practical needs, and the editorial help of Mrs Veronica Rainsford-Koechli.

K.D. Rainsford, PhD, MRCPath, FRSC
Professor of Pharmacology and Pathology
Director — Pharmacology of Rheumatic Diseases
McMaster University Faculty of Health Sciences
Hamilton, Ontario, Canada, L8N 3Z5

Azapropazone – 20 years of clinical use. Rainsford, KD (ed)
© Kluwer Academic Publishers. Printed in Great Britain

Section I
EXPERIMENTAL

Section 1
EXPERIMENTAL

1

Introduction to therapy with azapropazone

KD Rainsford

Azapropazone was one of the early representatives of the class of non-steroidal anti-inflammatory drugs (NSAIDs) to be introduced following phenylbutazone and indomethacin. In the true sense of the words it has certainly stood the test of time, especially in the wake of withdrawals of well over 15% of the 100 or so NSAIDs which appeared during the two decades[1] following its introduction. This period was one of discovering the intrinsic toxicities in man of the NSAIDs and of critical medico-legal and political issues which followed the withdrawal of a number of NSAIDs; all of those which survived have received critical evaluation, not the least of which has been azapropazone.

The drug was initially introduced into a number of European countries and there has found steady acceptance. Two attempts were made to introduce it into the USA, but without success. Initially, AH Robins Incorporated, in Richmond, performed some toxicological studies and found that the drug was relatively toxic to the gastrointestinal (GI) tract in pure bred dogs. This problem is not unusual, for species variations in GI ulcerogenicity and indeed other toxic reactions are not uncommon with the NSAIDs. Dogs in particular are particularly capricious. For this and for other reasons, the drug was not marketed by that company in the USA. However, perseverance by the UK branch of that company led to improved understanding of the toxicological profile, and with studies on the pharmacokinetics of the drug in different species by the parent company which developed the drug, Siegfried AG, as well as by AH Robins (UK) Co. Ltd., an improved understanding of what can be regarded as species-specific or rational toxicity was obtained. The clinical success and safety profile of this drug in humans have given ample justification of the considerable amount of preclinical data which was derived during the 1970s. Aspects of these preclinical studies have been comprehensively reviewed by Walker[2] and details of the preclinical and later clinical studies to date will be found in this book.

A second attempt to introduce the drug in the USA was made recently by EI duPont de Nemours (Wilmington, DE). Here it was considered for use in the therapy of gout and is being evaluated currently as a potential protective agent in ischaemic reactions accompanying myocardial infarction

Azapropazone – 20 years of clinical use. Rainsford, KD (ed)
© Kluwer Academic Publishers. Printed in Great Britain

and other forms of oxyradical-induced tissue injury. Oxygen radicals have found a particularly important place in the initiation of cell injury in a wide variety of conditions and the exciting prospect that their production can be controlled or effects limited by drugs such as azapropazone is an impetus for further research. It should not be forgotten, however, that there are complex consequences of a range of biochemical events (including oxyradical generation) and of various cellular manifestations, immune reactions and so forth which emanate from myocardial infarction. Thus, we should not be surprised if there are limited outcomes from the attempt to control such early events. We may also find that drugs may have multiple actions and this is certainly true with azapropazone. A number of chapters in this book address this respect.

A wealth of clinical studies has been performed on azapropazone, principally in European centres. The evaluation of these has been undertaken with diligence by authorities in the field who have had extensive experience with azapropazone and other NSAIDs. Comparing azapropazone with others of its class is important, for we wish to know what are the main features of the drug. How the balancing act of dealing with side-effects can be conjured to seek out the drug which is most suitable for the patient, especially those susceptible to side-effects (e.g. the elderly or infirm patient), is also important. Finally, it is important to understand the mode of action and pharmacokinetics of the drug so that it can be exploited to enable application to be optimized to reduce the occurrence of side-effects, improve its efficacy and possibly enable us to use the drug for inflammatory conditions other than arthritis. All these aspects are considered in this volume.

In the absence of a detailed account of the history of the development of azapropazone I feel bound to give a brief outline. The reader may wish to refer to the detailed review by Walker[2] which gives an overview of the early development of this drug.

Dr Georg Mixich, the chemist who developed azapropazone, was largely influenced in his thinking about the design of azapropazone by the preceding development of phenylbutazone, both being keto-enolic acids. In fact so close was the thinking, that azapropazone was misclassified as a pyrazolone by Mixich himself, a fallacy which has been corrected only recently[3], following re-evaluation of the chemical properties, especially by comparing the hydrolytic behaviour of azapropazone with that of phenylbutazone. Thus azapropazone is precisely catagorized as a benzotriazine. This is strictly correct from a historic context, since it was the experience of the chemistry of benzotriazines which led Mixich to consider their potential as anti-inflammatory drugs. One wonders why Mixich considered azapropazone as a pyrazolone in the first place when he had the evidence of the hydrolytic behaviour under acidic and alkaline conditions before his eyes! Perhaps the success of the Geigy product was all too great a lure for this modest man?

In determining the pharmacological, pharmacokinetic and toxicological profile of the drug there was clearly a need for undertaking detailed studies. The reader interested in these early studies is referred to the work of Jahn, Wagner–Jauregg and their co-workers[2,4–6], especially detailed structure–activity comparisons.

References

1. Rainsford, KD (1987). Introduction and historical aspects of the side-effects of anti-inflammatory analgesic drugs. In: Rainsford, KD and Velo, GP (eds). *Side Effects of Anti-Inflammatory Drugs.*, Vol. I (Lancaster, UK: MTP Press) pp. 3–26

2. Walker, FS (1985). Azapropazone and related benzotriazines. In: Rainsford, KD (ed.) *Anti-Inflammatory and Anti-Rheumatic Drugs*, Vol. II. (Boca Raton, Fl: CRC Press), pp. 1–32

3. Walker, FS (1987). Azapropazone is not a pyrazolidine derivative. In: Rainsford, KD and Velo, GP (eds) *Side Effects of Anti-inflammatory Drug* (Lancaster, UK: MTP Press), pp. 431–8

4. Jahn, U and Adrian, RW (1969). Pharmakologische und toxikologische Prüfung des neuen Antiphlogisticums Azapropazon = 3-dimethylamino-7-methyl-1,2-(n-propylmalonyl)-1,2-dihydro-1,2,4-benzotriazin. *Arzneim-Forsch*, **19**, 36–52

5. Wagner–Jauregg, Th, Jahn, U and Bürlimann, W (1973). Fibrinolytische Anti-rheumatika. Vergleich von Substanzen der Flufenamsäure-Reiche mit Trifluormethyl-Analogen des Azapropazon. *Arzneim-Forsch*, **23**, 911–3

6. Jahn, and Wagner–Jauregg, Th (1974). Wirkungsvergleich saurer Antiphlogistika im Bradykinin-, UV-Erythem- und Rattenpfotenödem-test. *Arzneim-Forsch*, **24**, 494–9

Azapropazon war einer der ersten Vertreter der Klasse der nicht-steroidalen Antirheumatika (NSAR) und wurde nach Phenylbutazon und Indometacin eingeführt. Es hat im wahrsten Sinne des Wortes die Zeit überdauert, wenn man bedenkt, daß über 15% der ca. 100 NSAR, die in den 20 Jahren nach seiner Einführung auf den Markt kamen, bereits wieder aus dem Verkehr gezogen worden sind. In dieser Zeit entdeckte man die intrinsische Toxizität der NSAR beim Menschen und setzte sich mit den kritischen medizinischen, rechtlichen und politischen Fragen auseinander, die sich nach dem Verbot mehrerer NSAR[1] ergaben. Die übriggebliebenen Arzneimittel wurden einer kritischen Prüfung unterzogen, so auch Azapropazon.

Das Arzneimittel wurde zunächst in einigen europäischen Ländern eingeführt und dort als Therapeutikum für eine Reihe rheumatischer und anderer schmerzhafter Erkrankungen anerkannt. Zwei Versuche, das Arzneimittel auch in den USA einzuführen, blieben erfolglos. Die ersten toxikologischen Studien wurden von A. H. Robins Co. Ltd. in Richmond durchgeführt, wobei sich herausstellte, daß die Substanz bei einer bestimmten Hunderasse eine relativ starke toxische Wirkung auf den Magen-Darm-Trakt hatte. Speziesspezifische Schwankungen sind bei der gastro-intestinalen Ulzerogenität nicht ungewöhnlich und bei den NSAR können durchaus auch andere toxische Wirkungen auftreten. Hunde haben sich in dieser Beziehung als besonders unberechenbar erwiesen. Das ist einer der Gründe, warum der Wirkstoff von dieser Firma nicht in den USA auf den Markt gebracht wurde. Die fortgesetzten Bemühungen der britischen Tochtergesellschaft dieser Firma führten jedoch zu einem wesentlich besseren Verständnis des toxikologischen Profils von Azapropazon. Durch pharmakokinetische Studien an verschiedenen Spezies, die vom Stammhaus der Siegfried AG, das die Substanz entwickelt hatte, und von A. H. Robins (U.K.) Co. Ltd. durchgeführt wurden, gelangte man zu einem besseren Verständnis dessen, was als speziesspezifische oder wissenschaftlich begründete Toxizität betrachtet werden kann. Der klinische Erfolg und das Sicherheitsprofil dieser Substanz beim Menschen haben das umfangreiche präklinische Datenmaterial, das während der 70er Jahre zusammengetragen wurde, als durchaus gerechtfertigt erscheinen lassen. Walker[2] beschäftigte sich ausführlich mit den Gesichtspunkten dieser präklinischen Studien; dieses Buch enthält auch Näheres zu den präklinischen Studien und den bisher durchgeführten klinischen Studien.

Vor kurzem unternahm E.I. duPont de Nemours (Wilmington, DE) einen zweiten Versuch, das Arzneimittel in den USA einzuführen. In diesem Fall sollte die Substanz bei der Gicht-Behandlung eingesetzt werden. Azapropazon wird gegenwärtig auch im Hinblick auf seine Eignung als Arzneimittel zur Vorbeugung ischämischer Reaktionen bei Myokardinfarkt und anderen Formen von Gewebsschädigung, die durch Sauerstoffradikale hervorgerufen werden, geprüft. Den Sauerstoffradikalen kommt eine besondere Bedeutung bei der Einleitung von Zellschädigungen bei verschiedenen Krankheitsbildern zu und die vielversprechende Aussicht, daß die Bildung dieser Sauerstoffradikale kontrolliert oder ihre Wirkung durch Substanzen wie Azapropazon zumindest eingeschränkt werden könnte, ist ein Anstoß für weitere Untersuchungen. Man darf jedoch nicht vergessen, daß biochemische Vorgänge komplexe Auswirkungen haben (wie z.B. die Bildung von Sauerstoffradikalen), und daß ein Myokardinfarkt verschiedene zelluläre Manifestationen, Immunreaktionen usw. nach sich zieht. Es sollte uns daher nicht überraschen, wenn Versuche, diese zu einem frühen Zeitpunkt auftretenden Ereignisse unter Kontrolle zu bringen, nur einen begrenzten Erfolg haben. Wir werden vielleicht auch feststellen, daß ein und dieselbe Substanz viele verschiedene Wirkungen haben kann. Im Fall von Azapropazon trifft das sicherlich zu. Einige Kapitel in diesem Buch befassen sich mit diesem Gesichtspunkt.

Mit Azapropazon wurden zahlreiche Studien durchgeführt, und zwar vor allem in Europa. Die Ergebnisse wurden von Experten, die große Erfahrung mit Azapropazon und anderen NSAR hatten, sorgfältig ausgewertet. Der Vergleich von Azapropazon mit anderen Substanzen dieser Klasse ist wichtig, weil wir die Hauptmerkmale der Substanz kennenlernen wollen. Weiterhin ist es wichtig, herauszufinden, wie das heikle Thema der Nebenwirkungen als Entscheidungshilfe für die Wahl der für bestimmte Patienten am besten geeigneten Arzneimittel nutzbar gemacht werden kann, wobei speziell Patienten, die für Nebenwirkungen sehr empfindlich sind (wie z.B. ältere oder sehr gebrechliche Patienten), im Vordergund stehen. Schließlich ist es wichtig, die Wirkungsweise und die Pharmakokinetik der Substanz zu verstehen, so daß dieses Wissen zur Optimierung der Arzneimittel-Anwendung genutzt werden kann, mit dem Ziel, die Nebenwirkungen zu verringern, die Wirksamkeit des Arzneimittels zu verbessern und es möglicherweise auch für andere entzündliche Krankheitsbilder neben der Arthritis einzusetzen. Viele dieser Gesichtspunkte werden in diesem Buch abgehandelt.

Die Geschichte der Entwicklung von Azapropazon soll hier nicht in allen Einzelheiten behandelt werden, aber ich möchte Ihnen trotzdem einen kurzen Abriß geben. Der interessierte Leser wird auf das Buch von Walker[2] verwiesen, das einen ausführlicheren Überblick über die frühen Entwicklungsstadien der Substanz gibt.

Der Chemiker Dr. Georg Mixich, der Azapropazons entwickelte, war hinsichtlich der Struktur des Azapropazons in seiner Denkweise stark von der vorausgegangenen Entwicklung des Phenylbutazons beeinflußt, da es sich bei beiden Substanzen um Keto-Enol-Säuren handelte. Die Annäherung an das Phenylbutazon war in der Tat so groß, daß Azapropazon zunächst von Mixich selbst fälschlicherweise als Pyrazolon eingestuft wurde. Dieser Irrtum wurde erst vor kurzem nach erneuter Überprüfung der chemischen Eigenschaften aufgeklärt, wozu insbesondere der Vergleich der hydrolytischen Eigenschaften von Azapropazon mit denen des Phenylbutazons beitrug. Danach wurde Azapropazon korrekterweise als Benzotriazin eingestuft. Vom historischen Kontext her ist das strenggenommen richtig, da Mixich durch die Kenntnis der chemischen Zusammensetzung der Benzotriazine auf den Gedanken kam, das Potential dieser Substanzgruppe als entzündungshemmende Arzneimittel zu untersuchen. Man fragt sich allerdings, warum Mixich Azapropazon überhaupt erst als Pyrazolon eingestuft hat, wo er doch die Beweise für die hydrolytischen Eigenschaften der Substanz unter sauren und basischen Bedingungen vor Augen hatte! Vielleicht war der Erfolg des Geigy Produktes für diesen bescheidenen Mann doch eine allzu große Versuchung?

Bei der Bestimmung des pharmakologischen, pharmakokinetischen und toxikologischen Profils der Substanz wurde deutlich, wie notwendig genauere Untersuchungen waren. Der Leser, der sich für diese ersten Studien interessiert, wird auf die Arbeiten von Jahn, Wagner-Jauregg und Mitarbeitern[2,4–6] und insbesondere auf den detaillierten Struktur/Wirksamkeits-Vergleich verwiesen. Diese Studien bereiteten eine wertvolle Basis für das Verständnis der Eigenschaften der Benzotriazine als Klasse antirheumatischer Substanzen. 20 Jahre weitreichender therapeutischer Anwendung sind Rechtfertigung genug für den Erfolg des Arzneimittels.

6

L'azapropazone est l'un des premiers produits de la classe des anti-inflammatoires non stéroïdiens (AINS) introduits après la phénylbutazone et l'indométacine. Littéralement, "elle a bien supporté l'épreuve du temps", particulièrement à la suite du retrait de plus de 15% des quelques 100 AINS qui ont fait leur apparition sur le marché pendant les deux décades consécutives à l'introduction de l'azapropazone. Cette période fut celle de la découverte de la toxicité intrinsèque des AINS chez l'homme et de sérieux problèmes médico-légaux et politiques qui découlèrent du retrait d'une série d'AINS[1]; ceux qui survécurent ont été sévèrement évalués, l'azapropazone n'étant pas le moindre d'entre eux.

Le produit fut introduit à l'origine dans un nombre de pays européens et y a trouvé une acceptation graduelle comme substance thérapeutique dans le traitement d'une série de maladies rhumatismales et autres affections douloureuses. On a tenté, à deux reprises, de l'introduire aux Etats-Unis, sans succès. Au début A.H. Robins Co. Ltd., de Richmond, ont réalisé des études de toxicologie et remarquèrent que le produit présentait un caractère relativement toxique au niveau des voies gastro-intestinales (GI) d'une certaine race de chiens. Ce problème n'est pas rare avec des espèces variées dans l'étude d'ulcérogénicité GI et, en fait, d'autres réactions toxiques ne sont pas inhabituelles avec les AINS. Les chiens sont particulièrement capricieux. Cette raison, parmi d'autres, a empêché la commercialisation du produit aux Etats-Unis. Toutefois, grâce à sa persévérance, la filiale britannique de cette société est parvenue à améliorer la compréhension du profil toxicologique de l'azapropazone. Des études pharmacocinétiques furent réalisées sur différentes espèces par la société principale qui développa le produit, la Siegfried SA, ainsi que par A.H. Robins (UK) Co. Ltd. Une meilleure compréhension de ce que l'on peut regarder comme toxicité spécifique de l'espèce ou toxicité rationnelle fut obtenue. Le succès clinique et le profil de sécurité de ce produit chez les êtres humains ont hautement justifié le grand nombre de données pré-cliniques que l'on a relevées au cours des années 70. Les aspects de ces études pré-cliniques ont été complètement révisés par Walker[2]; les études pré-cliniques et les études cliniques postérieures accomplies jusqu'à ce jour sont expliquées en détail dans le présent livre.

Une deuxième tentative d'introduction du produit aux Etats-Unis a récemment été réalisée par E.I. duPont de Nemours (Wilmington, DE) qui en étudia les possibilités dans le traitement de la goutte. On en examina aussi le potentiel en tant qu'agent protecteur dans les réactions ischémiques qui accompagnent l'infarctus du myocarde et d'autres formes d'affections tissulaires provoquées par les oxyradicaux. On a donné une place très importante aux radicaux oxygénés dans le processus d'initiation des lésions cellulaires sous de nombreuses conditions différentes, et la thèse captivante selon laquelle leur production pourrait être contrôlée ou leurs effets limités par des médicaments tel que l'azapropazone donne une motivation supplémentaire à la poursuite des recherches. On ne doit toutefois pas oublier les conséquences compliquées d'une série de phases biochimiques (y compris la génération oxyradicale) et les différentes manifestations cellulaires, réactions immunitaires etc. qui émanent d'un infarctus myocardiaque. Nous ne devons donc pas être surpris si les résultats de l'effort fait pour contrôler des phases aussi précoces sont limités. Nous découvrirons peut-être aussi que les médicaments ont des actions multiples, un fait certainement vrai en ce qui concerne l'azapropazone. Plusieurs chapitres de ce livre sont dédiés à cet aspect de la question.

Une grande variété d'études cliniques a été réalisée avec l'azapropazone principalement dans des centres européens. L'évaluation de ces études a été entreprise avec diligence par des autorités compétentes qui ont acquis une ample expérience dans le domaine de l'azapropazone et des AINS. La comparaison de l'azapropazone à d'autres produits de sa classe est un facteur important si nous voulons en connaître les principales caractéristiques. Il est aussi très important de savoir comment on peut arriver à un équilibre valable entre les effets secondaires d'un produit et ce même produit, s'il est aussi celui qui convient le mieux à des malades, particulièrement si ces derniers sont susceptibles aux effets secondaires (par exemple, les personnes âgées ou les infirmes). Enfin, il est important de comprendre le mode d'action et la pharmacocinétique du médicament pour qu'il puisse être exploité en permettant à son application d'être maximalisée grâce à la diminution de la fréquence des effets secondaires, l'amélioration de l'efficacité et, éventuellement, en favoriser l'emploi pour des affections inflammatoires autres que l'arthrite. Un grand nombre de ces aspects sont pris en considération dans ce livre.

Dans l'absence d'un compte-rendu détaillé de l'histoire du développement de l'azapropazone, je crois de mon devoir de donner quelques explications. Le lecteur aimera peut-être consulter la revue détaillée écrite par Walker[2] qui donne une idée d'ensemble des premiers développements de ce produit.

Dr. Georg Mixich, le chimiste qui a développé le produit, a été vivement influencé dans ses idées concernant la conception de l'azapropazone, par le développement préalable de la phénylbutazone, toutes deux étant des acides céto-énoliques. En fait, il fut tellement influencé par ces idées que l'azapropazone fut classifiée, à tort, comme pyrazolé par Mixich lui-même, une erreur qui n'a été corrigée[3] que récemment à la suite d'une ré-évaluation des propriétés chimiques, en particulier la comparaison du comportement hydrolytique de l'azapropazone avec celui de la phénylbutazone. Donc, l'azapropazone est spécifiquement classée comme benzotriazine. Ce fait est strictement correct, d'un point de vue historique, puisque c'est en analysant la chimie des benzotriazines que Mixich fut amené à considérer leur potentiel dans le traitement des affections anti-inflammatoires. On se demande pourquoi Mixich considéra l'azapropazone comme pyrazolé au départ, quand il avait devant lui la preuve du comportement hydrolytique sous des conditions acides et alcalines! Il se peut que le succès du produit Geigy était une trop grande tentation pour cet homme modeste!

En déterminant les aspects pharmacologique, pharmacocinétique et toxicologique du produit, on se rend compte qu'une recherche approfondie était nécessaire. Le lecteur que ces premières études intéressent est renvoyé aux travaux de Jahn, Wagner-Jauregg et leurs associés[2,4-6], particulièrement en ce qui concerne les comparaisons détaillées de la structure et de l'activité. Ces études ont servi de base importante dans la compréhension des propriétes des benzotriazines classifiées comme agents anti-inflammatoires. Vingt ans d'utilisation thérapeutique de l'azapropazone en justifient amplement le succès.

2

The chemical classification of azapropazone

FM Dean

I. NOMENCLATURE

The names of drugs are often formed by combining syllables taken from
chemical sources so as to produce chemical-sounding names which, however,
lack the meaning they would convey in a systematic context. Thus *aza, prop,*
and *one* are all well known syllables combined in *azapropazone* to produce
what is really a nonsense-word.

It is clear that such names are useless for classification purposes. To
supplement such names, therefore, it is common practice to classify drugs
by using subsections of the entire structure and naming them by one of the
systematic methods. Thus indomethacin (**1**; Figure 1) has been classified as
a 3-indolylacetic acid, more broadly as an arylacetic acid, and even very
broadly as just an acetic acid derivative. There are no rules about such
choices except that (where possible) the classifier is meant to indicate the
part(s) of the structure believed to influence the pharmacological activity.
Thus indomethacin (**1**) is not classified (as it certainly could be) as a derivative
of 4-chlorobenzamide or of *p*-anisidine merely because there is no current
interest in those substructures. Such choices may change as understanding
increases or even if fashion changes.

The names used for the substructures are commonly genuine chemical
names in current use and are correctly used as far as the context permits.
Here systematic nomenclature is defined by the pronouncements of IUPAC

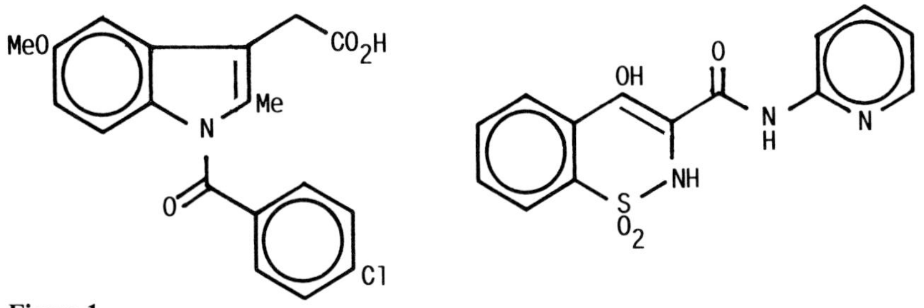

Figure 1

(1) (2)

Azapropazone – 20 years of clinical use. Rainsford, KD (ed)
© Kluwer Academic Publishers. Printed in Great Britain

and of *Chemical Abstracts* – particularly the latter, because most searches are made through its Indices and its Registry is increasingly employed to identify compounds. However, other systems are called upon if they are more familiar or more convenient. Difficulties arise when novelty is sought or where common usage differs from systematic usage. Thus the term 'oxicam' used to classify piroxicam (**2**; Figure 1) has no systematic meaning at all, while the term 'pyranocarboxylate' used to classify etodolac (**3**; Figure 2) conveys erroneous impressions when interpreted systematically.

It is important that modern systematic nomenclature is concerned only with formal structural relations; it is not itself meant to convey any chemical ideas. Indeed many practising chemists would not immediately recognize the systematic name 1,1'-oxybisethane as referring to their old friend, ether. Of course the time has long gone since names like butter of antimony, milk of magnesia, spirit of vinegar, muriate of potash . . . were used for scientific purposes, but it is still easy to expect (wrongly) that a structural name should reflect some aspect of chemistry or some kind of property. A very few words still survive that convey such ideas; we still talk about salts and acids and aromatic compounds, and the terms acid and salt still form a part of modern systematic nomenclature as well as describing groups of compounds of particular kinds. In extreme cases, systematic nomenclature makes use of names for compounds that cannot possibly exist; the Index Guide for Volume 76, Section IV, Sub-section 154, refers to 1,4-ethenonaphthacene and appends structure (**4**), for example (Figure 2). Much more common are examples where systematic nomenclature serves to obscure a simple chemical relation between well-known compounds. Whereas acetic anhydride is recognizably a derivative of acetic acid, it is not immediately obvious that 3,4-dihydrofuran-2,5-dione is a derivative (anhydride) of succinic acid or even of butandioic acid. In times past, succinic anhydride was indeed an indexed name, but nowadays it is confined to common parlance. Another example illustrating how systemization can sometimes actually separate two very closely related structures is seen in comparing (**5**) with (**6**) (Figure 3). Compound (**5**) is indexed as 4-dimethylaminobenzoic acid hydrochloride, while (**6**), far from being named as a derivative of benzoic acid, is found under 4-carboxytri-*N*-methylbenzeneaminium chloride. Evidently systematic nomenclature, excellent for its own purposes, cannot automatically provide good classifications

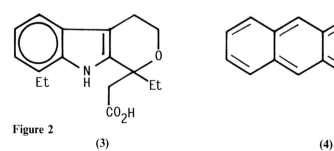

Figure 2

(3)   (4)

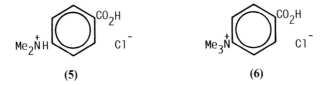

Figure 3

(5)   (6)

for pharmaceutical purposes.

A less obvious trap in classification is set by the fact that the presence in a structure of specified structural segments need not mean that the compound has certain chemical (or pharmacological) properties. The best-known example has carbonyl and hydroxy groups linked by methylene groups, i.e. $HO(CH_2)_n(C=O)R$. All such compounds do indeed behave as ketones and alcohols – except the first, with $n=0$, which is comparatively strongly acidic, difficult to oxidize, and loth to react with most carbonyl reagents. Such large differences have long persuaded chemists to put RCOOH compounds in a class of their own, the carboxylic acids. For the others in the series there are no such special classes, yet each one differs markedly from the others. Certainly, in all one can demonstrate carbonyl activity and alcohol behaviour, but when $n=1$, we have a group that confers outstanding reducing properties, when $n=2$ a group that eliminates water with ease, when $n=3$ a group that readily cyclizes to a ring like that in sugars, and so on. And all are named as x-hydroxyalkan-y-ones. Benzene provides an even more elementary example; anyone wishing to regard benzene as a triene has to justify himself very carefully, even though benzene is still commonly written as a triene with three distinguishable double bonds.

The difficulty for classification is that *any* conjunction of groups or systems is liable to produce effects in addition to, or instead of, the combined effects of the groups taken separately. Chemistry and pharmacology produce examples regularly; indeed, if that were not so, these subjects would cease to arouse so much interest or present so much difficulty. Yet some degree of classification is necessary, if only to promote economy in thought and discussion.

Turning to azapropazone (7) itself (Figure 4), we find it named in *Chemical Abstracts* as 5-dimethylamino-9-methyl-2-propyl-1*H*-pyrazolo[1,2-a][1,2,4]benzotriazine-1,3(2*H*)-dione. Although this name does not make overt reference to a pyrazolone nucleus, such a nucleus can be traced in structure (7) and so it is indisputable that the drug is *formally* a pyrazolone. Whether it is *chemically* reasonable to classify azapropazone as a pyrazolone in the same class as phenylbutazone (8; Figure 4) is a substantially different matter, to which we shall now address ourselves.

II. NMR SPECTRA

The proton NMR spectra of azapropazone and its hydrochloride in various solvents have been recorded and discussed by Fenner and Mixich[1] and by

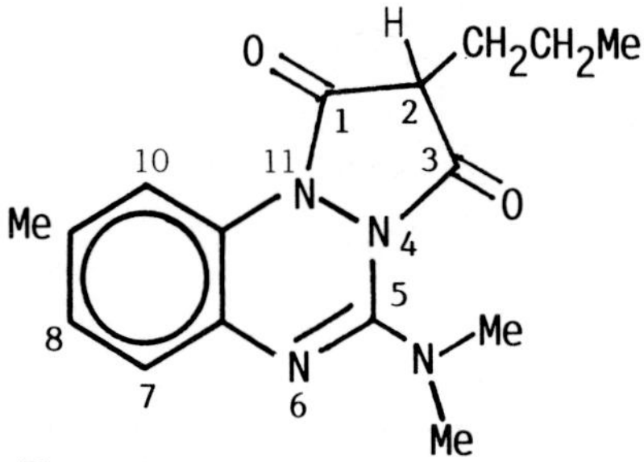

Figure 4

(7)

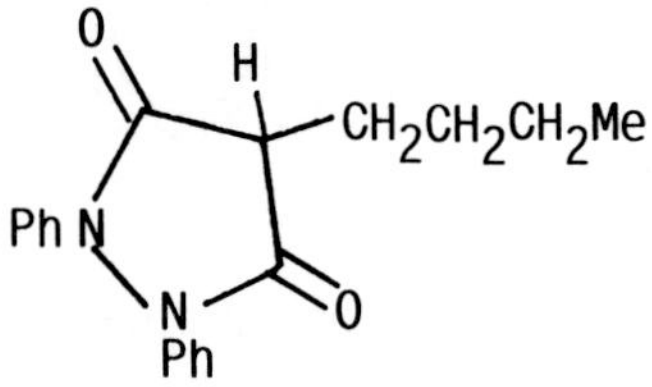

(8)

Mathieson (unpublished observations). The system is largely or entirely enolic, the two forms (9a) and (9b) being available (Figure 5). Briefly, the spectra show no signal for a proton at position 2 between the two carbonyl groups, and the signal for the adjacent methylene group is merely a triplet devoid of the extra splitting that a 2-proton would induce. The OH proton, which must be present, is not easily recognizable in the spectra, but exchange and hydrogen-bonding phenomena would account adequately for this lack. In contrast, phenylbutazone (8) gives spectra indicating that it does have a proton between the two carbonyl groups and is not enolized. Although the NMR method is not highly sensitive and azapropazone might contain a little of the non-enolized form, while phenylbutazone might contain a little of an enol, the main conclusion is supported by the UV changes that follow basification[2]. Azapropazone has long wavelength absorption which is not much changed by base, in agreement with a structure already enolic. Phenylbutazone has no such absorption until enolization is induced by alkali. In passing it should be noted that enols are normally indexed as the carbonyl tautomer; even if completely enolized, azapropazone would still be named as a pyrazolinedione derivative.

It is possible to distinguish between the two enols. The NMR spectrum of azapropazone displays a resonance for the isolated aromatic proton at position 10, which is considerably downfield (by about 1 ppm) of the two

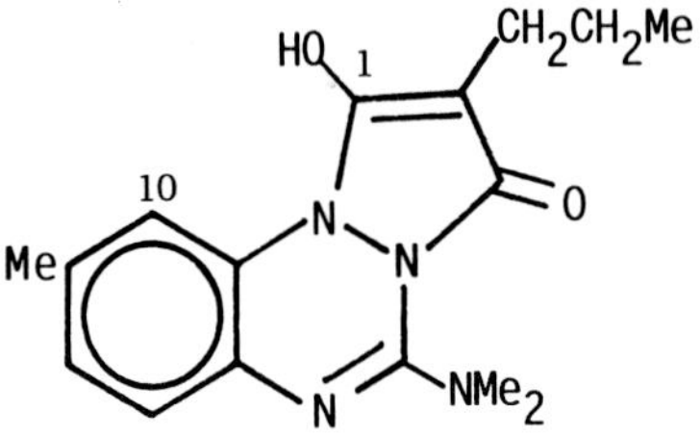

Figure 5

(9a)

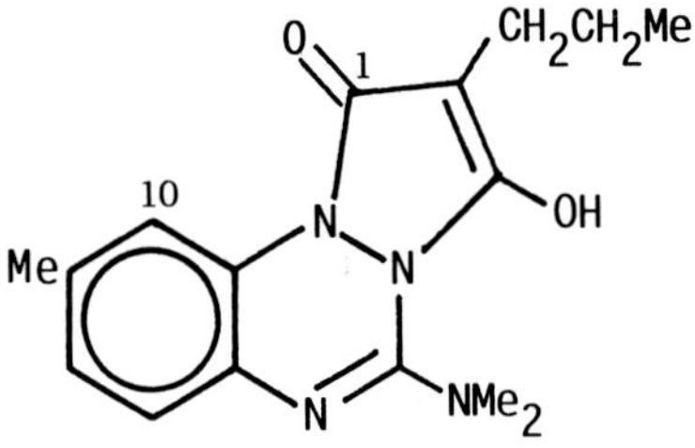

(9b)

12

other aromatic protons. This downfield shift is a strong indication that the proton lies in the deshielding cone of a carbonyl group which has to be that in position 1 of structure (**9b**). It is important that the whole ring system is flat and rigid so that the aromatic proton cannot escape the influence of this carbonyl group. Again phenylbutazone differs strongly. Structure (**10**) indicates that, if all the rings are held flat and coplaner, important collisions will result, mainly because the *ortho* hydrogens overlap seriously, and partly because they collide with the carbonyl oxygen atoms (Figure 6). Molecules generally relieve such collisions by allowing groups to rotate where possible, and here such rotation requires the two phenyl groups to move out of the pyrazolone plane and into their own planes more or less parallel to each other. Structure (**11**) attempts to show this (Figure 6). There will be chemical consequences, because the delocalization of electrons across the nitrogen–benzene link will be diminished. Some interpretations of the spectroscopic properties ignore this factor and may have to be revised[3]. Significantly, the proton NMR spectrum of phenylbutazone[1] shows that all its aromatic protons resonate at the same field; none is selectively affected by a carbonyl deshielding cone.

With azapropazone in the enolic form (**9b**) there is the possibility of hydrogen bonding between the hydroxy group and the dimethylamino nitrogen atom. This would account for the fact that only the one enol is observed. A broad signal at low field in the NMR spectrum accords with a proton in such a position[1], and the absence of this band from spectra of the hydrochloride or dihydrate supports the idea, since shifts and further broadening would result from rapid exchange phenomena.

If hydrogen bonding is to occur it must involve the nitrogen lone pair which must therefore lie in or close to the plane of the ring system. Models indicate that this is very likely even if there is no hydrogen bonding, because the methyl groups cannot remain in-plane without collisions, as shown in structure (**12**) in Figure 7. Again, the repulsive forces can be removed by allowing the dimethylamino group to rotate, bringing the methyl groups out

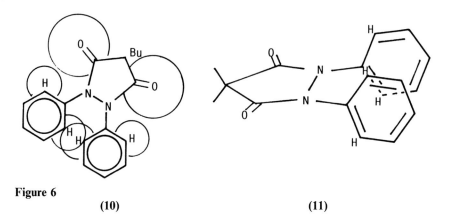

Figure 6

(**10**)   (**11**)

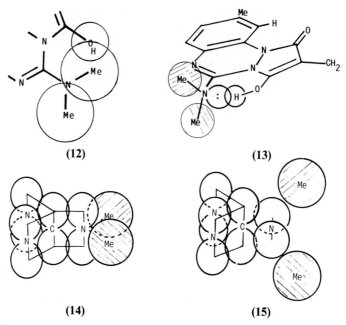

Figure 7

of the plane and putting the lone pair into it as shown in diagram **(13)** in Figure 7.

With a rotation through 90° (it might not be so large), the system is greatly altered in character; it ceases to be a guanidine system and becomes a (modified) amidine system. Diagram **(14)** shows the Y-shaped guanidine interactions before, and diagram **(15)** the V-shaped amidine interaction after, the rotation (Figure 7). A lesser consequence is that the dimethylamino nitrogen, which must be sp^2 in the guanidine arrangement, can change to sp^3 after rotation so as to improve the hydrogen bonding interaction with the OH group. Thus azapropazone must be regarded as a guanidine derivative in a formal, structural sense, while not necessarily showing guanidine behaviour.

III. IONIZATION CHARACTERISTICS

The most obvious chemical feature of guanidine derivatives is their high basicity, a fact that leads us to consider next the ionization characteristics to be expected from azapropazone. Perhaps a caution is needed here: although pK_a measurements can be made with considerable accuracy and reliability, they cannot be interpreted with a corresponding reliability. The reason is simply that one pK unit, usually regarded as a 'large' quantity, really corresponds to (say) an energy step of around 6.3 kJ/mole, a level at which many minor phenomena can contribute, so confusing every issue.

Except for situations under the closest control, even energy differences of 20 kJ/mole (about 3 pK units) can be extremely difficult to explain, not to speak of predicting them reliably. In such circumstances, it is usual to argue from the closest possible analogous situations in order to minimize the predictive element; in the case of azapropazone, no really close analogues are to hand. We are restricted to indicating trends rather than forecasting exact figures, but even this exercise is useful.

Six-membered alicyclic diones have pK_a values close to 5, a value not much altered by incorporating the carbonyl groups in ester linkages, as in meldrumic acids. Anilides tend to parallel esters in this respect. Reducing the ring size to five members has a small acidifying effect, so that tetronic acids have pK_a values near to 4 and phenylbutazone (8) with pK_a 4.5 fits neatly into this pattern. In azapropazone (7), only one of the relevant nitrogen atoms is of anilide type, leaving us to assess to contribution of the other. A simple amide nitrogen would lower the acidity, as seen in the lactam (16) which has pK_a 7.05 (Figure 8). The imine group connected to it would increase the acidity through its electron-withdrawing ability which, however, will be much smaller than that of a carbonyl group and possibly reduced further by the dimethylamino substituent which is normally electron-releasing (although, as already seen, the present situation is not normal). There is also hydrogen bonding to consider, which is another acid-weakening effect, though not a strong one except in circumstances not applicable here. We might reduce the value of 7.05 by 2 units to allow for the imine group and add 1 unit to allow for hydrogen bonding, thus arriving at a prediction of 6 for the pK_a of azapropazone. Though rough, this assessment allows us to identify the (titration) pK_a 6.5 for azapropazone as referring to the enolic dione system, notwithstanding the higher acidities of some other cyclic diones, including phenylbutazone.

Several authors have considered the possibility that azapropazone exists as some type of zwitterion. Obviously, the hydrogen bonding situation would at some point pass over into a zwitterion (17; Figure 8) depending upon the acidity of the enol and the basicity of the dimethylamino group. Even in a true guanidine system, this group would not be the basic centre; here it is disconnected as noted already. Again a very close model is elusive, but dimethylaniline with a 2-methyl substituent (to provide a steric cause

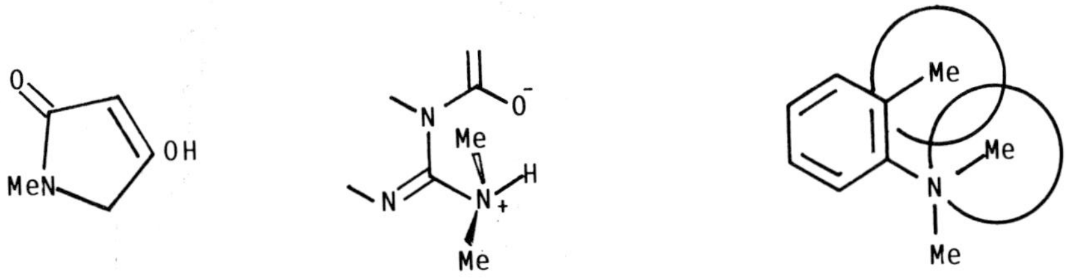

(16)   (17)   (18)

Figure 8

15

for rotation) (**18**) might be a reasonable one (Figure 8); its conjugate acid has pK_a 5.1 (in 50% ethanol). Again, an allowance has to be made for the electron-withdrawing imine group and again we lack a close precedent. Fortunately, that is not critical, because the groups concerned are directly connected and their interactions will be strong, and hardly less than the equivalent of 2 units of pK_a, from which we may conclude that the (protonated) dimethylamino group would have a pK_a substantially less than 5, making the zwitterion a stronger acid than the enol. It is unlikely, therefore, that azapropazone would exist to a significant extent as the zwitterion (**17**).

Azapropazone is obtainable as the hydrochloride. The obvious site for the protonation is the imine nitrogen at position 6, which would be the basic centre in the guanidine and also in the amidine grouping. From various tables of basicities it readily transpires that groups attached to the central carbon atom in an amidine have rather a small effect, those attached to the terminal nitrogen atoms have large one. Hence the phenylamidine (**19**; Figure 9) provides a starting-point for calculation; it has pK_a' 8.3. The centrally connected dimethylamino group will not matter much, but the terminal nitrogen is connected in various ways with the carbonyl group(s) of the enol. Yet again we have no proper parallel to call upon, but can note that acylation of guanidine causes major reductions in pK_a values (guanidine, 13.6; acetylguanidine, 8.2; diacetylguanidine, 4.9); on average, a fall of 4.5 units per acetyl group. Applied to the phenylamidine (**19**), such a fall leads to a value for azapropazone of 3.8 to which further though small corrections have to be made to allow for the two nitrogen substituents (NMe_2 and N-11) and their electronegativities. These corrections might amount to one unit in all, giving a predicted pK_a value for azapropazone hydrochloride of about 2.8.

The nitrogen atoms at positions 4 and 11 will probably be substantially less basic than the others, because they are both amidic in nature and at first sight neither is a likely contender for the protonation centre in the hydrochloride. On the other hand, we have had to make large approximations in assessing the basicity of both the imide nitrogen at position 6 and the dimethylamino nitrogen and we cannot really decide between them. Fortunately, the proton NMR spectrum provides a clear answer; in the spectrum of the hydrochloride, the signal assigned to the proton at position

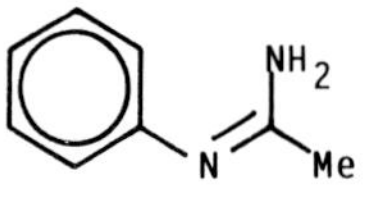

(19) 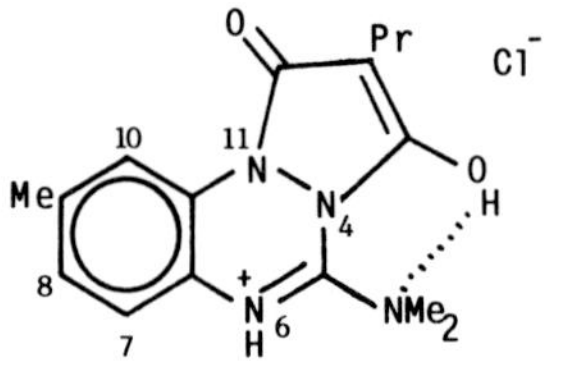   (20) 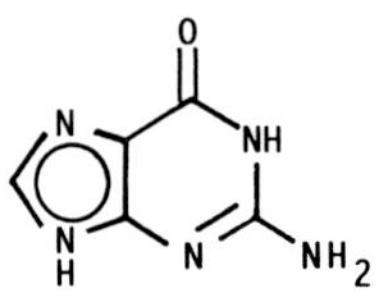   (21)

Figure 9

7 has moved downfield by about 1 ppm, leaving the other signals almost as they were. So large and specific a shift can only be attributed to protonation of the adjacent nitrogen atom at position 6, demonstrating that the structure of azapropazone hydrochloride is (20) (Figure 9). For aqueous solutions, however, the situation is less secure and there could be several equilibria in which several hetero-atoms are visited by protons, even while N-6 remains the favoured site.

As a cross-check, we can compare azapropazone component by component, or even atom by atom, with compounds such as guanine (21; Figure 9). Notwithstanding the initially dissimilar appearance, guanine maps quite well against azapropazone, except that the amino substituent is not hindered and can be fully conjugated within the guanidine grouping. The point is that guanine salts have pK_a 3.3 thus assuring us that azapropazone should have an acidity greater than this, a pK_a near 2 being quite in keeping.

IV. DIFFERENCES BETWEEN AZAPROPAZONE AND PHENYLBUTAZONE

Returning to the classification theme, we can review the differences between azapropazone and phenylbutazone and its related drugs. Though both drugs are enolic, the degree of enolization differs and, importantly, the degree of acidity differs. A major feature is the shape around the pyrazolinedione system, dictated by steric factors and not easily altered by thermal chaos or by site-fitting requirements. At higher acidities, azapropazone takes up a proton at a point that does not exist in the phenylbutazone drugs. The extra structural components in azapropazone interact with the pyrazolinedione sector which therefore cannot be considered as an entirely separate entity. There are two ways in which this consideration can be further illustrated. First, the amide link in azapropazone (a true amide link, not a disrupted one as in phenylbutazone) if written in its charge-separated canonical form as in diagram (22) can be regarded as having structural affinities with indolizine (23), one of the less common aromatic heterocyclic systems (Figure 10). Second, the enolic OH group along with the adjacent dimethylamino group offers a prime site for complexation with metals and perhaps metalloids like boron; however, this possibility has not yet been examined.

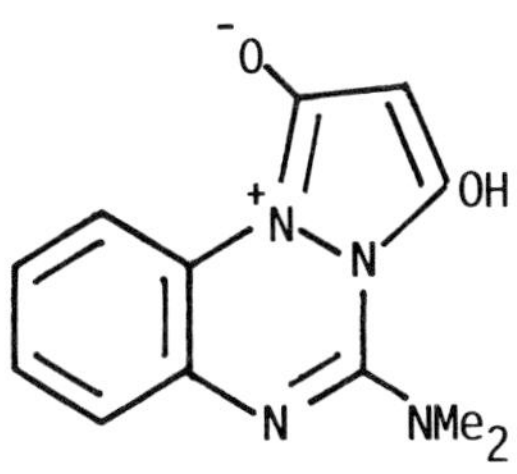

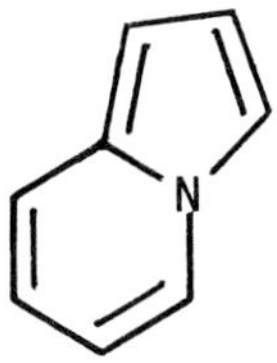

Figure 10

(22)   (23)

17

The last consideration is whether azapropazone might be degraded chemically or biologically to a compound or compounds with structures and properties more directly related to those in the phenylbutazone series. So far the evidence is against such transformations[4]. Both oxidation and hydrolysis destroy the pyrazolinedione part of azapropazone without destroying the triazine ring, which is entirely in agreement with general chemical considerations. Biological degradation involves other considerations, but to date no study appears to support the idea that the triazine ring could be modified so as to leave a (relatively) simple phenylpyrazolinedione product similar to phenylbutazone.

Acknowledgement

I thank Keith McCormack (McCormack Limited) for introducing me to the problem and assisting me with data and discussions.

References

1. Fenner, H and Mixich, G (1973). NMR studies of the molecular structure of azapropazone and interpretation of its pharmacokinetics and biotransformation. *Arzneim-Forsch*, **23**, 667–9
2. Sugiyama, H, Okazaki, T and Adachi, A (1966). Empirical studies on *in vivo* fate of azapropazone. Presented at 13th Congress of Japanese Rheumatism Society, May 16, 1966.
3. Singh, SP, Parmar, SS, Stenberg, SI and Farnum, SA (1978). Carbon-13 nuclear magnetic resonance spectra of anti-inflammatory drugs: phenylbutazone, oxyphenbutazone, and indomethacin. *J Heterocycl Chem*, **15**, 13–16
4. Mixich, G (1968). The chemical behaviour of the anti-phlogistic agent azapropazone (Mi 85). *Helv Chim Acta*, **51**, 532–8

Summary

According to the rules of nomenclature, azapropazone is a derivative of pyrazolinedione in much the same way as phenylbutazone and a resemblance between the two compounds seems obvious when their structures are written out in the usual manner. However, the rules of nomenclature are not primarily concerned with chemical properties, only with connectivity between atoms, while structures as ordinarily written often fail to indicate important electronic interactions and stereochemical features. A detailed comparison (structural, spectroscopic and chemical) of azapropazone with phenylbutazone reveals major differences.

Although azapropazone is more highly enolised than phenylbutazone it is less acidic for a variety of reasons. The two phenyl groups of phenylbutazone cannot attain planarity with the rest of the system whereas the (one) phenyl group of azapropazone is held rigidly planar; from this fact should flow both chemical (electronic) and biochemical (site fitting) differences. The dimethylamino substituent present *only* in azapropazone also has a special character; it probably has to rotate out of plane and will be able to interact with the enol that does not exist in phenylbutazone. The rotation would also probably prevent it from contributing fully to the guanidine system of which it is a part, so that this system should be less basic than the formal structure would suggest.

These considerations suggest that azapropazone should be classified separately from phenylbutazone.

Zusammenfassung

Gemäss den Regeln chemischer Nomenklatur ist Azapropazon ein Pyrazolindion-Derivat, ähnlich wie Phenylbutazon. Wird die Struktur dieser beiden Substanzen in üblicher Weise niedergeschrieben, scheint eine offensichtliche Ähnlichkeit zwischen ihnen zu bestehen. Die Regeln der Nomenklatur berücksichtigen jedoch nicht in erster Linie die chemischen Eigenschaften, sondern lediglich die Verbindungen zwischen Atomen, und aus der gewöhnlichen Niederschrift der chemischen Struktur gehen wichtige Elektronen-Interaktionen und stereochemische Eigenschaften häufig nicht hervor. Ein eingehender Vergleich von Azapropazon und Phenylbutazon bezüglich Struktur, Spektroskopie und Chemie fördert erhebliche Unterschiede zutage.

Obwohl Azapropazon stärker enolisiert ist als Phenylbutazon, ist es aus verschiedenen Gründen weniger säurebildend. Die zwei Phenylgruppen von Phenylbutazon können nicht planar zum Rest des Moleküls stehen, während sich die einzige Phenylgruppe von Azapropazon starr planar einteilt. Aus dieser Tatsache sollten sich sowohl chemische (elektronische) als auch biochemische Unterschiede (räumliche Einpassung) ergeben. Auch der *nur* bei Azapropazon vorhandene Dimethylamin-Substituent stellt ein besonderes Merkmal dar; er kann wahrscheinlich aus der Ebene rotieren und mit der Enol-OH-Gruppe in Wechselwirkung treten. Damit besteht die Möglichkeit der Chelatbildung mit Metallatomen, die bei Phenylbutazon nicht existiert. Diese Rotation hat vermutlich auch zur Folge, dass der Substituent nicht voll am Guanidin-System mitwirken kann, zu dem er gehört, so dass dieses System weniger basisch sein dürfte, als anhand der formalen Struktur zu vermuten wäre.

Aus diesen Überlegungen geht hervor, dass Azapropazon und Phenylbutazon getrennt klassifiziert werden sollten.

Resumé

Selon les règles de nomenclature, l'azapropazone est un dérivé pyrazolidine-dione très proche de la phénylbutazone, et la ressemblance entre les deux molécules semble évidente lorsque l'on compare leurs structures telles qu'elles sont reproduites habituellement. Cependant, les règles de la nomenclature ne sont pas intéressées, en principe, par les propriétés chimiques, mais seulement des liaisons entre atomes, alors que les structures habituellement représentées n'indiquent souvent ni les interactions importantes entre électrons, ni les caractéristiques stéréochimiques. Une comparaison détaillée (structurelle, spectroscopique et chimique) entre l'azapropazone et la phénylbutazone fait ressortir d'importantes différences.

Bien que l'azapropazone soit plus fortement énolisée que la phénylbutazone, elle est moins acidifiante, et ceci pour différentes raisons. Les deux groupes phényl- de la phénylbutazone ne peuvent être dans le même plan que le reste de la molécule, alors que le (seul) groupe phényl- de l'azapropazone se maintien rigidement dans le même plan; des différences chimiques (électroniques) et biochimiques (liaison au site) devraient donc en découler. Le substitutif diméthylamino- présent *uniquement* dans l'azapropazone a également un caractère particulier: il doit probablement effectuer une rotation hors du plan pour pouvoir interagir avec le groupe énol-OH et fournir un site pour les métaux chélateurs, possibilité qui n'est pas donnée dans la phénylbutazone. La rotation l'empêche probablement de contribuer entièrement au système guanine dont il fait partie, ce qui fait que ce système doit être moins basique que sa structure chimique ne le laisserait croire.

Ces considérations suggèrent que l'azapropazone devrait être classée différemment de la phénylbutazone.

3
Survey of toxicological investigations of azapropazone

U Jahn

I. INTRODUCTION

The development of azapropazone more than twenty years ago was initiated by the discovery of compounds of the 1,2-dihydro-1,2,4-benzotriazine group with marked anti-inflammatory effect. The majority of those compounds proved, however, to be rather toxic in investigations carried out in the rat. The observation that fusing alkylmalonic acids at the 1,2 position of benzotriazine reduces the toxicity of these substances without diminishing their anti-inflammatory effect was therefore a decisive step forward.

Azapropazone was selected for more detailed investigation because pharmacological screening showed it to have low toxicity and very little harmful effect on rat gastric mucosa, as well as a demonstrable anti-inflammatory effect in different animal inflammation models. The low toxicity and the mucosa-sparing effect are discussed below.

II. TOXICITY TESTS

Figure 1 shows the acute toxicity of the currently most common non-steroidal anti-inflammatory drugs (NSAIDs), in the form of their mean lethal doses (LD_{50}) after single-dose administration to rats. With an LD_{50} of 4200 mg/kg bodyweight, azapropazone is much less toxic than the reference substances.

Apart from piroxicam, which has to be given in very low doses in man on account of its long half-life, azapropazone is still in first position, even in a comparison of the LD_{50} as a multiple of the maximum therapeutic dose for a mean bodyweight of 65 kg. Table 1 shows that, with a quotient of 152, azapropazone ranks after piroxicam in front of all reference substances from different chemical classes.

Although the single-dose toxicity does not have a great bearing on long-term therapeutic administration, it is relevant for assessing the risk of accidental or intentional overdosage. In this context, it has been reported

Azapropazone – 20 years of clinical use. Rainsford, KD (ed)
© Kluwer Academic Publishers. Printed in Great Britain

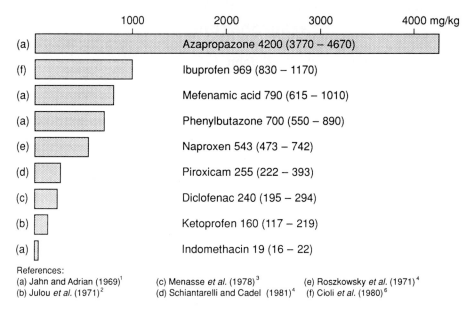

References:
(a) Jahn and Adrian (1969)[1]   (c) Menasse *et al.* (1978)[3]   (e) Roszkowsky *et al.* (1971)[4]
(b) Julou *et al.* (1971)[2]   (d) Schiantarelli and Cadel (1981)[4]   (f) Cioli *et al.* (1980)[6]

Figure 1 Acute toxicity of different NSAIDs in rats: LD_{50} values mg/kg (95% confidence limits) after single oral administration.

Table 1 LD_{50} values of NSAIDs in rats as multiples of maximum human dose in mg/kg (related to 65 kg body weight)

Compound	*LD_{50} in rats* (mg/kg) (a)	*Maximum human dose*		
		(mg/day) (b)	(mg/kg) (c)	(a)/(c)
Piroxicam	255	40	0.6	425
Azapropazone	4200	1800	27.7	152
Diclofenac	240	150	2.3	104
Phenylbutazone	700	600	9.2	76
Ketoprofen	160	300	4.6	35
Naproxen	543	1000	15.4	35
Mefenamic acid	790	1500	23.1	34
Ibuprofen	969	2400	36.9	26
Indomethacin	19	200	3.1	6

that ingestion of 15 g azapropazone by a 22-year-old man caused only repeated bloody vomiting, upper abdominal pain, and transient anuria. However, dizziness was the only symptom observed in a 30-year-old woman who received gastric lavage $3\frac{1}{2}$ hours after ingestion of 6 g azapropazone together with ethanol and flurazepam[7].

The toxicity of azapropazone on repeated oral administration in different animal species was investigated over different periods. Subacute and chronic toxicity tests involving daily dosages of 20–600 mg/kg, were carried out in rats, dogs and monkeys (Table 2).

In the rat, the 'no effect level' determined was 80 mg/kg daily over 1–2 years and 150 mg/kg daily over 8 weeks. Higher daily dosages resulted in slowing down of weight increase and in gastrointestinal damage associated with increased mortality. No changes attributable to azapropazone were observed in other organs. In view of the fact that the rat is most comparable with man with regard to the pharmacokinetics of azapropazone[15,16], and that the daily dosage of azapropazone in long-term treatment in human subjects is 600–1200 mg, i.e. only 9–18 mg/kg, a relatively satisfactory safety margin is assured, in so far as any such direct comparison is valid.

Azapropazone is less well tolerated in dogs than in other animal species, a phenomenon also known with some other NSAIDs. Purebred beagles are apparently more sensitive than mongrels. Well-tolerated daily dosages are 50 mg/kg for 12 weeks (mongrels), 25 mg/kg for six months (beagles) and less than 25 mg/kg for twelve months (beagles). Here, too, toxicity took the form of dose-dependent damage to the gastrointestinal tract. This species-specific sensitivity is possibly due to the unique kinetics of azapropazone observed in the dog. Dog plasma, for instance, binds azapropazone to a much lesser extent than plasma in the rat, monkey and man; elimination of azapropazone via the kidney is much less than in the rat and man, and peak serum levels of azapropazone are reached in the dog 6–8 hours after oral administration, compared with 3–6 hours in the rat and in man. The dog must be considered the animal species that is least comparable with man[15].

The long-term experiments conducted in monkeys have shown that azapropazone is particularly well tolerated by this animal species. Daily administration of 500 mg/kg to baboons for 6 months and 600 mg/kg to rhesus monkeys for 12 months did not cause any appreciable pathological changes. In this context, azapropazone was much better tolerated than phenylbutazone, which at a daily dosage of 80 mg/kg brought about the death of one baboon in the 6-month test and increased liver and kidney weights in the surviving animals. In a special tolerance test carried out in baboons given a daily intravenous injection of azapropazone ampoule solution, with doubling of the dosage every second day, azapropazone was well tolerated up to a daily dosage of 340 mg/kg[17]. Since azapropazone is as strongly bound to protein in the rhesus monkey and baboon plasma as in human plasma, the results obtained in the primates are possibly more relevant for human subjects[15].

III. TESTING FOR REPRODUCTIVE TOXICITY

Table 3 is a survey of the reproductive toxicology tests performed with azapropazone.

23

Table 2 Toxicity tests with repeated oral administration of azapropazone

Species	Duration of study	Doses (mg/kg) daily	No effect level (mg/kg/day)	Parameters affected by high doses	Reference
Rat	8 weeks	100, 150, 200, 300, 400	150	Retarded body-weight gain, stomach haemorrhage, increased deaths	Wazeter and Goldenthal (1974)[8]
Rat	12 months	80, 160, 200	80	Decreased body-weight, GI lesions, increased deaths	Wazeter and Goldenthal(1977)[9]
Rat	24 months	80, 160	80	As in 12 months test	Wazeter and Goldenthal (1977)[9]
Mongrel dog	12 weeks	50	50	No adverse changes	Jahn and Adrian (1967)[10]
Beagle dog	26 weeks	25, 50	25	Vomiting, diarrhoea, gastric irritation and ulceration	Adrian (1970)[11]
Beagle dog	12 months	25, 50, 100	< 25	Damage to the gastrointestinal tract	Wazeter and Goldenthal (1975a)[12]
Baboon	26 weeks	20, 200–500	500	2/6 animals small gastric erosions	Heywood et al. (1972)[13]
Rhesus monkey	12 months	100, 300, 600	600	No adverse changes	Wazeter and Goldenthal (1975b)[14]

Table 3 Studies on reproductive toxicology of azapropazone

Type of study	Species	Oral dose (mg kg^{-1} day^{-1})	Duration of treatment	Reference
Teratogenicity	Mouse	100, 300, 600	7th–12th day of gestation	Ito et al. (1969)[18]
Teratogenicity	Rat	100, 200	9th–14th day of gestation	Ito et al. (1969)[18]
Teratogenicity	Rat	100, 200	1st–14th day, 8th–12th day of gestation	Adrian (1970a)[19]
Teratogenicity	Rat	75, 150, 300	6th–16th day of gestation	Wazeter and Goldenthal (1975c)[20]
Teratogenicity	Rabbit	100, 400	6th–18th day of gestation	Adrian (1970b)[21]
Teratogenicity	Rabbit	50, 100, 200, 400	6th–18th day of gestation	Wazeter and Goldenthal (1975d)[22]
Reproduction	Rat	50, 100	Males for 20 weeks, females from 16th day before mating until end of lactation	Adrian (1973)[23]
Fertility and reproduction	Rat	50, 100, 200	Males for 80 days, females from 14th day before mating until end of weaning	Wazeter and Goldenthal (1975e)[24]
Peri- and post-natal toxicity	Rat	75, 150, 300	From 15th day of gestation until end of weaning	Wazeter and Goldenthal (1975f)[25]

The teratological investigations carried out in mice, rats and rabbits did not reveal any signs of a teratogenic effect of azapropazone. The substance had no effect on the fertility or reproductive performance of rats and did not impair normal development of the young animals.

IV. CARCINOGENICITY TESTS

Carcinogenicity tests were carried out with azapropazone in mice and rats (Table 4). In none of the four tests performed did azapropazone exhibit a carcinogenic effect, although it was administered in the maximum tolerated daily doses. The recent, particularly carefully performed test in rats is of relevance for purposes of comparison in that the rat is closest to man with regard to the pharmacokinetics of azapropazone[15,16].

V. SPECIAL TESTS OF GASTRIC TOLERANCE

With all NSAIDs, the dominant undesired, serious side-effect is lesions of the gastrointestinal tract. With azapropazone, too, the organ most specifically affected by toxicity after high doses in animal experiments proved to be the gastrointestinal tract. It was therefore an obvious step to compare this side-effect with those of other NSAIDs and to evaluate it in relation to the anti-inflammatory action[30,31,32].

The rat is particularly eligible for such comparisons, since both the ulcerogenic and anti-inflammatory actions are easy to demonstrate in this animal species. Very large-scale comparative studies were performed, also in our laboratory, which included some standard NSAIDs[33]. In these studies, rats were sacrificed $3\frac{1}{2}$ hours after a single oral dose of the test substances and the dose-dependent inhibition of rat paw oedema induced by subplantar injection of carrageenan was assessed graphically, as was the presence of gastric ulcers. It was found that the intensity of the ulcerogenic effect of the test substances in the rat had no direct bearing on the anti-inflammatory effect. The relative severity of the gastrointestinal toxicity of the test substances

Table 4   Carcinogenicity studies with azapropazone

Species	Dose (mg/kg) and administration	Duration of study	Reference
Newborn mouse	1.25 mg subcutaneously on 1st day of life	1 year	Adrian and Jahn (1969)[26]
Mouse	80, 160, 320 daily in the feed	18 months	Wazeter and Goldenthal (1976)[27]
Mouse	80, 160, 320 daily in the feed	18 months	Stadler (1988)[28]
Rat	50, 100, 150 daily by gastric tube	124 weeks	Prejean (1981)[29]

in relation to a given anti-inflammatory effect was determined on the basis of a ranking list derived from the quotients ED_{50} oedema inhibition/ED_{50} ulcerogenic effect (ulcerogenic index). Table 5 shows that azapropazone ranks as one of the substances with the least gastric toxicity.

Table 5 Comparison of anti-inflammatory and ulcerogenic actions of various NSAIDs after single oral administration in rats

Compound	ED_{50} (mg/kg) carrageenan paw oedema (a)	ED_{50} (mg/kg) ulcerogenic activity (b)	Ulcerogenic index (a)/(b)
Azapropazone	62	690	0.09
Carprofen	2.3	19	0.12
Pirprofen	0.6	4.5	0.13
Indoprofen	1.9	7.5	0.25
Piroxicam	1.2	2.9	0.41
Ketoprofen	1.6	3.5	0.46
Bumadizone	54	118	0.46
Flurbiprofen	0.5	1.0	0.50
Naproxen	1.9	3.2	0.59
Niflumic acid	10	14	0.71
Diclofenac	6.2	6.5	0.95
Alclofenac	54	46	1.17
Ibuprofen	42	15	2.80

According to Jahn, U (1985)[33]

VI. CONCLUSIONS

When azapropazone was selected 20 years ago for introduction into clinical practice, only a small number of standard substances such as acetylsalicylic acid, phenylbutazone, indomethacin and mefenamic acid were available for comparative studies, and the requirements with regard to preclinical documentation were still relatively modest. The recent avalanche of new NSAIDs on the drug market and the extension of the toxicological document-ation requirements of the authorities mean that preclinical testing of azapropazone continues unabated. As can be seen from the investigation material presented in this context, even in the current situation, the anti-rheumatic drug azapropazone, which has been used successfully for a long time, must be regarded as having been subjected to comprehensive and meticulous toxicological investigation and as possessing a tolerance that surpasses that of other substances, including more recent ones, in animal studies.

References

1. Jahn, U and Adrian, RW (1969). Pharmakologische und toxikologische Prüfung des neuen Antiphlogistikums Azapropazon = 3-Dimethylamino-7-

methyl-1,2-(n-propylmalonyl)-1,2-dihydro-1,2,4-benzotriazin. *Arzneim-Forsch/ Drug Res*, **19**, 36–52

2. Julou, L, Guyonnet, J–C, Ducrot, R *et al.* (1971). Etude des propriétés pharmacologiques d'un nouvel anti-inflammatoire, l'acide (benzoyl-3-phenyl)-2-propionique (19583 RP). *J Pharmacol (Paris)*, **2**, 259–86

3. Menassé, R, Hedwall, PR, Kraetz, J *et al.* (1978). Pharmacological properties of diclofenac sodium and its metabolites. *Scand J Rheumatology*, Suppl. **22**, 5–16

4. Schiantarelli, P and Cadel, S (1981). Piroxicam pharmacologic activity and gastrointestinal damage by oral and rectal route. Comparison with oral indomethacin and phenylbutazone *Arzneim-Forsch/Drug Res*, **31**, 87–92

5. Roszkowski, AP, Rooks, WH, Tomolonis, AJ and Miller, LM (1971). Anti-inflammatory and analgesic properties of d-2(6'-methoxy-2'-naphthyl)-propionic acid (naproxen). *J Pharmacol Exp Ther*, **179**, 114–23

6. Cioli, V, Putzolu, S, Rossi, V and Carradino, C (1980). A toxicological and pharmacological study of ibuprofen guaiacol ester (AF 2259) in the rat. *Tox Appl Pharmacol*, **54**, 332–9

7. Vale, JA and Meredith, TJ (1986). Acute poisoning due to non-steroidal anti-inflammatory drugs. Clinical features and management. *Medical Toxicology*, **1**, 12–31

8. Wazeter, FX and Goldenthal, EI (1974). AHR-3018, eight week tolerance study in rats. *Unpublished data on file Siegfried Ltd.*, Doc. No. 4779

9. Wazeter, FX and Goldenthal, EI (1977). AHR-3018, twenty-four month oral toxicity study in rats. *Unpublished data on file Siegfried Ltd.*, Doc. No. 1892

10. Jahn, U and Adrian, RW (1967). Toxicological studies in dogs with Mi85-Di. *Unpublished data on file Siegfried Ltd.*, Doc. No. 1206

11. Adrian, RW (1970). Bericht über eine orale 6 montatige Toxizitätsprüfung mit Mi85-Di an Beagle-Hunden. *Unpublished data on file Siegfried Ltd.*, Doc. No. 0705

12. Wazeter, FX and Goldenthal, EI (1975a). AHR-3018, twelve month oral toxicity study in dogs. *Unpublished data on file Siegfried Ltd.*, Doc. No. 2444

13. Heywood, R, Squires, PF, Street, AE and Hague, PH (1972). Oral toxicity study in baboons (repeated dosage for 26 weeks). *Unpublished data on file Siegfried Ltd.*, Doc. No. 1211

14. Wazeter, FX and Goldenthal, EI (1975b). AHR-3018, twelve month oral toxicity study in monkeys. *Unpublished data on file Siegfried Ltd.*, Doc. No. 4777

15. Jahn, U, Reller, J and Schatz, F (1973). Pharmakokinetische Untersuchungen mit Azapropazon bei Tieren. *Arzneim-Forsch/Drug Res*, **23**, 660–6

16. Klatt, C and Koss, FW (1973). Pharmacokinetics of ^{14}C-azapropazone in rats. *Arzneim-Forsch/Drug Res*, **23**, 913–9

17. Varney, P (1981). Azapropazone: 14 day (intravenous administration) tolerated dose study in the baboon. *Unpublished data on file Siegfried Ltd.*, Doc. No. 4070

18. Ito, R, Nakagawa, S and Daikuhava, K (1969). A study on teratogenic activity of azapropazone, a new anti-inflammatory agent. *Medical Treatment*, **2**, 38–47

19. Adrian, RW (1970a). Report on teratologic testing of Mi85 in rats. *Unpublished data on file Siegfried Ltd.*, Doc. No. 0538

20. Wazeter, FX and Goldenthal, EI (1975c). AHR-3018, teratology study in rats. *Unpublished data on file Siegfried Ltd.*, Doc. No. 2150

21. Adrian, RW (1970b). Teratological tests conducted with Mi85 on rabbits. *Unpublished data on file Siegfried Ltd.*, Doc. No. 0539

22. Wazeter, FX and Goldenthal, EI (1975d). AHR-3018, teratology study in

rabbits. *Unpublished data on file Siegfried Ltd.*, Doc. No. 2149

23. Adrian, RW (1973). Reproduktionstoxikologische Untersuchungen mit Azapropazon an Ratten. *Arzneim-Forsch/Drug Res*, **23**, 658–60

24. Wazeter, FX and Goldenthal, EI (1975e). AHR-3018, fertility and general reproductive performance study in rats. *Unpublished data on file Siegfried Ltd.*, Doc. No. 2148

25. Wazeter, FX and Goldenthal, EI (1975f). AHR-3018, perinatal and postnatal study in rats. *Unpublished data on file Siegfried Ltd.*, Doc. No. 1503

26. Adrian, RW and Jahn, U (1969). Prüfung von Dimetacrin und Azapropazon in einem Carcinogentest an Mäusen. *Arzneim-Forsch/Drug Res*, **19**, 1997–8

27. Wazeter, FX and Goldenthal, EI (1976). AHR-3018, eighteen month oral carcinogenic study in mice. *Unpublished data on file Siegfried Ltd.*, Doc. No. 1891

28. Stadler, JC (1988). Oncogenicity study with azapropazone, eighteen-month feeding study in mice. *Unpublished data on file Siegfried Ltd.*, Doc. No. 6196

29. Prejean, JD (1981). A carcinogenicity bioassay of apazone in the rat. *Unpublished data on file Siegfried Ltd.*, Doc. No. 4052

30. Rainsford, KD (1977). Comparison of the gastric ulcerogenic activity of new non-steroidal anti-inflammatory drugs in stressed rats. *Br J Pharmacol*, **73**, 79c–80c

31. Peskar, BM, Rainsford, K, Brune, K and Gerok, W (1981). Effekt nichtsteroidartiger Antiphlogistika auf Plasma- und Magenmukosakonzentrationen von Prostaglandinen. *Verh Dtsch Ges Inn Med*, **87**, 833–8

32. Rainsford, KD (1982). An analysis of the gastro-intestinal side effects of non-steroidal anti-inflammatory drugs, with particular reference to comparative studies in man and laboratory species. *Rheumatol Int*, **2**, 1–10

33. Jahn, U (1985). Vergleich der antiphlogistischen und ulzerogenen Wirkung von Azapropazon und von neueren nichtsteroiden Antiphlogistika bei Ratten. *Arthritis & Rheuma*, **7**, 21–7

Summary

The material presented in this survey shows that azapropazone has been subjected to comprehensive and careful toxicological investigation and that its tolerance surpasses that of other nonsteroidal antiinflammatory drugs, including recent ones, in animal studies.

Zusammenfassung

Die in dieser Übersicht vorgestellten Ergebnisse zeigen auf, dass Azapropazon einer umfassenden und sorgfältigen toxikologischen Prüfung unterzogen wurde. Es wird auch gezeigt, dass die Verträglichkeit von Azapropazon in tierexperimentellen Studien diejenige anderer, auch neuer nichtsteroidaler Antirheumatika übertrifft.

Resumé

Les résultats présentés dans cet exposé montrent que l'azapropazone à été soumis à des examens toxicologiques étendus et soigneux et que sa tolérance, lors d'études expérimentales chez l'animal, est supérieure à celle des autres anti-inflammatoires non-stéroïdiens, y compris les plus récents.

4

The mode of action of azapropazone in relation to its therapeutic actions in rheumatic conditions and its major side-effects

KD Rainsford

I. INTRODUCTION

Azapropazone* is a moderately potent anti-inflammatory analgesic agent when compared, on a dose-for-weight basis in animal models and man, with standard drugs, such as aspirin, indomethacin and phenylbutazone[1,2]. In some of the standard acute and chronic animal models of inflammatory conditions, the potency of azapropazone is between that of ibuprofen and phenylbutazone[1,2] (see Tables 1 and 2). In man, the dose range for the control of pain and inflammation in most rheumatic diseases is 1200–1800 mg daily[1]. At this dose, its efficacy is roughly comparable to most other non-steroidal anti-inflammatory drugs (NSAIDs) at their respective recommended daily doses.

One of the generally held beliefs widely promulgated in the clinical and pharmacological literature, and also by drug regulatory authorities

Table 1   Effects of azapropazone compared with standard NSAIDs, given orally in a therapeutic treatment regime, on the progress of adjuvant-induced arthritis in Sprague-Dawley rats

Drug	ED_{50} (mg kg^{-1} d^{-1})
Azapropazone	150
Aspirin	200
Clobuzarit (Clozic®)	20
Indomethacin	2.0

Drugs were dosed from day + 14 post-induction of arthritis (from tail-base injection of heat killed and delipidated *Mycobacterium tuberculosis*) for a period of 14 days. Data from Ref. 2.

*A comprehensive review of the chemistry, pharmacology, toxicology and clinical uses of azapropazone up to 1985 has been reported by Walker[1].

Azapropazone – 20 years of clinical use. Rainsford, KD (ed)
© Kluwer Academic Publishers. Printed in Great Britain

Table 2 Comparative acute anti-inflammatory and analgesic activity of azapropazone

Drug	ED_{50} (mg/kg, p.o.) rat paw oedema induced by				ED_{50} (mg/kg, p.o.) UV erythema in guinea pigs	ED_{50} (mg/kg) bradykinin bronchospasm (Collier test) in guinea pigs after administration:		ED_{50} (mg/kg, p.o.) anti-nociceptive tests in:	
	Carrageenan	Aerosil	Kaolin	C + A + K		i.v.	i.d.	Randall–Selitto model in rats	Koster model in mice
Azapropazone	82	160	130	84	150 110 (Na salt)	3	>100	43 (as Na salt)	240 (as Na salt)
Aspirin				223	[52–200]	1	128		
Flufenamic				77	10 (Na salt)	2	>10		
Ibuprofen				32	7	>2	7		
Indomethacin	7		6	6	[0.9–10]	0.6	>10	2	
Mefenamic acid				63	18 (Na salt)	3	>10		7
Phenylbutazone	50	30	50	82	10 (Na Salt) 16	3	>10	30 (as Na salt)	240 (as Na salt)

is that (i) all NSAIDs act by inhibiting the synthesis of inflammatory prostaglandins (PGs), and (ii) the differing potencies of these drugs can be ascribed to their differential effects on the production of PGs and their pharmacokinetics[3]. Mostly, the differences in gross pharmacokinetics of NSAIDs are compensated by adjustment of the frequency and dose so as to achieve approximate equal efficacy.

While there are variations in the uptake of NSAIDs into synovial tissues which may influence the therapeutic effects in the arthritic joint, the order of magnitude of drug concentrations in synovial tissues is up to half or more of the plasma levels[4], and these may vary according to drug dosage and frequency.

Thus the question focuses on whether there is a relationship between inhibition of PG production by the NSAIDs to their therapeutic actions *in vivo* or if there are other biochemical or cellular actions of these drugs which are of equal or greater importance. The short answer to this question is that we do not know the full story. However, the picture is emerging, largely from investigations on the actions of NSAIDs in cellular systems *in vitro* or *ex vivo* that there are marked differences in the actions of various NSAIDs on the synovial accumulation and functions of leucocytes and, especially, their production of novel inflammatory mediators (e.g. superoxide anions, cytokines)[3,5-7]. The end effect of these observations may be that some NSAIDs can be shown to have a range of actions on these prostaglandin-independent leucocyte functions such that this forms a greater component of actions, compared with those drugs which more or less act by the inhibition of PGs[3,5]. It is possible that azapropazone is among the representatives of those drugs having a wide range of actions on leucocytes and that its PG synthesis inhibitory effects, which are relatively weak, are only one component of the mode of action of this drug. The present chapter will address these differing actions of azapropazone as far as can be thought relevant to its actions as an anti-rheumatic drug, especially in comparison with other NSAIDs.

A second aspect of the actions of azapropazone which may have potential significance concerns the relation of its anti-inflammatory and analgesic actions to the occurrence of the more frequent side-effects, i.e. its therapeutic index. As with other NSAIDs, the major side-effects include dermatological reactions (principally skin rashes), gastrointestinal (GI) symptoms (epigastric pain, diarrhoea, etc.) and, less frequently, upper GI irritation and bleeding. While the basis for development of side-effects in the GI tract, skin and the renal system for most NSAIDs involves a variety of complex reactions, one of the main features underlying these effects is the capacity of these drugs to inhibit the prostaglandin (PG) cyclo-oxygenase system. In this respect, azapropazone is a relatively weak PG synthesis inhibitor and this, together with certain pharmacokinetic properties of the drug, may account for the low degree of GI irritation and renal injury evident with this drug in controlled experimental or clinical studies (except in elderly subjects – see

Ref. 8 and discussion later). Thus, when it comes to comparing the therapeutic actions with side-effect profiles, it could be argued that drugs such as azapropazone, which are weak PG synthesis inhibitors but which also have added actions on a range of non-PG related inflammatory reactions, may well have more favourable therapeutic indices compared with those drugs which exert their effects by being potent inhibitors of the PG synthesis system alone.

II. PHARMACOLOGICAL ACTIONS

1. *In vivo* actions in laboratory animal models

A. Acute anti-inflammatory, anti-nociceptive and other properties

The basic pharmacological properties of azapropazone and structure-activity investigations of the benzotriazines, which led to the selection of azapropazone, were originally reported by Jahn and his co-workers[9,10]. A summary of some of the principal findings of these authors concerning the anti-inflammatory and analgesic properties of azapropazone compared with other NSAIDs, as determined in standard acute animal model systems, is shown in Table 2.

As noted at the beginning of this chapter, azapropazone exhibits moderate anti-inflammatory and analgesic activity in most of these test systems. To some extent the slow absorption of azapropazone (given orally as a suspension) from the upper gastrointestinal tract limits the full development of acute anti-inflammatory and analgesic activity by this drug. The slow or limited response in the carrageenan oedema model has been observed with some other NSAIDs, especially those drugs which, like azapropazone, are thought to act largely on non-PG dependent pathways[11]. Procedures for overcoming this problem employed by some authors include multiple dosing[11] or the administration of the more aquo-soluble sodium salts of the acidic NSAIDs. The latter method was employed by Jahn and co-workers and the results obtained[9,10] showed that the sodium salts exhibited about 20–30% greater anti-inflammatory activity than the acidic form of the drugs. Unfortunately, in preparing the sodium salts, the authors employed sodium hydroxide, and since azapropazone, indomethacin and phenylbutazone all degrade at the high pH of sodium hydroxide solutions, it is possible that a certain amount of chemical degradation could have occurred during the preparation of these drug solutions. There were no details mentioned in the reports from Jahn and co-workers of any checks on the degradation of the drug solutions they employed.

The relationship of timing of administration of the drug to the duration of anti-oedemic action was investigated by Militzer and Hirche[12]. In their studies, these authors unfortunately used relatively low doses of azapropazone (12.5–50 mg/kg p.o.) and thus clearly obtained data at the low end of the

34

dose-response curve. However, even under these conditions this drug had effects which persisted up to 6–24 hours (depending on the dose). In their system, high doses (10 mg/kg) of indomethacin, as well as flufenamic acid and aspirin, showed similar persistent effects. When the drugs were given 24 hours after induction of oedema, it was found that azapropazone, aspirin and phenylbutazone failed to exhibit any appreciable effects, whereas indomethacin, flufenamic acid and prednisolone did show some anti-oedemic activity, though not well related to dosage. The effects of the former two NSAIDs may be related to the pronounced enterohepatic recirculation of these drugs in the rat such that the drug effects relate to their long residence times in this species.

These results[12] show that the acute anti-inflammatory effects of azapropazone are of relatively long duration. The persistence of anti-oedemic effects with azapropazone may be considered approximately intermediate in comparison with other anti-rheumatic agents and probably relates to the plasma concentration profile of this drug in rats[1].

It should be noted that the basic pathophysiological reactions underlying the development of the inflammatory and algesic conditions elicited in the acute animal models as employed by Jahn et al.[9,10] were not well understood at the time that these studies were performed. Essentially, the models employed were empirical, and were regarded as among the best available to determine the influences of drugs on soft tissue inflammation. Now, however, with information available on the range of mediators and leucocyte reactions which develop during the expression of the inflammatory or algesic reactions, it is possible to make some tentative predictions of the mode of action of azapropazone in comparison with some standard NSAIDs in these animal models.

In the conventional carrageenan rat paw oedema model, it appears that during the initial primary phase, 1–2 hours after administration of the inflammagen, there is release of amines, kinins, various protein chemotactic factors, accompanied by the release of autolytic lysosomal enzymes, vascular injury and consequent extravasation of plasma proteins and polymorphonuclear leukocytes (PMNs)[13–16]. The secondary phase, at approximately 2.5–7 hours, involves the generation of large quantities of prostaglandins: principally PGE_2, to a lesser extent $PGF_{2\alpha}$[16,17] and there is probably also production of the leukotrienes[18], with further accumulation of PMNs[14]. A tertiary phase, from 7–24 hours or even longer, is accompanied by extensive accumulation of monocytes[14] and there may be other accompanying immune reactions from the diverse immunological actions of carrageenan[19,20].

NSAIDs exert their effects principally on the second phase of the carrageenan oedema[21], although aspirin and phenylbutazone (but not indomethacin) have some weaker inhibitory effects on the primary phase[21]. The inhibition of the second phase is related, in part, to their inhibitory actions on the production of PGs[5], although it is clear that inhibition of leucocyte migration also plays a major role[5,14]. Thus any interpretation of the inhibitory effects of azapropazone in this model will necessarily implicate effects on both inhibition of PG production and leucocyte emigration, and may also even involve influences on the production of other mediators in the primary and secondary phases. There is obviously little influence on the tertiary macrophage accumulation phase such as is evident with cortico-steroids.

It will be seen from Table 2 that azapropazone inhibits the kaolin oedema but at higher doses than those which were observed with its effects on carrageenan-induced inflammation. Kaolin oedema is thought to involve production of kinins and PGs, and complement activation, but there is little influence of 5-HT nor of the pronounced cellular accumulation seen with carrageenan[22]. Most NSAIDs have weaker effects in this model than in either the carrageenan or other paw inflammation models[22]. Thus it is tempting to suggest that comparison of the results obtained in the carrageenan paw oedema model with those in kaolin oedema may mean that some of the acute anti-inflammatory effects of azapropazone, as well as of other NSAIDs, could be attributed to their influence on leucocyte accumulation and activation of these cells which would be expected to predominate in the carrageenan model. The anti-bradykinin effects of azapropazone seen in the Collier bronchoconstriction model in guinea pigs after intravenous, but not intradermal administration of the drug (Table 2), suggests that where concentrations of this drug accumulate at or near the sites of receptor actions for this kinin there could be some antagonism of this peptide. It is curious that the potencies of the i.v.-administered NSAIDs are about equal in this model and well outside those for the inhibition of PG synthesis, a known consequence of the actions of bradykinin[23,24]. The anti-bradykinin action of azapropazone may well underly, in part, its anti-nociceptive effects as revealed in the Randall–Selitto and Koster tests (Table 2), although it is known that a variety of effects on the peripheral nervous system and possibly even higher centres underlies the complexity of these behavioural tests.

The ultraviolet (UV) erythema model in guinea pigs probably involves predominantly the stimulation of PG production[25]. Certainly the results obtained with a range of NSAIDs of varying potency as PG synthesis inhibitors suggest that the anti-erythema actions of these drugs are likely to be more pronounced with the more potent inhibitors of PG production, and there is a pronounced favouring of selection of drugs based on this screening test for the latter effects[25,26]. Since little or no leucocyte accumulation is observed in this model[25], it probably represents among the most selective screens for inhibitory actions on PG production. The results in Table 2 show that azapropazone exhibits very weak inhibitory actions in the UV erythema in comparison with other NSAIDs, in particular phenylbutazone, ibuprofen and flufenamic acid, with which it is roughly comparable in anti-inflammatory actions in other leucocyte-dependent inflammatory models (c.f. data in Ref. 25). These give further support to the suggestion that the weak effect on PG production probably constitutes only a minor action of azapropazone.

B. Chronic anti-inflammatory models

Azapropazone given orally inhibits the progress of the established mycobact-
erial adjuvant-induced polyarthritis in rats, which, in comparison with
published data, is in the range of potency comparable with that of ibuprofen,
mefenamic acid and phenylbutazone[27,28] (Table 1). Unpublished data (quoted
in Ref. 1) suggests that the drug inhibits the secondary paw inflammation
(presumed to occur from paw injection of the adjuvant) and that the
erythrocyte sedimentation rate (ESR) was also reduced. However, none of
the details of the experiment, including those of the dosage was reported.
Intraperitoneal administration of the drug (20 or 40 mg/kg) has also been
reported to inhibit the paw swelling[29]. Szanto and co-workers[30] have also
shown that 500 μg azapropazone i.p. (in rats weighing 150–200 g) reduced
the arthritis induced by local injections in the paws with formalin alone or
with PGE_2, concomitant with reduced histochemical staining for succinic
and malate dehydrogenases[30]. The exact significance of the latter effect was
not explained by the authors, although it may be drug related, since other
NSAIDs have been reported to inhibit the activities of these mitochondrial
enzymes.

It could be argued that the dosages required for establishing anti-
arthritic activity in the adjuvant model in rats are high. However, the doses
for anti-inflammatory effects have to be reconciled against the rates of
clearance of the drugs. For azapropazone, this is rapid (plasma elimination
half life circa 3–4 hours in rats; c.f. man, where it is circa 12–16 hours) and
is probably related to the appreciably lower protein binding of the drug in
rats[1,31].

Detailed morphological and histological investigations of the effects of
azapropazone and comparator NSAIDs have been reported[2]. In the range
of comparable drug effects on the control of swelling in the soft tissues of the
subplantar region of the hind paws and the tibio-tarsal region, azapropazone
exhibited similar control of pannus, cartilage destruction, periostitis and new
bone development as that of indomethacin and clobuzarit (Clozic®)[2]. None
of the drugs totally prevented the joint damage characteristic of this vigorous
and highly destructive disease.

The control of joint destruction exhibited by azapropazone and
comparator NSAIDs is illustrated by radiological and histopathological
observations, as shown in Figures 1 and 2 respectively. Radiological
observations have been considered to be among the most sensitive means of
determining the response to drug therapy in the joint injury in arthritic
conditions and this is most evident also with the adjuvant arthritis model[32-34].
It can be seen that azapropazone is as effective as the comparator drugs in
controlling the bone and cartilage destruction, as well as the proliferation of
pannus, which occurs in this disease.

In the standard croton oil granuloma model induced in rats, the effects
of azapropazone on granuloma weight were less than with phenylbutazone,

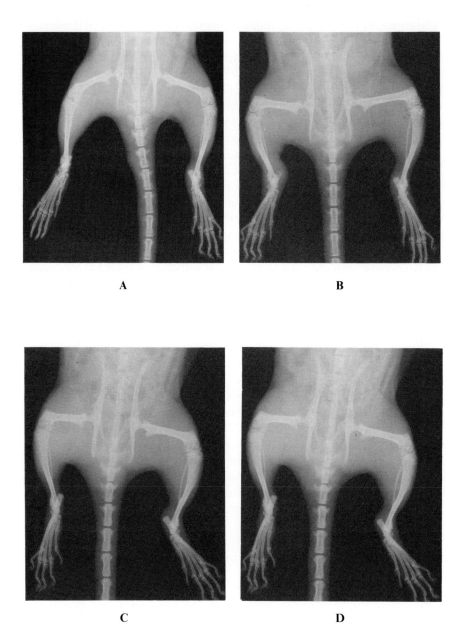

A

B

C

D

Figure 1 X-Radiographs of the hind limb regions of adjuvant arthritic rats who had received (**A,B**) azapropazone (150 mg kg^{-1} d^{-1}), (**C**) indomethacin (2 mg kg^{-1} d^{-1}), or (**D**) water (1 ml/d) – control for 19 days from the day of induction of the disease. Two radiographs are shown from azapropazone-treated rats to give representative views of the spectrum of response to this drug

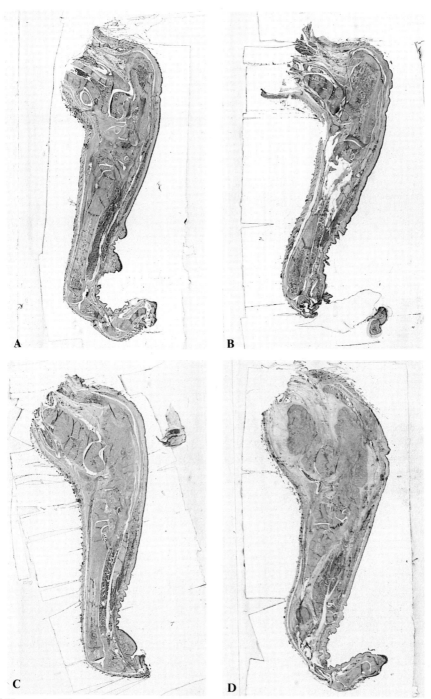

Figure 2 Histological sections (haematoxylin and eosin-stained) of the decalcified hind limbs of adjuvant arthritic rats treated from days $+14$ to $+28$ post-induction with (**A**) azapropazone ($150\,mg\,kg^{-1}\,d^{-1}$), (**B**) indomethacin ($2\,mg\,kg^{-1}\,d^{-1}$), (**C**) clobuzarit ($20\,mg\,kg^{-1}\,d^{-1}$) or (**D**) control ($1\,ml/d$). Indomethacin and clobuzarit were included for comparison; clobuzarit being a weak PG synthesis inhibitor like that of azapropazone. Based on studies in ref. 2

but in the cotton pellet granuloma, azapropazone was more potent in inhibiting granuloma formation[9]. Such crude models of granuloma development give only indications of general drug influences on either growth or cellular infiltration accompanying the inflammatory reactions, which are indeed diverse.

2. *In vitro* actions

A. Relevant drug concentrations

It is a general practice to evaluate the *in vitro* actions of drugs including the NSAIDs in relation to the plasma concentrations of the drugs or metabolites which are achieved during therapy. While of some help in interpreting the actions on circulation leucocytes and possibly the immune system, this does not give a very accurate representation of the range of drug concentrations to which the cells in the inflamed or damaged joints will be exposed. Thus steady state plasma concentrations achieved during therapy of rheumatoid arthritis (RA) with 600 mg azapropazone b.d. for 5 days are in the order of 60–150 μg/ml = 0.2–0.5 mmol/L (trough to peak values)[36,37]. The highest plasma concentrations recorded under steady state conditions achieved following ingestion of 2.4 g/day of the drug (rarely used except in gout) are in the order of 240 μg/ml = 0.8 mmol/L[37], so this may be considered the uppermost, though not a generally applicable limit. Synovial fluid concentrations in RA patients after a single dose of 300 mg of the drug are about 10 μg/ml = 30 μmol/L (peak at 3–24 hours)[38] and range between 7–106 μg/ml = 23–350 μmol/L at steady state after 5 days administration of 1.2 g of the drug in RA subjects[36]. Synovial tissue concentrations in these subjects range between 7–33 μg/ml = 23–100 μmol/L[36].

Thus for practical purposes relevant drug concentrations for cells in the synovium, and possibly cartilage as well, are of the order of 20–100 μmol/L, with an upper limit 300 μmol/L where it is possible these cells could be exposed to synovial fluids. For circulating leucocytes the levels could range up to 200–500 μmol/L. Within these ranges, a discussion follows of the *in vitro* actions of azapropazone compared with other NSAIDs.

B. Pharmacological actions

A summary is shown in Tables 3 and 4 of the principal findings reported of the *in vitro* actions of azapropazone. It is clear that there are a variety of actions of the drug on the production of inflammatory mediators, the actions of leucocytes and on cartilage biochemistry all of which are, in their way, somewhat relevant to the overall spectrum of anti-inflammatory actions of the drug. It is obvious that while many of these biochemical and cellular effects of the drug seem logical for its anti-inflammatory actions *in vivo*, it has not been established just under what circumstances or conditions these individual effects are relevant in the control of inflammatory and

40

Table 3 *In vitro* and/or *in vivo* **pharmacological properties of azapropazone relevant to its anti-inflammatory activities**

Actions on:	Approximate concentration or dose-range
Inhibitory effects	
1. Prostaglandin synthesis	See Table 4 for *in vitro* data. 200 mg/kg (gastric mucosa[76].
2. Superoxide generation (also xanthine oxidase inhibition – see refs. 40, 41)	$IC_{50} = 15\mu M$ (polyhistidine, phorbol ester stimuli). Variation according to stimulus[2,39,40]
3. Lysosomal stabilization	1.0 nM–1.0mM range. 250–500 mg/kg p.o. × 5d[38]
4. Accumulation and degranulation of leucocytes	$100\,\mu M$[39,40]
5. Production of interleukin-1 (IL-1)	10–200 μM[2]
Negative effects	
1. Platelet aggregation induced by ADP, collagen	No effect on second phase with 10 nM drug[2] or with single oral dose of 300 mg drug*
2. IL-1-induced resorption of cartilage	20–100 μM[2]
Stimulatory effects	
1. Proteoglycan synthesis	25–250 μM[2]

*Unpublished studies by M. Aylward in 1978 provided by A.H. Robins (UK) Ltd.

Table 4 **Comparative effects of azapropazone on prostaglandin production in various cellular systems**

Drug	PGE production SSV microsomes IC_{50} (μM)[a]	System PGE$_2$ production macrophage IC_{50} (μM)[b]	PGF$_{2\alpha}$ production guinea pig lung[c] IC_{50} (μM)
Azapropazone	3.0	11.2	156
Aspirin	83	6.6	52.8
Diclofenac	0.3	0.01	NT
Indomethacin	0.4	0.002	0.56
Phenylbutazone	12.9	5.5	16.2

[a] From Humes *et al.*
[b] From Brune *et al.*—quoted in Ref. 35.
[c] From Luscombe and Nicholls (1973)—quoted in Ref. 1.

immunological actions in the various arthritic diseases, and this is probably a comment applicable to most, if not all of the NSAIDs!

It would seem that, given the above caveat, azapropazone may exert its major inflammatory effects by inhibiting (i) the production of tissue-destructive oxygen radicals (such as represented by the effects of the drug on superoxide anion production by PMNs), (ii) the biosynthesis of PGs (in which it is, as previously indicated, a weak inhibitor, (iii) the accumulation and possibly degranulation of leucocytes, (iv) the release of autolytic enzymes from lysosomal bodies, (v) the production by synovial tissues of interleukin 1, and (iv) the physical interaction (by stabilization) with plasma proteins, including the acute phase protein, alpha$_1$ acid glycoprotein[2,39-45].

Azapropazone does not appear to inhibit the synthesis of cartilage proteogylcans (PrGns) and glycosaminoglycans (GAGs)[2,47] such as is evident with some NSAIDs such as aspirin or phenylbutazone[48-60]; indeed it may, like benoxaprofen[61], at some drug concentrations may even stimulate the synthesis of these macromolecules[2]. Some authors[52-58,62,63] have claimed that the absence of inhibitory effects of certain NSAIDs on the biosynthesis or even turnover of PrGns and GAGs can be conceived as being an advantageous feature of these NSAIDs for the therapy of osteoarthritis (OA). Some evidence in support of this thesis may be derived from the studies in OA reported by Rashad, Walker, the author and colleagues[64] (see also Chapter 17). While this is an attractive hypothesis, it may be an oversimplification of the potential of these drug effects on otherwise complex biochemical changes in cartilage during the genesis and progression of OA. Thus the resorption of cartilage, and possibly stimulation of new PrGn synthesis, that occurs around chondrocytes during those stages of OA in which proliferation of these cells occurs, may in fact represent desirable events to be modulated or inhibited by certain NSAIDs capable of modulating PrGn and collagen biosynthesis. Even if this is not the case for this class of compounds, it is possible, in contrast to the situation in OA, that inhibition of the synthesis of PrGns may be a desirable feature in rheumatoid arthritis where there is a proliferation of pannus and stimulation of the synthesis of PrGns and GAGs. Finally, as noted by Walker (see Chapter 17) it is also possible that by depressing the synthesis of vasodilatatory PGs, certain NSAIDs with potent inhibitory effects of the cyclo-oxygenase enzyme system may impair the vascular perfusion through bone. Clearly the relevance of these manyfold drug effects deserves further investigation, especially in human models of the various arthritic diseases.

III. MAJOR SIDE-EFFECTS

While it is not intended to give a detailed review of the development of side-effects compared with other NSAIDs (see chapters in Refs. 65–67 and Refs. 68–72, and the chapters in this volume by Jahn, Hort and others for more details), some of the more important of these untoward effects will be considered, especially in relation to the actions of these drugs.

1. Gastrointestinal ulceration and haemorrhage

Detailed investigations in man (summarized in Refs. 68, 71, 72, and studies in Refs. 73, 74) together with extensive studies in a variety of laboratory animal models[75-80] indicates that azapropazone has a relatively low propensity for producing GI ulceration and haemorrhage. Data compiled from reports to European drug regulatory authorities (see chapters in Refs. 65–67) indicates, however, a much higher incidence of these adverse effects than would be otherwise indicated from the clinical and laboratory animal studies. It has been suggested that one reason for the high incidence observed in these agency reports is that they may have occurred in elderly individuals given an inappropriate high dosage of the drug[8]. This is a moot point with all the NSAIDs, as indeed are the potential complications which can arise from the drugs interacting with concurrent antidiuretics, antihypertensives and anticoagulants[65-67].

The intrinsically low GI irritancy probably has a basis in a multiplicity of actions of the drug (see Refs. 77, 78 and 81). These can be summarized by:

(i)   the slow rate of gastric absorption of the drug[44,76,78] and unique physico-chemical properties (see chapters by Dean and McCormack, this volume), which combine to minimize the irritation to the surface mucosal cells as seen with those rapidly absorbed NSAIDs that are carboxylic acids;

(ii)   its weak inhibitory actions on the synthesis of mucosal protective prostaglandins[76-79];

(iii)   the possibility that the drug may, at high concentrations, inhibit the production of 5-lipoxygenase products[77], which in the case of 5-hydroperoxyeicosatetraenoic acid (5-HPETE) and the peptido-leuko-trienes appear to contribute to vascular injury[81]. Thus, in the presence of cyclo-oxygenase inhibition, the diversion of arachidonic acid through the lipoxygenase pathway, as observed with potent cyclo-oxygenase inhibitors[81], would, in effect, be prevented by azapropazone;

(iv)   the lack of inhibitory effects on the biosynthesis of the protective mucus layer in the GI tract[82];

(v)   the apparent stabilizing effect the drug has on the release of lysosomal enzymes[39], which may have consequences in not only causing autolysis, but where there is any small local injury this could possibly be minimized;

(vi)   the possibility that the drug exhibits anti-oxidant actions and inhibitory effects on the generation of oxygen radicals[2,42,77].

Thus by comparison with the more ulcerogenic NSAIDs, which inhibit a wide variety of biochemical and cellular mechanisms underlying the normal protective processes in the GI mucosa, azapropazone may spare many of these biochemical and cellular processes. There is still much which has to be done to establish how the NSAIDs affect various biochemical and cellular functions underlying gastro-ulcerogenesis, and this is true also for azapropazone. It is especially important to know what effects this drug has on the biochemical and cellular processes underlying mucosal defences in man.

2. Skin reactions

Rashes and photosensitivity reactions occur with azapropazone[3,83-85]; in this respect the drug shares a common side-effect with that of a number of other NSAIDs[3]. There have also been occasional reports of skin eruptions with this drug[86,87], a feature which is also associated, infrequently, with ingestion of other NSAIDs[3].

Curiously, *in vivo* evaluation of the phototoxic potential of azapropazone using the ultraviolet (UV) exposed tail technique in mice was found to yield negative results[88]. *In vitro* assays of phototoxicity revealed that exposure of azapropazone-treated erythrocytes to UV-A light caused haemolysis, whereas growth inhibition of UV-treated *Candida albicans* (another suggested *in vitro* test for phototoxicity by NSAIDs) was found to be unaffected by azapropazone[89]. These inconsistent results (i.e. with respect to clinical findings) contrast with the frequent association of positive reactions in both the abovementioned *in vivo*[88] and *in vitro*[89] assays with the propionic acid derivatives (e.g. benoxaprofen, naproxen).

Detailed investigations of the phototoxicity by azapropazone have not yet been performed such as to draw conclusions as to the mechanism. Photo-products have been identified and their mode of action determined for benoxaprofen and piroxicam[3]. Pulse radiolysis studies of azapropazone, compared with phenylbutazone and oxyphenbutazone have been performed by Jones and co-workers[90]. These authors found that azide (N_3^-) and bromide (Br_3^-) radicals react in a one-electron removal process to form a putative, but as yet unidentified positive azapropazone species (Az^+).

The authors also found that the 8-hydroxy metabolite and carboxylic acid derivative (Mi307) of azapropazone also underwent the same reactions as did the three phenylbutazone derivatives[90]. That the carboxylic acid derivative, Mi307, was of about the same order of reactivity as that of azapropazone itself suggests that the reactive species is not restricted to being a keto-enolate. It is also of interest to note that the reactivity of propionic acids (e.g. benoxaprofen) is about the same as that of the keto-enolic acids[91]. Since benoxaprofen, like that of other propionic acids, also shows phototoxic reactions to isolated cells *in vitro*[91-93] it is possible that there are common features about the 3 or 4-carbon moiety attached to the carbonyl (carboxyl) moieties of both the keto-enolates (azapropazone, phenylbutazone) and the propionic acids leading both these groups of drugs to have similar propensity for phototoxic reactions. The phototoxic product derived from benoxaprofen was found to be its decarboxylated derivative, 2-(4-dichloro-phenyl)-5-ethyl benzoxazole (DPEB)[92,93]. It is, therefore, possible that the attachment of a long carbon chain could somehow favour the elimination of the carboxyl moiety during photolysis of the propionic acids. It is of interest also that the phototoxic metabolite of piroxicam 'metabolite C', is a product of the removal at a carbonyl moiety. Thus, it is suggested that the long carbon chain of the propyl moiety attached to the carbonyl-enolic acid structure of both azapropazone and phenylbutazone may favour attack by whatever means leading to the removal of attachment at one of the carboxyl moieties, probably at position 1 (since Mi307 which is susceptible to photolysis is opened to form the carboxylic acid at this portion).

Thus the following reactions for azapropazone are envisaged:

Further aspects of this theory will be developed elsewhere[94].

From a practical viewpoint, this theory does not give direct practical implications. It is, however, known that the phototoxicity from NSAIDs is reversible upon removal of the subject from sources of ultraviolet light. Even sunscreen agents were promoted in the period when benoxaprofen was first shown to exhibit phototoxicity, but their efficacy was unproven up to the time this drug was withdrawn.

3. Renal and hepatic injury

There have been some reports of renal impairment or even failure associated with ingestion of azapropazone[95–97]. Most cases have proven reversible, i.e. return to normal renal function was observed upon cessation of the drug[96], a feature which azapropazone shows with a number of other NSAIDs[65,66,69,70]. Renal concentrating ability was unaffected by long-term azapropazone therapy in arthritic subjects[98]. Plasma protein binding of the drug (as reflected by the free fraction) is, however, markedly reduced in subjects with kidney and liver disease[99]. Azapropazone can also exhibit accumulation in elderly subjects[100] and the susceptibility in elderly arthritic subjects towards reduced renal function[70–72] raises the possibility that, as with other NSAIDs, serious attention should be given to reducing the dosage of azapropazone in elderly frail arthritic subjects.*

The triad of reduced renal elimination of the drug leading to systemic accumulation and potential for liver injury has been suggested as a major problem in elderly subjects receiving NSAIDs[70-72]. The occasional reports of hepatitis[101] may have origins in this triad of drug–disease–age interactions. Interactions with drugs used frequently in the elderly, e.g. frusemide[102], tolbutamide[103] and warfarin[104,105] may have important consequences for the pharmacokinetics and/or pharmacodynamic properties of azapropazone (though notably not with digoxin[106]).

4. Conclusions

The spectrum of therapeutic and side-effects of azapropazone is, in some respects, not unlike that of other NSAIDs though there may be some notable differences. Compared with azapropazone, these include the appreciably lower incidence of blood dyscrasias (see chapter by Hort), low GI ulceration and haemorrhage in low-middle aged arthritic subjects. Though the risk of GI and other side-effects increases in the elderly, the precise reasons for this have not been fully established.

References

1. Walker, FS (1985). Azapropazone, and related benzotrianzes. In: Rainsford, KD (ed), *Anti-Inflammatory and Anti-Rheumatic Drugs*, Vol. II. (Boca Raton, FL.: CRC Press), pp. 1–32
2. Rainsford, KD, Davies A, Mundy, L and Ginsburg, I (1989). Comparative effects of azapropazone on cellular events at inflamed sites. Influence on joint pathology in arthritic rats, leucocyte superoxide and eicosanoid production, platelet aggregation, synthesis of cartilage proteoglycans, synovial production and actions of interleukin-1 in cartilage resorption correlated with drug uptake into cartilage *in-vitro. J Pharm Pharmacol*, **41**, 322–30
3. Rainsford, KD (1989). Concepts of the mode of action and toxicity of anti-inflammatory drugs. A basis for safer and more selective therapy, and for future drug developments. In: Rainsford, KD and Velo, GP (eds), *New Developments in Anti-Rheumatic Therapy*. (Lancaster, UK: Kluwer Academic Publishers), pp. 37–92
4. Famaey, J–P (1987). Synovial anti-inflammatory and anti-rheumatic drug levels: importance in therapeutic efficacy. In: Lewis, AJ and Furst, DE (eds), *Nonsteroidal Anti-Inflammatory Drugs, Mechanisms and Clinical Use*. (New York & Basel: Marcel Dekker), pp. 201–14
5. Kitchen, EA, Dawson, W, Rainsford, KD and Cawston, T (1985). Inflammation and possible modes of anti-inflammatory drugs. In: Rainsford, KD (ed), *Anti-Inflammatory and Anti-Rheumatic Drugs*, Vol. I. (Boca Raton, FL: CRC Press), 21–87
6. Lewis, AJ and Furst, DE (eds) (1987). *Non-steroidal Anti-Inflammatory Drugs. Mechanisms and Clinical Use*. (New York & Basel: Marcel Dekker)

---

*The European distributors of this drug recommend in the package insert adjustment of dosage for the elderly with respect to renal function.

7. Paulus, HE, Furst, DE and Dromgoole, SH (eds) (1987). *Drugs for Rheumatic Disease*. (New York: Churchill Livingstone)
8. Anon (1987). Which NSAID? *Drug Therapeutics Bulletin*, **25**, 21
9. Jahn, U and Adrian, RW (1969). Pharmakoligische und toxikologische Prüfung des neuen Antiphogisticums Azapropazon = 3-Dimethylamino-7-methyl-1-2-(2-propylmalonyl)-1, 2-dihydro-1, 2, 4-benzo-triazin. *Arzneim-Forsch*, **19**, 36–52
10. Jahn, U and Wagner–Jauregg, Th (1974). Wirkungsvergleich sauer Antiphlogistika im Bradykinin-, UV-Erythem-und Rattenpfotenödem-Test, *Arzneim-Forsch*, **24**, 494–9
11. Dawson, W (1979). Models of acute inflammation — a commentary. In: Rainsford, KD and Ford-Hutchinson, AW (eds). *Prostaglandins and Inflammation* AAS6. (Basel: Birkhauser), pp. 83–9
12. Militzer, K and Hirche, H (1981). Prophylaktische und therapeutische Anwendung von Antiphlogistika — untersucht am Carrageenin — Pfotenödem der Ratte. *Arzniem-Fosch*, **31**, 26–32
13. DiRosa, M and Sorrentino, L (1970). Some pharmacodynamic properties of carrageenin in the rat. *Br J Pharmacol*, **38**, 214–20
14. DiRosa, M, Papadimitriou, JM and Willoughby, DA (1971). A histopathological and pharmacological analysis of the mode of action of non-steroidal anti-inflammatory drugs. *J Path*, **105**, 239–56
15. Bolam, JP, Elliott, PNC, Ford–Hutchinson, AW and Smith, MJH (1974). Histamine, 5-hydroxytryptamine, kinins and the anti-inflammatory activity of human plasma fraction in carrageenan-induced paw oedema in the rat. *J Pharm Pharmacol*, **26**, 434–40
16. Vinegar, R, Truax, JF and Selph, JL (1976). Quantitative studies on the pathway to acute carrageenan inflammation. *Fed Proc*, **35**, 2447–56
17. Willis, AL (1970). Identification of prostaglandin E_2 in rat inflammatory exudate. *Pharmacol Res Commun*, **2**, 297–304
18. Blackham, A, Norris, AA and Woods, FAM (1985). Models for evaluating the anti-inflammatory effects of inhibitors of arachidonic acid metabolism. *J. Pharm Pharmacol*, **37**, 787–93
19. Thompson, AW, Fowler, EF and Pugh-Humphreys, RGP (1979). Review/commentary. Immunopharmacology of the macrophage toxic agent carrageenan. *Int J Immunopharmacol*, **1**, 247–61
20. Thompson, AW and Fowler, EE (1981). Carrageenan: A review of its effects on the immune system. *Agents & Actions*, **11**, 265–73
21. Vinegar, R, Schrieber, W and Hugo, R (1969). Biphasic development of carrageenan edema in rats. *J Pharmacol Expt Therap*, **266**, 96–103
22. Gemmell, DK, Cottney, J and Lewis, AJ (1979). Comparative effects of drugs on four paw oedema models in the rat. *Agents & Actions*, **9**, 107–16
23. Moncada, S, Ferriera, SH and Vane, JR (1975). Inhibition of prostaglandin synthesis as a mechanism of analgesia of aspirin-like drugs in the dog knee joint. *Europe J Pharmacol*, **31**, 250-60
24. Juan, H and Lembeck, F (1976). Release of prostaglandins from the isolated perfused rabbit ear by bradykinin and acetylcholine. *Agents & Actions*, **6**, 642–5
25. Otterness, IG, Wiseman, EH and Gans, DJ (1979). A comparison of the carrageenan edema test and ultraviolet light-induced erythema test as predictors for the clinical dose in rheumatoid arthritis. *Agents & Actions*, **9**, 177–83
26. Woodward, DF, Rowal, P, Pipkin, MA and Owen, DAA (1981). Re-evaluation of the effect of non-steroidal anti-inflammatory drugs on U.V.-induced cutaneous inflammation. *Agents & Actions*, **11**, 711–7
27. Winter, CA and Nuss, GW (1966). Treatment of adjuvant arthritis in rats with anti-inflammatory drugs. *Arth Rheum*, **9**, 394–404
28. Maeda, M, Tanaka, Y, Suzuki, T and Nakamura, K (1979). Pharmacological studies on carprofen, a new non-steroidal anti-inflammatory drug, in animals.

Folia Pharmacol Japon, **73**, 757–77

29. Lewis, DA, Best, R and Bird, J (1977). Anti-inflammatory action of azapropazone. *J Pharm Pharmacol*, **29**, 113–4

30. Szanto, L, Tanka, D and Kellner, M (1976). Inhibitions of prostaglandin potentiated formalin induced arthritis with non steroid antiphlogistics. *Int J Clin Pharmacol*, **13**, 113–9

31. Jahn, U, Reller, J and Schatz, F (1973). Pharmacokinetische Untersuchungen mit Azapropazon bei Tieren. *Arzneim-Forsch*, **23**, 660–6

32. Ackerman, NR, Rooks, WH, Shott, HL, Genant, H, Maloney, D and West, E (1979). Effects of naproxen on connective tissue changes in the adjuvant arthritic rat. *Arth Rheum*, **22**, 1365–74

33. Bensley, DN and Nickander, R (1982). Comparative effects of benoxaprofen and other anti-inflammatory drugs on bone damage in the adjuvant arthritic rats. *Agents & Actions*, **12**, 313–9

34. Fukawa, K, Kanezuka, T. Ohba, S and Irino, O (1985). Studies on anti-inflammatory agents (5). Specific characteristic of bone changes in adjuvant arthritic rats with passage of time. *Folia Pharmacol Japon*, **85**, 407–14

35. Brune, K, Rainsford, KD, Wagner, K and Peskar, BA (1981). Inhibition by anti-inflammatory drugs of prostaglandin production in cultured marcrophages. Factors influencing the apparent drug effects. *Naunyn-Schmiedebergs Arch Pharmacol*, **315**, 269–76

36. Spahn, H, Thabe, K, Mutschler, E, Tillmaner, K and Gikaloo, I (1987). Concentration of azapropazone in synovial tissues and fluid. *Europ J Clin Pharmacol*, **32**, 303–7

37. Rainsford, KD (1985). Distribution of azapropazone and its principal 8-hydroxy-metabolite in plasma, urine and gastrointestinal mucosa determined by HPLC. *J Pharm Pharmacol*, **37**, 341–5

38. Aylward, M, Bater, PA, Davies, DE, *et al.* (1980). Simultaneous pharmacokinetics of azapropazone in plasma and synovial fluid in patients with rheumatoid disease. Report to AH Robins (UK) study RE3/5122 [report and data on their files]

39. Lewis, DA, Capstick, RB and Ancill, RJ (1971). The action of azapropazone, oxyphenbutazone and phenylbutazone on lysosomes. *J Pharm Pharmacol*, **23**, 931–5

40. Mackin, WM, Ratich, SM and Marshall, CL (1986). Inhibition of rat neutrophil functional responses by azapropazone, an anti-gout drug. *Biochem Pharmacol*, **35**, 917–22

41. Gans, KR, Mackin, WM and Galbraith, W (1985). Effect of azapropazone on xanthine oxidase, PMN function and macrophage arachidonate metabolism. *The Pharmacoligist*, **27**, 243

42. Jahn, U and Thiele, K (1988). *In vitro* inhibition on xanthine oxidase by azapropazone and 8-hydroxyazapropazone. *Arzneim-Forsch*, **38**, 507–8

43. Montor, SG, Thoolen, MJ, Makin, WM and Timmermans, PB (1987). Effects of azapropazone and allopurinol on myocardial infarct size in rats. *Europ J Pharmacol*, **140**, 203–7

44. Wagner–Janregg, Th, Burlimann, W and Fischer, J (1969). Vergleich antiphlogistischer Substanzen in Plasmaeiweiss-Trübungs-Test nach Mizushima. *Arzneim-Forsch*, **19**, 1532–6

45. Urien, S. Albengres, E, Pinquier, JL and Tillerment, JP (1986). Role of alpha$_1$acid glycoprotein, albumin, and nonesterified fatty acids in serum binding of azapropopazone and warfarin. *Clin Pharmacol Ther*, **39**, 683–9

46. Mutschler, E, Jahn, U and Thiele, K (1985). 2. Positions of azapropazone relative to the category of nonsteroidal anti-rheumatic agents. In: Eberl, R and Fellmann, N (eds), *Rheuma Forum Special Issue* 2. (Karlsruhe: G. Braun), pp. 13–17

47. Jahn, U (1985). 3. Azapropazone and the problems of damage to cartilage by NSA. In: Eberl, R and Fellmann, N (eds), *Rheuma Forum Special Issue* 2.

(Karlsruhe: G. Braun), pp. 19–23
48. Bostrom, H, Berntsen, K and Whitehouse, MW (1964). Biochemical properties of anti-inflammatory drugs II. Some effects on sulphate^{-35}S metabolism *in vivo*. *Biochem Pharmacol*, **13**, 413–20
49. Whitehouse, MW (1965). Some biochemical and pharmacological properties of anti-inflammatory drugs. *Progress in Drug Research*, **8**, 321–429
50. Denko, CW (1964). The effect of phenylbutazone and its derivatives oxyphenyl-butazone and sulfinpyrazone on ^{35}S-sulphate incorporation in cartilage and stomach. *J Lab Cin Med*, **63**, 953–8
51. Kalbhen, DA, Karzel, K and Domenjoz, W (1967). The inhibitory effects of some antiphlogistic drugs on the glucosamine incorporation into mucopolysaccharides synthesized by fibroblast cultures. *Med Pharmacol Exp*, **16**, 185–9
52. Kleine, TO and Hild, W (1972). Effect of anti-inflammatory drugs on the biosynthesis of Ch-4-peptides in aging bovine cartilage. *Scan J Clin Lab Invest*, **29**, (Suppl. 123), 21
53. Palmoski, MJ and Brandt, KD (1980). Effects of some non-steroidal anti-inflammatory drugs on proteoglycan metabolism and organization in canine articular cartilage. *Arth Rheum*, **23**, 1010–20
54. Brandt, KD and Palmoski, MJ (1983). Relationships between matrix proteoglycan content and the effects of salicylate and indomethacin on articular cartilage. *Arth Rheum*, **26**, 528–31
55. Brandt, KD and Palmoski, MJ. Effects of salicylates and other non-steroidal anti-inflammatory drugs on articular cartilage. *Am J Med*, **77**, 65–9
56. Palmoski, MJ and Brandt, KD (1985). Proteoglycan depletion, rather than fibrillation, determines the effects of salicylate and indomethacin on osteoarthritic cartilage. *Arth Rheum*, **28**, 548–53
57. Carney, SL (1987). A study of the effects of NSAIDs on proteoglycan metabolism in cartilage explant cultures. In: *Focus on tiaprofenac acid. Proc Int Symp on Rheumatol*. Huskisson, EC and Shiokawa, Y (eds) *New Trends in Rheumatology*, Vol. 5. (Amsterdam: Excerpta Medica), pp. 24–34
58. Iwata, H (1987). Effect of anti-arthritic drugs for articular cartilage and synovial fluid. In: *Focus on tiaprofenic acid. Proc Int Symp on Rheumatol*, Huskisson, EC and Shiokawa, Y (eds.) *New Trends in Rheumatology*, Vol. 5. (Amsterdam: Excerpta Medica), pp. 35–46
59. McKenzie, L. Horsburgh, B and Gosh, P (1976). Effect of anti-inflammatory drugs on sulphated glycosaminoglycan synthesis in aged human articular cartilage. *Ann Rheum Dis*, **35**, 487–97
60. Herman, J, Appel, A and Khosea, R (1986). The *in vitro* effect of select classes of non-steroidal anti-inflammatory drugs on normal cartilage metabolism. *J Rheumatol*, **13**, 1014–8
61. Palmoski, MJ and Brandt, KD (1983). Benoxoprofen stimulates proteogycan synthesis in normal canine knee cartilage *in vitro*. *Arth Rheum*, **26**, 771–4
62. Franchimont, P, Gysen, Ph, Lecomte–Yern, MJ and Malaise, M (1983). Non-steroidal anti-inflammatory agents and articular proteoglycans. In: Tiaprofenic acid. *Proc Symp Xth European Congress of Rheumatology*, Moscow, 26th June–2nd July 1983. Huskisson, EC and Franchimont, P (Amsterdam: Excerpta Medica), pp. 3–14
63. Saxne, T, Heinegard, D and Wollheim, FA (1987). Cartilage proteoglycans in synovial fluid and serum in patients with inflammatory joint disease. *Arth & Rheum*, **30**, 972–9
64. Rainsford, KD, Rashad, S, Revell, P and Walker, F (1988). Effect of NSAIDs on joint arthropathy in osteoarthritic patients at arthroplasty: relation to inhibition of prostanoids and proteoglycans. In: *4th International Meeting of the Inflammation Research Association*, Abstracts, White Haven, PA
65. Rainsford, KD and Velo, GP (eds) (1983). *Side-Effects of Anti-Inflammatory /Analgesic Drugs*. (New York: Raven Press)
66. Rainsford, KD and Velo, GP (eds) (1987). *Side-Effects of Anti-Inflammatory*

Drugs. Clinical and Epidemiological Agents. Pt.I. (Lancaster, UK: MTP Press)

67.   Rainsford, KD and Velo, GP (eds) (1987). *Side-Effects of Anti-Inflammatory Drugs. Studies in Major Organ Systems.* Pt.II. (Lancaster, UK: MTP Press)

68.   Rainsford, KD (1982). An analysis of the gastrointestinal side-effects of non-steroidal anti-inflammatory drugs, with particular reference to comparative studies in man and laboratory species. *Rheumatol Internat,* **2,** 1–10

69.   Rainsford, KD (1984). Side-effects of anti-inflammatory/analgesic drugs. Epidemiology and gastrointestinal tract. *Trends in Pharmacological Sciences,* **5,** 156–9

70.   Rainsford, KD (1984). Side-effects of anti-inflammatory/analgesic drugs. Renal, hepatic and other systems. *Trends in Pharmacological Sciences,* **5,** 205–8

71.   Rainsford, KD (1987). Toxicity of currently used anti-inflammatory and anti-rheumatic drugs. In: Lewis, AJ and Furst, DE (eds). *Nonsteroidal Anti-inflammatory Drugs. Mechanisms and Clinical Use.* (New York: Marcel Dekker) 215–244.

72.   Rainsford, KD (1987). Side-effects of anti-inflammatory/analgesic and anti-rheumatic drugs. In: Williamson, WRN (ed), *Anti-Inflammatory Drugs.* (New York: Marcel Dekker) pp. 359–406

73.   Mintz, FG and Fraga, A (1976). Gastrointestinal bleeding in patients with rheumatoid arthritis: effect of azapropazone treatment. *Curr Med Res Opin* **4,** 89–93

74.   Hradsky, M and Bruce, L (1987). Endoscopic evaluation of the effect of azapropazone on the gastric mucosa. *Scan J Gastroenterol,* **7,** 31–2

75.   Rainsford, KD (1981). Comparison of the gastric ulcerogenic activity of new non-steroidal anti-inflammatory drugs in stressed rats. *Brit J Pharmacol,* **73,** 79c–80c

76.   Rainsford, KD and Willis, C (1982). Relationship of gastric mucosal damage induced in pigs by anti-inflammatory drugs to their effects on prostaglandin production. *Dig Dis Sci,* **27,** 624–35

77.   Rainsford, KD, Fox, SA & Osborne, DJ (1984). Comparative effects of some non-steroidal anti-inflammatory drugs on the ultrastructural integrity and prostaglandin levels in the rat gastric mucosa. Relationship to drug uptake. *Scand J Gastroenterol,* **19,** (Suppl. 101), 55–68

78.   Rainsford, KD, Fox, SA and Osborne, DJ (1985). Relationship between drug absorption, inhibition of cyclooxygenase and lipoxygenase pathways and the development of gastric mucosal damage by non-steroidal anti-inflammatory drugs in rats and pigs. In: Bailey, MJ (ed), *Advances in Prostaglandins, Leukotrienes and Lipoxins.* (New York: Plenum Press), pp. 639–53

79.   Rainsford, KD (1986). Structural damage and changes in eicosanoid metabolites in the gastric mucosa of rats and pigs induced by anti-inflammatory drugs in varying ulcerogenicity. *Int J Tiss React,* **8,** 1–14

80.   Rainsford, KD (1987). Gastric ulcerogenicity of non-steroidal anti-inflammatory drugs in mice with mucosa sensitized by cholinomimetic treatment. *J Pharm Pharmacol,* **39,** 669–72

81.   Rainsford, KD (1987). Effects of 5-lipoxygenase inhibitors and leukotriene antagonists on the development of gastric mucosal lesions induced by non-steroidal anti-inflammatory drugs in cholinomimetic treated mice. *Agents & Actions,* **21,** 316–9

82.   Rainsford, KD (1978). The effects of aspirin and other non-steroidal anti-inflammatory drugs on the gastrointestinal mucus glycoprotein biosynthesis *in vivo.* Relationship to ulcerogenic actions. *Biochem Pharmacol,* **27,** 877–85

83.   Thune, S (1976). A comparative study of azapropazone and indomethacin in the treatment of rheumatoid arthritis. *Curr Med Res Opin,* **4,** 70–5

84.   Thune, S (1976). Long-term use of azapropazone in the treatment of rheumatoid arthritis. *Curr Med Res Opin,* **4,** 80–8

85.   Diffey, BL, Pal, B and Robson, J (1986). Azapropazone therapy and photosensitivity. *Photodermatol,* **3,** 304–5

86. Barker, DJ and Cotterill, JA (1977). Skin eruptions due to azapropazone. *Lancet*, **1**, 90

87. Barker, DJ and Cotterill, JA (1977). Azapropazone induced bullous drug eruptions. *Acta Derm Venereol*, **57**, 461–2

88. Ljunggren, B and Lundberg, K (1985). *In vivo* phototoxicity of non-steroidal anti-inflammatory drugs evaluated by the mouse tail technique. *Photodermatol*, **2**, 377–88

89. Llunggren, B (1985). Proprionic acid-derived non-steroidal antiinflammatory drugs are phototoxic *in vitro*. *Photodermatol*, **2**, 3–9

90. Jones, RA, Navaratnam, S, Parsons, BJ and Phillips, GO (1988). One-electron oxidation and reduction of azapropazone and phenylbutazone derivatives in aqueous solution: a pulse radiolysis study. *Photochem Photobiol*, **48**, 401–8

91. Navaratnam, S, Hughes, JL, Parsons, BJ and Phillips GO (1985). Laser flash and steady-state photolysis of benoxaprofen in aqueous solution. *Photochem Photobiol*, **41**, 375–80

92. Sik, RH, Pashall, CS and Chignall, CF (1983). The phototoxic effect of benoxaprofen and its analogues on human erythrocytes and rat peritoneal mast cells. *Photochem Photobiol*, **38**, 411–5

93. Reszka, K and Chignall, CG (1983). Spectroscopic studies of cutaneous photosensitizing agents—IV. The photolysis of benaxoprofen, an anti-inflammatory drug with phototoxic properties. *Photochem Photobiol*, **38**, 281–91

94. Rainsford, KD (1989). Mechanism of phototoxic reactions by some NSAIDs. *In preparation*

95. Atkinson, LK, Goodship, TH and Ward, MK (1986). Acute renal failure associated with pyelonephritis and consumption of non-steroidal anti-inflammatory drugs. *Br Med J*, **292**, 97–8

96. Sipila, R, Skrifrars, B and Tornroth, T (1986). Reversible non-oliguric impairment of renal function during azapropazone treatment. *Scand J Rheumatol*, **15**, 23–6

97. Adams, DH, Howie, AJ, Richard, J, McConkey, B, Bacon, PA and Adu, D (1986). Non-steroidal anti-inflammatory drugs and renal failure. *Lancet*, **1**, 57–60

98. Templeton, JS (1978). Azapropazone and renal function. *Rheumatol Rehab*, **17**, 219–21

99. Jahucen, E, Blanck, KJ, Breuing, KH, Gilfrinch, HJ, Meinertz, T and Trenk, D (1981). Plasma protein binding of azapropazone in patients with kidney and liver disease. *Br J Clin Pharmacol*, **11**, 361–7

100. Ritch, AE, Perera, WN and Jones, CJ (1982). Pharmacokinetics of azapropazone in the elderly. *Br J Clin Pharmacol*, **14**, 116–9

101. Lo, TC and Dymock, IW (1988). Azapropazone induced hepatitis. *Br Med J*, **297**, 1614

102. Williamson, PJ, Eve, MD and Roberts, CJ (1984). A study of the potential interactions between azapropazone and frusemide in man. *Br J Clin Pharmacol*, **18**, 619–23

103. Waller, DG and Waller, D (1984). Hypoglycaemia due to azapropazone – tolbutamide interaction. *Br J Rheumatol*, **23**, 24–5

104. McElnay, JC and D'Arcy, PF (1978). Interaction between azapropazone and warfarin. *Experientia*, **34**, 1320–1

105. McElnay, JC and D'Arcy, PF (1978). The effect of azapropazone on the binding of warfarin to human serum protein. *J Pharm Pharmacol*, **30** (Suppl.), 73P

106. Faust–Tinnenfeldt, G and Gilfrich, HJ (1977). Digitoxin-Kinetik unter antirheumatischer Therapie mit azapropazone. *Arzneim-Forsch*, **27**, 2009–11

Summary

Azapropazone is, in comparison with other NSAIDs, a moderately potent anti-inflammatory and analgesic agent with relatively low gastrointestinal irritancy. The drug may exert its anti-inflammatory actions by inhibiting a variety of cellular systems manifesting production of inflammatory mediators (superoxide anion, prostaglandins, release of lysosomal enzymes, interleukin-1) as well as inhibiting the accumulation of leucocytes with inflamed sites and their degranulation. It should be noted, however, that these *in vitro* actions of the drug have not in some cases, been established *in vivo*. Further work is also wanting to determine if the reported stimulatory actions of azapropazone on proteoglycan synthesis *in vitro* have any significance in the maintenance of cartilage integrity especially in osteoarthritis.

Of the major side-effects (aside from those in the gastrointestinal tract) skin rashes notably from photosensitivity reactions are, as with many other NSAIDs, most common. They are of low grade and invariably are reversible. The mechanisms of the production of rashes might involve formation of a reactive or phototoxic metabolite according to a postulated reaction sequence. This reaction requires further investigation to confirm the basis for its formation.

Zusammenfassung

Azapropazon ist ein im Vergleich zu anderen nichtsteroidalen Antirheumatika (NSAID) mässig potentes Antiphlogistikum und Analgetikum mit relativ schwacher Reizwirkung auf den Gastrointestinaltrakt. Die Substanz übt ihre entzündungshemmende Wirkung wahrscheinlich über die Hemmung verschiedener zellulärer Systeme aus, welche Entzündungsmediatoren produzieren (Superoxid-Anionen, Prostaglandine, Freisetzung lysosomaler Enzyme, Interleukin-1); daneben hemmt sie die Ansammlung von Leukozyten am Entzündungsort sowie deren Degranulation. Es muss jedoch angemerkt werden, dass diese *in vitro*-Wirkungen in manchen Fällen *in vivo* nicht bestätigt werden konnten. Es sind auch weitere Forschungsarbeiten zur Klärung der Frage nötig, ob die *in vitro* beobachtete stimulierende Wirkung von Azapropazon auf die Synthese von Proteoglycanen irgendeine Bedeutung für die Aufrechterhaltung der Knorpelintegrität hat, insbesondere bei Arthrosen.

Unter den bedeutenden Nebenwirkung ausserhalb des Gastrointestinaltrakts treten wie bei zahlreichen anderen NSAID am häufigsten Hautexantheme auf, vorwiegend als Folge von Photosensitivitäts-Reaktionen. Diese Exantheme sind wenig ausgeprägt und ohne Ausnahme reversibel; bei ihrer Entstehung könnte die Bildung eines reaktiven oder phototoxischen Metaboliten gemäss einer postulierten Reaktionskette eine Rolle spielen. Zur Erarbeitung der Grundlagen dieser Reaktionskette sind weitere Forschungsarbeiten nötig.

Resumé

L'azapropazone, comparativement aux autres AINS, est un médicament anti-inflammatoire et analgésique de puissance modérée, irritant relativement peu la muqueuse gastro-intestinale. Le médicament peut développer ses effets anti-inflammatoires en inhibant toute une série de systèmes cellulaires produisant des médiateurs de l'inflammation (anions superoxides, prostaglandines, libération d'enzymes lysosomiaux, interleukine-1), de même qu'en prévenant l'accumulation de leucocytes aux sites de l'inflammation, et leur dégranulation. Il faut cependent relever que dans certains cas, ces effets du médicament *in vitro* n'ont pas été prouvés *in vivo*. D'autres travaux sont encore nécessaires pour déterminer si les effets stimulateurs de l'azapropazone sur la synthèse de protéoglycanes, observés *in vitro*, ont une importance quelconque dans la sauvegarde de l'intégrité du cartilage, particulièrement dans l'arthrose.

Parmi les principaux effets secondaires (ceux au niveau du tractus gastro-intestinal mis à part), les éruptions cutanées, sur réactions de photosensibilisation notamment, sont les plus fréquentes, tout comme avec beaucoup d'autres AINS. Elles sont discrètes et, sans exception, réversibles. Les mécanismes impliqués dans ces exanthèmes peuvent faire intervenir la formation d'un métabolite réactif ou phototoxique, si l'on en croit une séquence de réactions qui a été postulée. Ceci exige d'autres recherches pour confirmer l'origine de cette réaction.

5
Pharmacokinetics of azpapropazone in comparison to other NSAIDs

K Brune

I. INTRODUCTION

Azapropazone has been in clinical use as an NSAID for two decades[1]. During this time the mode of action and the pharmacokinetic behaviour of this compound have been carefully evaluated[2-5]. The results obtained are of therapeutic relevance. There are, however, some areas of clinical importance which have not been investigated in detail so far. Since azapropazone is believed to display some advantages which may be of therapeutic relevance, the known data as well as the data lacking should be carefully evaluated in order to extrapolate on the optimal use of this compound.

II. PHYSICAL CHEMISTRY OF AZAPROPAZONE

The physicochemical data on the molecule azapropazone have been investigated repeatedly[7-11] and will be discussed in detail in another chapter of this symposium[12]. For clinical use, it may be of importance that this compound comprises a slight yellowish crystalline powder with a weak odour of acetic acid. It has no adverse taste as many other NSAIDs. Moreover, it has a relatively high melting point and forms salts in alkaline aqueous solutions (Table 1). These characteristics are of major pharmaceutical importance allowing for the different types of formulations which, in turn, may cause slightly different pharmacokinetic behaviour of the active compounds in humans (Table 1).

1. Absorption

Azapropazone is almost completely absorbed from the gastrointestinal tract following oral administration[13-19], ensuring a bioavailability of approximately 80%[6,18]. Despite its relatively good solubility in aqueous solutions even at acidic pH conditions, it is now widely accepted that azapropazone is only marginally absorbed in the stomach (for details, see other chapters of this book[11,20]). Consequently, azapropazone is absorbed in the small

Azapropazone – 20 years of clinical use. Rainsford, KD (ed)
© Kluwer Academic Publishers. Printed in Great Britain

Table 1 Pharmacokinetic characteristics of azapropazone

Names	Physicochemical data	Structure(s)
Generic name: azapropazone Trade names: Cinnamin® Prodisan® Prolix® Prolixan (A)® Rheumox® Tolyprin® Xani®	Molecular weight: 336 Melting point: 233 pK_a (aqua + alc.): 6.3 S (ng/ml): 73 P (n-octanol/buffer): 6.2 P_b human%: 99%	

Drug = (I) Metabolite = (II)

DI-KETO CATION   ZWITTERION   ENOLATE ANION

(I) R=H   (II) R=OH

References
Index Nominum[50]

Brune and Lanz[6]
Herzfeldt and Kümmel[9]

Brune and Lanz[6]
McCormack and Brune[5]

Lombardino et al.[8]
McCormack and Brune[10]
Templeton[4]

ˣdepending on the formulation

Absorption	Distribution	Elimination
Time-to-peak: p.o.: 3–6 h rect.: 4–7 h Bioavailabil. p.o. 80–90% rect. ~60%	App. rel. vol. distr.: (1/kg) Volunt.: 0.14–0.22 Elderly: unchanged ren. dysf.: unchanged hep. dysf.: unchanged	$t_{50\%}$ Volent: α: 0.3 h β: 3–4 h γ: vol. 12–25 h

γ: Elderly: up to 73 h γ: ren. dys.: up to 32 h γ: hep. dys.: up to 62 h |
| AUC: linear up to 1200 mg/sing. dose | deept comp.: inflamed tissue | |
| Brune and Lanz[6] | Breuing et al.[18] Gikalov et al.[21] Woodhouse and Wynne[34] Ritch et al.[33] Spahn et al.[25] | Breuing et al.[18] Brune and Lanz[6] Gikalov et al.[21] Ritch et al.[33] |

S = solubility, buffer at pH 7.0
P_b = protein binding

intestine over prolonged periods of time. The available data are compiled in Table 1. It is apparent that after oral and rectal administration of different galenic forms, the time-to-peak plasma concentration is reached only after 3–5 h. Aspirin, for example, in most formulations is absorbed faster with the absorption being predominantly in the stomach[6]. It is obvious that the retarded absorption of azapropazone has advantages and disadvantages. On the one hand, if fast pain relief of inflammatory pain is required, an oral or rectal administration of azapropazone may not satisfy the patient. If ethical, possibly an intravenous injection of azapropazone may be used, guaranteeing high plasma concentration of the drug[18,21]. On the other hand, sparing the stomach as a site of absorption may have advantages, i.e. it may reduce the incidence of blood-loss and stomach ulceration.

2. Distribution

Plasma protein binding of azapropazone is more than 99%[6,22,23]. The distribution behaviour of the zwitterion of azapropazone is not very well investigated (for data on the rat, see reference 15). In comparison to other NSAIDs, the volume of distribution (Table 1) appears relatively large. This may be due to the relatively high pK_a-value allowing for an apparent volume of distribution which includes more than the easily accessible body water space[24]. Data on the uptake of azapropazone into some compartments (e.g. the cerebrospinal fluid) are not available. Azapropazone does however accumulate in inflamed tissue in man similarly to many other NSAIDs and displays a prolonged elimination half-life[6,25,26]. The question as to whether azapropazone accumulates in other compartments apart from deep inflamed tissues cannot be answered with certainty. Interestingly, the data available from patients suffering from impaired renal and kidney function (Table 1) do not indicate an increase in the apparent volume of distribution in these disease states[27,28]. This is somewhat surprising because serious liver damage often causes a reduction of available protein binding sites for highly protein bound NSAIDs. It might therefore be expected that an increased apparent volume of distribution (V_d) would be evident in these patients. The data (Table 1) do not support this reasoning.

3. Elimination

More than 60% of azapropazone is eliminated via the kidney in an unchanged form[6,13,16,18]. In addition, 8-hydroxy-azapropazone (formerly called 6-hydroxy-azapropazone) has been recovered in the urine (ca. 20% of the dose)[29,30] and recently also in the plasma (up to 10% of the parent substance)[31]. It may, consequently, be assumed that much less than half of the dose administered is eliminated by hepatic metabolisation and the predominant part by renal excretion of unchanged azapropazone. In agreement with this finding and interpretation is the fact that both serious renal damage and considerable hepatic damage increases the elimination half-life significantly[27,28]. Interestingly, and somewhat at variance with the data on the elimination, is the fact that serious hepatic damage results in a much higher prolongation of the elimination half-life than serious renal damage.

This may be brought about by a diminished albumin concentration and consequently increased free fraction of azapropazone in the plasma as well as impaired renal clearance in these patients[23,27,28]. The principal metabolite 8-hydroxy-azapropazone has no known toxic and only very weak anti-inflammatory action[32]. It is obvious that in patients with seriously impaired renal function as well as in patients with severe hepatic damage azapropazone should either not be used, or the dose decreased considerably. This drug dosage should be related to the degree of renal or hepatic dysfunction. The same precautions should be taken in the elderly, where diminished renal and liver function frequently occur[33,34].

4. Drug interactions

Azapropazone has been extensively investigated for its interactions with other compounds[24,35-45]. In these studies it showed no interactions with usual antirheumatic agents like aurothioglucose[39], prednisolone[39], chloroquine[37], D-penicillamine[36] and some immunosuppressive drugs[36]. Azapropazone can also be given together with antacids and laxatives since there is no significant clinically important interaction[38]. The relevant interactions may be categorized as pharmacokinetic or pharmacodynamic. They are all listed in Table 2. Most of them are similar to those observed and described for salicylates and phenylbutazone. Azapropazone clearly shows interactions with phenytoin[45] as well as with widely used Vitamin K-antagonists[41-43] and tolbutamide[44]. Individual cases of interactions with digitoxin[35] have been found. In analogy to interactions observed with many other NSAIDs[6] caution has to be exercized when azapropazone is administered together with lithium, methotrexate and thiazide diuretics. It cannot be excluded that the elimination of lithium and methotrexate is retarded under the influence of azapropazone, and that the pharmacodynamic effect of thiazide diuretics is reduced but the elimination retarded. It is also possible that other NSAIDs (particularly salicylates) and also aluminium-containing antacids, reduce the AUC of azapropazone either by interfering with the absorption or enhancing the elimination of this compound. These effects may be pertinent to the clinical effectiveness of azapropazone, but are unlikely to cause problems although it has been postulated that in renal insufficiency the combined effect of thiazide diuretics and NSAIDs may cause electrolyte disturbances involving sodium, potassium and chloride which may add to the risk of cardiovascular failure[46]. Again, additional studies should help to clarify these questions.

III. CONCLUSION

It may be stated that azapropazone shows somewhat different pharmacokinetics from other NSAIDs. The specific behaviour of the zwitterion may offer advantages as to the gastrointestinal toxicity[10,11,20,47-49]. The relative

Table 2 Drug interactions of azapropazone

Pharmacokinetic interactions		Pharmacodynamic interactions	
Absorption	*Distribution and Elimination*	*Effects of azapropazone on other drugs*	*Effects of other drugs on azapropazone*
Antacids: Al: $C_{PL. aza.}$ (4/6)[a] Al+Mg: $C_{PL.aza.}$ (2/3)[a]	digitoxin, $t_{50\%}$ (2/8)[a] diuretics, $t_{50\%}$?↑[b] lithium, $t_{50\%}$?↑[b] methotrexate, $t_{50\%}$?↑ phenytoin, $t_{50\%}$ ↑ salicylates, $t_{50\%}$?[b] tolbutamide, $t_{50\%}$ → warfarin, $t_{50\%}$?↓[c]	diuretics, effect ?↓[b]	salicylates, effect ?↓[b]
Laxatives (Bisacodyl): effect C_{aza}			

[a] fraction showing the effect but differences of mean-values being not statistically significant

[b] no data, assumed from reports on other NSAIDs

[c] indirect evidence comp. references

[b] no data, but effects reported for other NSAID

References:
Faust-Tinnefeld et al.[38]

Andreasen et al.[44]
Faust-Tinnefeld et al.[38]
Gaeney et al.[45]
Green et al.[24]
McElnay and D'Arcy[41,42]
Daly et al.[51]

[b] *cf.* Brune and Lanze[6]

high amounts of azapropazone necessary for the treatment of inflammatory rheumatic diseases may add to the risk of drug interactions. Some potentially risky interactions have not been investigated so far. These points require further investigation in the future.

References

1. Bach, GL (1985). Clinical Aspects, In Eberl, R and Fellman, N (eds.). *Determination of the Classification of Azapropazone*, Reuma Forum, Special Issue 2 (Karlsruhe: G Braun)
2. Brooks, PM and Buchanan, WW (1976). Azapropazone – its place in the management of rheumatoid conditions. *Curr Med Res Opin*, **4**, 94–100
3. Sondervorst, M (1979). Azapropazone. *Clin Rheum Dis*, **5**, 465–480
4. Templeton, JS (1983). Azapropazone. In Huskisson, EC (ed.). *Anti-Rheumatic Drugs*, pp. 97–116 (New York: Praeger)
5. Walker, FS (1985). Azapropazone and related Benzotriazines. In Rainsford, KD (ed.) *Anti-Inflammatory and Anti-Rheumatic Drugs*, **Vol. II**, p. 1–32 (Boca Raton: CRC Press, Inc.)
6. Brune, K and Lanz, R (1985). Pharmacokinetics of non-steroidal antiinflammatory drugs. In: Bonta IL, Bray MA, Parnham, MJ (eds.). *Handbook of Inflammation. The pharmacology of Inflammations*, **5**, pp. 413–450. (Elsevier)
7. Fenner, H and Mixich, G (1973). NMR-Untersuchungen zur Molekülstruktur von Azapropazon und Deutung seiner Pharmakokinetik und Biotransformation. *Arzneim Forsch/Drug Res.*, **23**, 667–669
8. Lombardino, JG, Otterness, IG and Wiseman, EH (1975). Acidic antiinflammatory agents – correlations of some physical, pharmacological and clinical data. *Arzneim Forsch/Drug Res*, **25**, 1629–1635
9. Herzfeldt, CD and Kümmel, R (1983). Dissociation constants, solubilities and dissolution rates of some selected nonsteroidal antiinflammatories. *Drug Dev and Indust Pharmacy*, **9**, 767–793
10. McCormack, K and Brune, K (1987). Classical absorption theory and the development of gastric mucosal damage associated with the non-steroidal antiinflammatory drugs. *Arch Toxicol*, **60**, 261–269
11. McCormack, K and Brune, K (1989). Amphiprotic non-steroidal anti-inflammatory drugs and the gastric mucosa. *Arch Toxicol*, (in press)
12. Dean, FM (1989). The clinical properties of azapropazone. In Rainsford, KD (ed.). *Azapropazone: 20 Years of Clinical Use*, Chap. 2. (Lancaster: Kluwer Academic Publishers)
13. Schatz, F, Adrian, RW, Mixich, G, Molnarowa, G, Reller, J and Jahn, U (1970). Pharmakokinetische Untersuchungen mit dem Antiphlogistikum Azapropazon (Prolixan 300) am Menschen. *Therapiewoche*, **20**, 2327–2333
14. Jahn, U, Reller, J and Schatz, F (1973). Pharmakokinetische Untersuchungen mit Azapropazon bei Tieren. *Arzneim Forsch/Drug Res*, **23**, 660–666
15. Klatt, L and Koss, FW (1973). Pharmakokinetische Untersuchungen mit ^{14}C-Azapropazon-Dihydrat an der Ratte. *Arzneim Forsch/Drug Res*, **23**, 913–920
16. Klatt, L and Koss, FW (1973). Humanpharmakokinetische Untersuchungen mit ^{14}C-Azapropazon-Dihydrat. *Arzneim Forsch/Drug Res*, **23**, 920–921
17. Jones, CJ (1976). The pharmacology and pharmacokinetics of azapropazone – a review. *Curr Med Res Opin*, **4**, 3–16
18. Breuing, KH, Gilfrich, HJ, Meinertz, T and Jähnchen, E (1979). Pharmacokinetics of azapropazone following single oral and intravenous doses. *Arzneim Forsch/-Drug Res*, **29**, 971–972

19. Verbeek, RK, Blackburn, JL and Loewen, GR (1983). Clinical pharmacokinetics of non-steroidal anti-inflammatory drugs. *Clin Pharmacokinet*, **8**, 297–331
20. McCormack, K (1989). Mathematical model for assessing risk of gastro-intestial reactions to NSAIDs. In Rainsford, KD (ed.). *Azapropazone*: 20 *Years of Clinical Use*, Chap. 7. (Lancaster: Kluwer Academic Publishers)
21. Gikalov, I, Kaufmann, R and Schuster, O (1982). Humanpharmokokinetik verschiedener i.v. Dosen von Azapropazon (HPLC-Bestimmung). *Arzneim Forsch/Drug Res*, **32**, 423–426
22. Fehske, KJ, Jaehnchen, E, Mueller, WE and Stillbauer, A (1980). Azapropazone binding to human serum albumin. *Naunya Schiedeberg's Arch Pharmacol*, **313**, 159–163
23. Jaehnchen, E, Blanck, KJ, Breuing, KH, Gilfrich, HJ, Meinertz, T and Trenk, D (1981). Plasma protein binding of azapropazone in patients with kidney and liver disease. *Br J Clin Pharmacol*, **11**, 361–367
24. Green, AE, Hort, JF, Korn, HET and Leach, H (1977). Potentiation of warfarin by azapropazone. *Br Med J*, **1**, 1532
25. Spahn, H, Thabe, K, Mutschler, E, Tillman, K and Gikalov, I. (1982). II – 12 Untersuchungen zur Pharmakokinetik von Azapropazon in Synovialgewebe und – flüssigkeit. DphH – Vortragsveranstaltung. *Sonderbeilage zu DAZ*, **39**, 10
26. Spahn, H, Thabe, K, Mutschler, E, Tillman, K and Gikalov, I (1987). Concentration of azapropazone in synovial tissues and fluid. *Eur J Clin Pharmacol*, **32**, 303–307
27. Gilfrich, HJ, Breuing, KH, Blanck, KJ and Jaenchen, E (1980). *Verh Dtsch Ges Rheumatol*, **6**, 325–326
28. Breuing, KH, Gilfrich, HJ, Meinertz, T, Wiegand, UW and Jaehnchen, E (1981). Disposition of azapropazone in chronic renal and hepatic failure. *Eur J Clin Pharmacol*, **20**, 147–155
29. Mixich, G (1972). Zum Metabolismus des neuen Antiphlogistikums Azapropazon. *Chimia*, **26**, 1031
30. Mixich, G (1972). Isolierung, Struktur und Synthese des Metaboliten von Azapropazon – Dihydrat. *Helv Chim Acta*, **55**, 1031–1038
31. Rainsford, KD (1985). Distribution of azapropazone and its principal 8-hydroxy-metabolite in plasma, urine and gastrointestinal mucosa determined by HPLC. *J Pharm Pharmacol*, **37**, 341–345
32. Jahn, U (1973). Pharmakologische Prüfung von 6-Hydroxy-Azapropazon. *Arzneim Forsch/Drug Res*, **23**, 666–667.
33. Ritch, AES, Perera, WNR and Jones, CJ (1982). Pharmacokinetics of azapropazone in the elderly. *Br J Clin Pharmacol*, **14**, 116–119
34. Woodhouse, KW and Wynne, H (1987). The pharmacokinetics of non-steriodal anti-inflammatory drugs in the elderly. *Clin Pharmacokinet*, **12**, 111–122
35. Faust-Tinnefeldt, G and Gilfrich, HJ (1977). Digitoxin-Kinetik unter antirheumatischer Therapie mit Azapropazon. *Arzneim Forsch/Drug Res*, **27**, 10, 2009–2011
36. Faust-Tinnefeldt, G, Geissler, HE and Mutschler, E (1977). Azapropazon-Plasmaspiegel unter rheumatologischer Kombinationstherapie mit D-Penicillamin und Immunosuppressiva. *Arzneim Forsch/Drug Res*, **27**, 2153–2157
37. Faust-Tinnefeldt, G and Geissler, HE (1977). Azapropazon und rheumatologische Basistherapie mit Chloroquin unter dem Aspekt der Arzneimittelinteraktion. *Arzneim Forsch/Drug Res*, **27**, 2170–2174
38. Faust-Tinnefeldt, G, Geissler, HE and Mutschler, E (1977). Azapropazon-Plasmaspiegel unter Begleitmedikation mit einem Antacidum oder Laxans. *Arzneim Forsch/Drug Res*, **27**, 2411–2414
39. Faust-Tinnefeldt, G and Geissler, HE (1978). Azapropazon und rheumatologische Kombinationstherapie unter dem Aspekt der Arzneimittelinteraktionen: Azapropazon/Aurothioglukose und Azapropazon/Prednisolon. *Arzneim Forsch/Drug*

Res, **28**, 337–341
40. Faust-Tinnefeldt, G, Geissler, HE and Gilfrich, HJ (1979). Azapropazon-Plasma-spiegel während kombinierter Anwendung mit Digitoxin. *Med Welt*, **30**, 181–182
41. McElnay, JC and D'Arcy, PF (1978). Interaction between azapropazone and warfarin. *Experientia*, **34**, 1320–1321
42. McElnay, JC and D'Arcy, PF (1977). Interaction between azapropazone and warfarin. *Br Med J*, **2**, 773–774
43. Powell-Jackson, PR (1977). Interaction between azapropazone and warfarin. *Br Med J*, **1**, 1193–1194
44. Andreasen, PB, Simonsen, K, Brocks, K, Dimo, B and Bouchelouche, P (1981). Hypoglycaemia induced by azapropazone-tolbutamide interaction. *Br J Clin Pharmacol*, **12**, 581–583
45. Geaney, DP, Carver, JG, Davies, CL and Aronson, JK (1983). Pharmacokinetic investigation of the interaction of azapropazone with phenytoin. *Br J Clin Pharmacol.*, **15**, 727–734
46. Zimran, A, Kramer, M, Plaskin, M and Hershko, C (1985). Incidence of hyperkalaemia induced by indomethacin in a hospital population. *Br Med J*, **291**, 107–108
47. Peskar, BM, Rainsford, KD, Brune, K and Gerok, W (1981). Effekt nichtsteroidar-tiger Antiphlogistika auf Plasma- und Magenmukosakonzentrationen von Pro-staglandin. *Verh Dtsch Ges Inn Med*, **87**, 833–838
48. Rainsford, KD (1982). An analysis of the gastro-intestinal side effects of non-steroidal anti-inflammatory drugs, with particular reference to comparative studies in man and laboratory species. *Rheumatol Int*, **2**, 1–10
49. Rainsford, KD (1989). The mode of action of azapropazone in relation to therapeutic action in rheumatic conditions and its major side-effects. In Rainsford, KD (ed.). *Azapropazone*: 20 *Years of Clinical Use*, Chap. 4. (Lancaster: Kluwer Academic Publishers)
50. Laboratory of the Swiss Pharmaceutical Society (1984). *Index Nominum*, p. 110 (Geneva: Swiss Pharmaceutical Society)
51. Daly, HM, Scott, GL, Boyle, J and Roberts, CJ (1986). Methotrexate toxicity precipitated by azapropazone. *Br J Dermatol*, **114**, 733–735

Summary

The non-steroidal anti-inflammatory drug (NSAID) azapropazone belongs to the class of substituted benzotriazines. The substance comprises a unique molecule which behaves in most body compartments like a weak acid, in some others, including the stomach, as its zwitterion. This behaviour results, on the one hand, in a pharmacokinetic behaviour as most NSAIDs, in particular as many other keto-enolate compounds. In addition, there are some unique features pertinent specifically to the absorption of azapropazone. The available data on absorption distribution and elimination of this compound in volunteers and patients are compiled and discussed.

Zusammenfassung

Das nicht-steroidale Antirheumatikum (NSAR) Azapropazon gehört in die Klasse der substitu-ierten Benzotriazine. Die Substanz ist ein einzigartiges Molekül, das sich in den meisten Körperkompartimenten wie eine schwache Säure verhält, in anderen, wie z.B. dem Magen, dagegen wie ein Zwitterion. Dieses Verhalten führt einerseits zu demselben pharmakokinetischen Verhalten, das die meisten NSAR, insbesondere viele andere Keto-Enol-Verbindungen, zeigen. Andererseits weist die Absorption von Azapropazon einige ganz spezifische Merkmale auf. Abschließend soll das über die Absorption, Verteilung und Elimination von Azapropazon bei freiwilligen Probanden und Patienten gesammelte Datenmaterial diskutiert werden.

Resumé

L'azapropazone est un anti-inflammatoire non stéroïdien (AINS) qui appartient au groupe de benzotriazines substituées. La substance est une molécule unique qui agit dans la plupart des parties du corps comme un acide faible; dans d'autres parties, y compris l'estomac, comme son zwittérion. Ce comportement aboutit, à un comportement pharmacocinétique semblable à celui de la plupart des AINS, particulièrement comme beaucoup d'autres composés céto-énolates. En outre, on observe des caractéristiques uniques, spécifiquement associées à l'absorption de l'azapropazone. Les données disponibles relatives à l'absorption, la distribution et l'élimination de ce composé chez des volontaires et des malades sont rassemblées et discutées.

6
The pharmacokinetics of azapropazone

JC McElnay and FS Walker

I. INTRODUCTION

The subject of pharmacology can conveniently be divided into two subsections, namely pharmacodynamics and pharmacokinetics. While pharmacodynamics deals with the therapeutic effects (both desirable and undesirable), i.e. what the drug does to the organism, pharmacokinetics deals with the kinetics of the processes of absorption, distribution and elimination of the drug, i.e. how the organism treats the drug. A careful study of the pharmacokinetic profile of a drug is desirable since the magnitude of both the desired therapeutic response and toxicity are often closely related to the concentration of the drug at its site(s) of action. This latter concentration can often be correlated with serum concentrations of the drug and it is via careful evaluation of serum drug concentrations, post administration, that the preliminary pharmacokinetic profile of a drug can be established.

Initial pharmacokinetic information for a new drug is often first obtained by administration of single doses of the drug to an animal species by the intravenous route. Since selective assay procedures may not be fully developed at this stage in the drug's development, administration is often of the radiolabelled drug. If the final route of administration is to be oral, further animal studies are often carried out with the drug administered to animals as an oral solution or suspension. When favourable results of initial toxicology studies are available the drug can be given to man, either as an oral liquid or in a solid dosage form. As well as evaluating circulating drug concentrations, when a selective assay method is available, urine samples can be quantitated to determine the elimination of unchanged drug and metabolites.

The aim of the early pharmacokinetic studies is to quantify the important pharmacokinetic parameters of absorption rate constant (ka), the distribution half-life ($t_{1/2\alpha}$), the elimination half-life ($t_{1/2\beta}$), the elimination rate constant (ke), the clearance (Cl) of drug from the serum, the apparent volume of distribution (Vd) and the oral bioavailability (F). The latter term, i.e. the percentage of drug absorbed after administration by the oral route, can only be calculated accurately if serum concentrations after both oral and

Azapropazone – 20 years of clinical use. Rainsford, KD (ed)
© Kluwer Academic Publishers. Printed in Great Britain

intravenous administration are known.

Although these data allow the mathematical estimation of steady-state serum concentrations after multiple dosing, it is advisable to carry out separate multiple dosing studies both in human volunteers and in the patient groups likely to receive the drugs, since the elimination kinetics may become non-linear at higher serum concentrations.

Using such an approach the drug's absorption, distribution and elimination (both metabolism and excretion) can be characterised. Additional *in vitro* evaluations will help to clarify the profile obtained e.g. for oral absorption, the determination of the physicochemical characteristics of pKa, lipid and aqueous solubility will greatly enhance the interpretation of results. Concerning distribution, the plasma and tissue protein binding characteristics of the drug are important. The chemical characteristics and the affinity for drug metabolising enzyme systems will also be major determinants of the drug's metabolic fate while the plasma protein binding and physicochemical characteristics of the drug (and its metabolites where applicable) will have a major influence on kidney elimination.

The aim of the present review is to document and evaluate currently available pharmacokinetic data on the drug azapropazone, a non-steroidal anti-inflammatory analgesic introduced into clinical practice in Europe in the early 1970s. The review is divided into five main sections, namely, animal pharmacokinetic data, human pharmacokinetic data, pharmacokinetics in disease states, pharmacokinetics in the elderly and distribution of azapropazone into synovial fluid. Finally a short discussion on pharmacokinetic drug interactions involving azapropazone is included. Prior to discussion of the pharmacokinetic profile of azapropazone it is, however, worthwhile considering some of the chemical and physicochemical characteristics of the drug which have a major bearing on pharmacokinetic events.

II. CHEMICAL AND PHYSICOCHEMICAL PROPERTIES OF AZAPROPAZONE

Azapropazone is 5-dimethylamino-9-methyl-2-propyl-1*H*-pyrazolo[1,2-α] [1,2,4]benzotriazine-1,3 (2*H*)-dione dihydrate (Figure 1). The name 'azapropazone' was given to the compound on the recommendation of the World Health Organisation. A detailed account of the synthesis and chemistry of

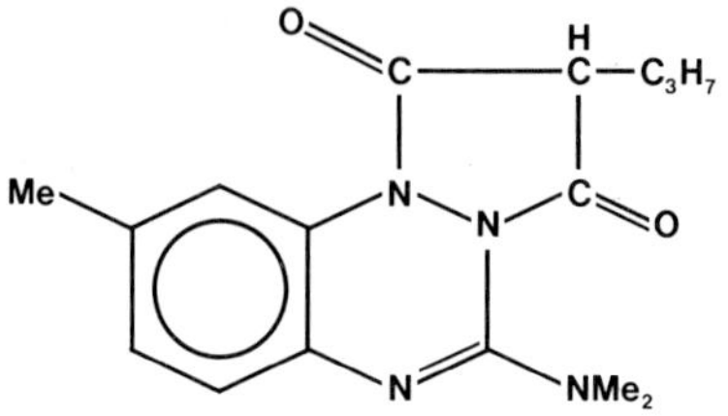

Figure 1 Structural formula of azapropazone

64

azapropazone has been published by Walker[1]. Much of the chemistry depends on the fact that it contains a 3,5-dioxo-pyrazolidine ring fused to the 1,2,4-benzotriazine ring structure. Azapropazone is easily attacked by a variety of hydrolysing and oxidising agents, all of which open the 3,5-dioxo-pyrazolidine ring[2]. Based on NMR data Fenner and Mixich[3] have shown that azapropazone in solution is best represented by a Zwitterion structure. Because of this azapropazone undergoes very little biotransformation, since an oxidative metabolism is limited by the electron deficiency of the benzotriazine system and a low lipophilic activity[1]. The drug's molecular structure promotes binding at the warfarin binding site on human serum albumin and indeed some authors have used the term warfarin/azapropazone to describe the area on human serum albumin to which the drug binds[4].

The pKa value of azapropazone is 6.3 at 25°C. The compound has low aqueous solubility at low pH values (135 mg/L in 0.1N HCl). High aqueous solubility is however achieved at more alkaline pHs, e.g. 13 g/L at pH 6.8. The lipid solubility is low (89 mg/L in isopropyl myristate). These characteristics obviously influence the absorption of azapropazone from the gastrointestinal tract; i.e. since the drug is virtually insoluble in gastric juice, dissolution and therefore absorption can only take place after the drug has passed through the stomach. Absorption is likely to take place in the duodenum. Distally rising pH of the gastrointestinal tract will lead to azapropazone being almost fully ionised as the enolate, which is likely to be poorly absorbed. Aqueous solubility at urinary pHs promotes the excretion of azapropazone and the inactive 8-hydroxy metabolite in the kidney.

III. PHARMACOKINETIC STUDIES IN ANIMALS

Early studies using ^{14}C-labelled azapropazone (labelled at the two carboxyl positions 1,3) in rats were carried out by Klatt and Koss[5]. Due to poor aqueous solubility, azapropazone was suspended in a 0.2% w/v suspension of gum tragacanth in water (concentration 10 mg/ml). An aliquot of this suspension (1.5 ml) was administered to non-fasting female Wistar rats via a stomach tube (i.e. 100 mg/kg); the radioactivity administered was approximately 0.7 mCi per rat. Urine and faeces were collected separately using specially designed metabolism cages. Bile excretion was also measured in anaesthetised rats (1 g urethane/kg, i.p.) after catheterisation of the bile duct. Animals were sacrificed at intervals over 24 hours and the azapropazone concentrations were measured in plasma and various tissues by scintillation counting. Bile excretion was quantified over a seven hour period.

Absorption was assessed by following the decrease in administered radioactivity in the gastrointestinal tract. Little azapropazone was absorbed from the stomach; however, once the drug reached the small intestine it was readily absorbed with about 50% of the administered dose being absorbed after four hours. The biological half-life for the biliary elimination of azapropazone was 2.2 hours but it was estimated that the biliary excretion was diminished in the anaesthetised animals studied. Radioactivity was detected in the plasma within 30 minutes. Serum protein binding studies were carried out using human serum, since it was known that binding of azapropazone in human and rat plasma was similar[6]. It was shown in these early experiments that 84% of azapropazone was bound to serum proteins. Radioactivity was detected in all organs studied. The highest content of azapropazone was found in the kidney and indeed the content of azapropazone in plasma, kidney and liver were considerably higher than in the other organs and tissues (adrenals, lung, heart, thyroid, spleen, muscle, brain and fatty tissue).

Concerning drug elimination, the kidney was found to be the principal organ for the excretion of azapropazone and that excretion took place by filtration rather than by active transport. The elimination half-life was 8.9 hours. Approximately 27.9% of the drug was eliminated in the faeces, part of this amount due to enterohepatic recycling. TLC studies indicated that excretion was primarily of unchanged drug (more than 95%). Two other metabolites were isolated the most abundant of which had the same Rf value as 8-hydroxy azapropazone.

This initial set of experiments clearly quantified the basic pharmacokinetic activity of azapropazone in the rat. Jahn and co-workers[6] were the first workers to publish pharmacokinetic data on azapropazone in a range of animal species. Azapropazone concentrations were determined spectrophotometrically (λ 255 nm) in plasma after first precipitating plasma proteins with methanol. Urine concentrations were determined after oxidative decomposition (H_2O_2) to the parent benzotriazine; the yellow colouration of this product was measured at 436 nm. The animal species studies included Wistar rats, mixed breed guinea pigs, New Zealand White rabbits and mongrel dogs. Animals of both sexes were employed in the experiments and both intravenous and oral routes of administration were used. Marked interspecies variations in pharmacokinetic parameters were noted (Table 1). This led to

Table 1 Absorption and elimination of azapropazone in four animal species (Data from Jahn et al., 1973)[6].

	Rat		Guinea pig		Rabbit		Dog	
Azapropazone dose	t_{max} (h)	$t_{1/2}$ (h)	t_{max} (h)	$t_{1/2}$ (h)	t_{max} (h)	$t_{1/2}$ (h)	t_{max} (h)	$t_{1/2}$ (h)
Intravenous								
10 mg/kg		3.3		4 +		2		2.8
25 mg/kg		2.1		4 +		2		2.5
Oral								
10 mg/kg		3[b]						< 2[c]
100 mg/kg	0.5[a] 3[b]	3.9[b]	6–8[b]	8.7[b]	6–8[b]	2[b]	4–8[c]	5.5[c]

[a] dose dissolved in equivalent NaOH
[b] aqueous suspension of drug
[c] drug given as capsule

marked variation in peak plasma concentrations in the various species after both oral and intravenous administration; for example, after oral administration (single dose, 100 mg/kg) peak plasma concentrations (μg/ml) were 158, 72, 9 and 60 in the rat, guinea pig, rabbit and dog respectively. These variations in peak serum concentrations correlated with the degree of protein binding (Sephadex® gel filtration) of azapropazone in serum from the various species (Figure 2). In this figure, for comparative purposes the serum protein binding of human and primate are also shown[7]. Such a correlation is expected since increased serum protein binding leads to a retention of drug within the plasma compartment and in turn leads to a reduction in the apparent volume of distribution. It is interesting that serum protein binding was considerably lower (than in man) in all the animal species examined, with the binding in dog serum being approximately half that of man. It is clear therefore that the dog, which is often considered a good animal model for use in kinetic studies, is an unsuitable species for examination of azapropazone's disposition and therefore its pharmacology and toxicology. Major species differences have been reported in the protein binding of other non-steroidal anti-inflammatory agents, e.g. salicylate binding differs in serum from baboon, dog, rat and man[8].

It is clear that there are major differences between species in the absorption and distribution of azapropazone. The metabolism of the drug seemed to be qualitatively similar in the species studied but quantitatively different. While it was possible to demonstrate only unchanged azapropazone using TLC in serum samples from rats and dogs, a metabolite was identified

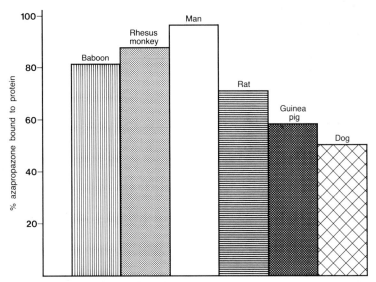

Figure 2 Serum protein binding of azapropazone in man* and a range of animal species. After Jones, 1976[7]
*Even higher values for the protein binding of azapropazone (> 99%) have been reported in more recent studies.

in urine. This metabolite, 8-hydroxy azapropazone (Figure 3), accounted for about 3% of the given dose in the rat and over 25% in the dog.

An investigation of the urinary excretion of azapropazone was carried out in rats and dogs[6]. In rats up to 87% of a 50 mg/kg dose was excreted within 24 hours; increasing the dose to 250 mg/kg led to a 42–69% recovery over the first 24 hours post administration. In dogs a much lower recovery of azapropazone (maximum 26%) was achieved over a 24 hour period at an oral dosage level of 25–250 mg/kg. This was probably due to a decreased absorption of azapropazone, and indeed administration of azapropazone by the intravenous route resulted in a recovery of 37.9% over 35 hours. Prolongation of the urine collection period did not increase the recovery after oral administration of the drug in either the rat or the dog.

IV. PHARMACOKINETICS IN HUMANS

The first published pharmacokinetic studies of azapropazone in human subjects were carried out by Schatz et al.[9]. The plasma concentrations of azapropazone (determined using UV absorption at 255 nm in methanolic solution) in five subjects were followed for 48 hours following single oral doses of 600 mg. Peak plasma concentrations were obtained after four hours in all cases, however, there were significant differences in Cp_{max} with measured values ranging from $\sim 30\,\mu g/ml$ to $\sim 70\,\mu g/ml$. This is approximately six times the maximum plasma concentration achieved in the dog at a similar dosage[7]. Dose ranging studies were also carried out in volunteer subjects who received doses of 200, 400, 600, 800 and 1600 mg. A wide variation in measured $t_{1/2}$ values were reported (range 4.5–16.5 h; mean 8.6 h), however, there was a good correlation between dose (mg/kg) and serum concentrations achieved at four hours post dosing, suggesting linearity in the kinetics of the drug over the dosage range examined (Figure 4).

Multiple dose studies at dosage levels of 200 mg t.i.d. or 300 mg morning and noon with 600 mg in the evening, each over a two day period, were also carried out in six volunteer subjects. Again the data obtained suggested that no unpredictable accumulation of the drug occurred (i.e. linear kinetics were obeyed). Two metabolites were isolated from urine samples but they were not identified. The authors, using urinary excretion data, estimated that more than 60% of the administered oral dose was excreted via the kidneys in the

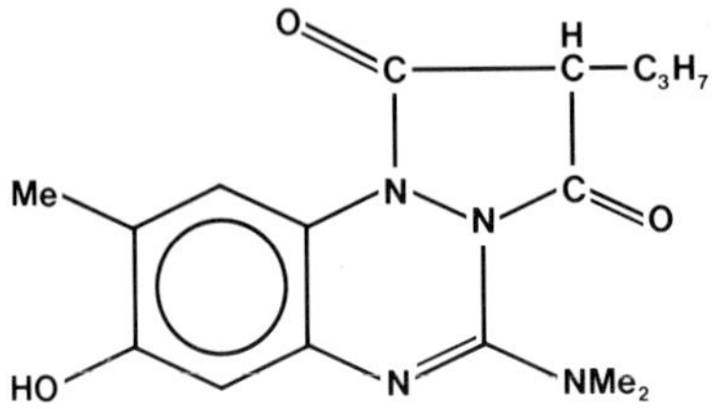

Figure 3 The metabolite of azapropazone, 8-hydroxy azapropazone

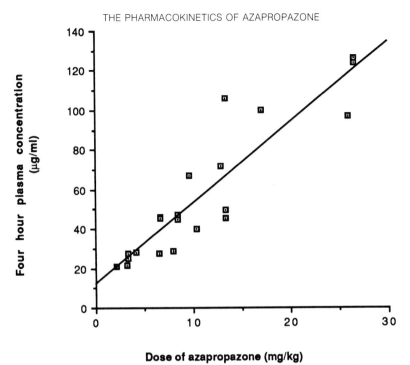

Figure 4 Correlation in humans between four-hour serum concentrations and dose (mg/kg as a single oral administration. $r^2 = 0.824$; $y = 4.08x + 11.96$) Data from Schatz *et al.* 1970

first 24 hours post dosing, mainly as unaltered substance.

Klatt and Koss in 1973[10] repeated some of their ^{14}C-azapropazone studies, this time in human subjects. The dose of radioactivity received by each person, irrespective of dose was $5\,\mu\text{Ci}$. Healthy male volunteers (aged 20–38 years) were given the azapropazone in the form of 200 mg hard gelatine capsules, at a dosage level of 200, 600 and 1000 mg. Plasma samples were collected over a 48 hour period while urine was collected up to 100 hours. To calculate the metabolite profile the urine samples were subjected to TLC. In some subjects stool samples were assessed to obtain a measure of unabsorbed azapropazone. Azapropazone was already detectable in the first blood sample taken (1 hour); Cp_{max} values were reached by six hours post dosing. These latter values varied according to the dose given and were approximately 20, 50 and $100\,\mu\text{g/ml}$ for doses of 200, 600 and 1000 mg respectively. The measured area under the plasma concentration versus time curve (AUC) also correlated with the dose administered. Using a single exponential to account for elimination of drug from the plasma, a mean plasma half-life of approximately 12 hours was calculated. This elimination of the drug was due in the most part to renal excretion. There appeared to be a somewhat lower excretion of drug at the 200 mg dosage level (75% when compared with the 600 and 1000 mg doses). The authors felt that this

69

may have been due to dose-related variations in serum protein binding of azapropazone. Chromatographic evaluation of the urine indicated that approximately 60% of the drug was excreted unchanged. This is somewhat lower than the value these same workers found in the rat (95%[10]). The metabolite 8-hydroxy azapropazone accounted for about 20% of the remaining radioactivity. Further metabolites were isolated but not identified.

Evans[11] also investigated the pharmacokinetics of azapropazone after single doses of drug (100 mg and 600 mg) in healthy volunteer subjects. Unlabelled drug was used and blood sampling was more frequent ($\frac{1}{2}$ hour intervals initially). This author was able to detect a bifid peak in the plasma concentration profile of several subjects between 7.5 and 10 hours following drug administration, suggesting the possibility of biliary recycling. Urinary recovery ranged from 31–93%. Chromatographic separation of the parent drug and metabolites, followed by mass spectrometric analysis indicated that approximately 67% of the azapropazone administered was excreted unchanged, 16% was 8-hydroxy azapropazone and 6% (originally observed but not identified by Klatt and Koss[10]) was shown to be Mi307, a compound not found by other investigations. Further pharmacokinetic data were published by Leach[12] in his paper on the determination of azapropazone in plasma.

A definitive study on the pharmacokinetics of azapropazone following single oral and intravenous doses was published by Breuing and his colleagues in 1979[13]. The research involved administration of azapropazone (600 mg) both orally and intravenously to seven healthy male volunteers (age 24–28 years) in a randomised cross-over fashion. A four-week wash-out period was allowed between doses. Oral medication was administered as capsules (Prolixan® 300 mg) on an empty stomach, while intravenous drug was administered as lyophilised sodium azapropazone dissolved in water. Heparinised blood samples were taken frequently over a three day period. Plasma concentrations of azapropazone were determined by quantitative TLC. Additionally plasma protein binding of azapropazone was quantified for six of the volunteers.

Plasma drug concentrations declined biexponentially after intravenous administration. The mean $t_{1/2\alpha}$ was 2.17 h (with fivefold intersubject differences) while the $t_{1/2\beta}$ ranged from 8.8 to 16.6 h (mean 13.6 h). Since data were available for both intravenous and oral doses of drug, the volume of distribution, clearance and % bioavailability could be calculated. Mean values ($\pm$ SD) for AUC, Vd and total clearance were $1037 \pm 281 \mu g.h/ml$, $11.9 \pm 3.5L$ and $10.1 \pm 2.1 ml/min$ respectively after intravenous administration. After oral administration peak plasma concentrations of $44.0 \pm 18.9 \mu g/ml$ occurred between 3–6 hours post dosing (mean 4.4 ± 1.3 h). AUC ($918 \pm 340 \mu g.h/ml$) was slightly reduced after oral dosage when compared with intravenous administration, leading to a mean calculated bioavailability (%) value of $83 \pm 19\%$. The calculated elimination half-life was slightly longer after oral dosage and had a value of 14.3 ± 2.8 h. Plasma

70

protein binding ranged from 98.67 to 99.64%. These high binding values are undoubtedly responsible for the low Vd and the low total clearance of azapropazone. The authors suggested that since the half-life was in the order of 14 hours after oral administration, b.i.d. dosing would be sufficient to maintain adequate serum concentrations of the drug in patients, assuming their disease condition did not influence the drug disposition.

It is of interest therefore that Rainsford[14] has measured plasma concentrations of azapropazone in 21 patients receiving repeated oral doses of 900–2400 mg of the drug daily for two to five days for the treatment of gout. All but two of these patients were receiving no other acidic NSAID but some patients were receiving antibiotics, azathioprine, steroids or cimetidine. A reverse phase HPLC assay procedure (with indomethacin as internal standard) was used; this separated azapropazone from its 8-hydroxy metabolite. Only one patient's plasma showed evidence of interfering components; (the interference appeared to be due to dihydrocodeine, although this patient was also receiving azapropazone and prednisolone). In the study three healthy volunteer subjects took a single dose 600 mg and unlike the patients, who gave early morning samples only, volunteers gave multiple blood samples over a 24 hour period. The peak plasma concentrations achieved in the volunteers were approximately 40 μg/ml and the elimination half-life was approximately 8 hours.

The main metabolites identified in the urine of the volunteers were thought to be 8-hydroxy-azapropazone and its glucuronide/sulphate conjugate. The 8-hydroxy-azapropazone accounted for approximately 55% of the total azapropazone + metabolites. This value is much higher than the 16% value for 8-hydroxy-azapropazone (GC mass-spec) reported by Jones[7]. It is interesting to note that Kline et al.[15] failed to observe conjugates of 8-hydroxy-azapropazone in their study; however, this may have been due to problems with sample preparation. In the studies of Rainsford[14] which indicated for the first time that metabolite conjugation does take place, Mi307 was not isolated.

The plasma concentration of azapropazone (mean $\pm$ SE) in gouty patients, two to five days after repeated daily ingestion of azapropazone are shown in Figure 5. Although no 8-hydroxy azapropazone was found in plasma after single doses it was evident on repeated dosing.

V. PHARMACOKINETICS IN DISEASE STATES

There is no evidence that rheumatoid arthritis, osteoarthritis or gout themselves change the pharmacokinetic profile of azapropazone but it has been clearly shown that chronic renal and hepatic disease can have a marked influence[13]. In this study the disposition of azapropazone after intravenous administration in six healthy male subjects (aged 26 to 29 years), 13 patients with cirrhosis (aged 28 to 63 years) and eight patients with chronic renal failure (aged 47 to 76 years) was investigated. The cirrhosis patients (alcoholic

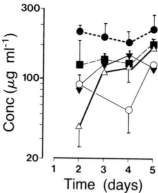

Figure 5 Plasma levels of azapropazone (mean ± SE) in gouty patients 2–5 days after repeated ingestion of 600–2400 mg azapropazone (● 2.4, ■ 1.8, △ 0.9, ▼ 1.2, ○ 0.6 g/day). After Rainsford 1985[14].

and posthepatitic) were divided into two groups according to the severity of impairment as judged by their clinical status, prothrombin complex activity and total serum bilirubin. Group I were considered to have modest and Group II severe impairment of liver function. One patient in Group II had also markedly impaired renal function. The renal patients had various degrees of impairment with serum creatinine values ranging from 1.5 to 6.4 mg% and creatinine clearance from 1.0–70 ml/min. Their renal failure was due to hypertension, glomerulonephritis and glomerulosclerosis. The intravenous dose was administered to all patients over a one minute period (600 mg lyophilised sodium azapropazone dissolved in 5 ml water). Plasma and urine samples were collected over a three to four day period. Azapropazone concentrations in plasma and urine were measured using quantitative TLC. In healthy volunteer subjects the elimination half-life was 12.2 ± 2.1 h (mean ± SD) while the Vd(area) was 10.6 ± 3.3 L. The values for total clearance, renal clearance and non-renal clearance were respectively 597 ± 135, 373 ± 130 and 224 ± 32 ml/h. The fraction of the administered dose which was excreted unchanged in the urine after 96 h was 0.62 ± 0.08. Azapropazone was shown to be 99.55% bound to plasma proteins (free fraction 0.0045 ± 0.0006) in healthy volunteer subjects. In Group I cirrhosis patients there was an approximate 2.5-fold increase in the free fraction of azapropazone. This decreased plasma protein binding led to an increased Vd of 14.9 ± 2.9 L. Although the half-life was markedly prolonged in three of the six subjects in the group and the mean value increased by 44%, variations between subjects meant that the difference was not stastistically significant. The portion of the dose eliminated in the urine after 96 h was 0.41 ± 0.24. Clearance of free drug from the plasma was reduced to a statistically signifiant degree, while total and renal clearance were not significantly different from control patient values. In Group II hepatic patients there was a highly significant ($p < 0.001$) increase in the percentage

72

of unbound azapropazone in plasma when compared with healthy subjects and Group I patients. The half-life in Group II patients was markedly increased to 61.5 h ($p < 0.005$) and total ($p < 0.001$), renal ($p < 0.01$) and non-renal clearances ($p < 0.005$) were markedly lower than in patients in Group I.

Renal disease, as expected, also had a marked influence on the disposition of azapropazone. In four of the patients the free fraction of azapropazone in plasma was higher than normal, while in the remaining four subjects the free fraction was normal. Vd values in the renal patients were normal. The $t_{1/2}$ was considerably prolonged to 31.7 h ($p < 0.005$ vs normal subjects). This prolonged half-life was due to decreased total and renal clearances of 230 ± 78 and 25.1 ± 19.9 ml/h respectively. Non-renal clearance was normal but clearance of the free drug from the plasma was only 22% of that in normal healthy subjects. Combining data from both the renal and the hepatic patient groups there was a clear relationship between the renal clearance of azapropazone and creatinine clearance. This appeared to be approximately linear until a plateau in renal clearance was reached at a corresponding creatinine clearance value of approximately 90 ml/min. A linear relationship was noted between renal clearance and total clearance in patients with liver disease and in normal subjects. A linear relationship also existed between total clearance and creatinine clearance when data from all subjects were computed, and in this case no plateau value was reached. Collectively the results led the authors to conclude that patients with cirrhosis and modest impairment of liver function may require about half the normal dose of azapropazone; however, patients with more severe hepatic impairment will be highly suceptible to dose related adverse-effects due to marked drug accumulation and decreased plasma protein binding. In renal disease, the authors suggested that the dose of azapropazone should be reduced according to the degree of kidney impairment and plasma protein binding of the drug.

Detailed study of the plasma protein binding (equilibrium dialysis) of azapropazone in patients with kidney and liver disease has been carried out by Jähnchen et al.[16] They found that the free fraction of azapropazone in healthy volunteer plasma ($n = 37$) ranged from 0.0027 to 0.0070 (0.0044 ± 0.0009, mean $\pm$ SD). The principal azapropazone binding protein was found to albumin. In a total of 27 renal failure patients there was an up to 12-fold increase in the free fraction values (0.0260 ± 0.0239) when compared with the upper normal range found in healthy volunteers. The degree of impairment of binding in the renal patients was not significantly correlated to the concentration of albumin, creatinine, uric acid or urea nitrogen in the serum. There was, however, a weak but statistically signifiant ($p < 0.05$) correlation between the free fraction values of azapropazone and creatinine clearance. Protein binding in the plasma of 32 patients with chronic liver disease was also measured and was found to be markedly reduced (free fraction values were 0.0210 ± 0.0242). The free fraction values were significantly correlated to the prothrombin complex activities ($r = 0.40$, $p < 0.05$) and the total bilirubin concentrations ($r = 0.90$, $p < 0.001$) in the plasma of the patients with chronic liver disease. No such correlations was found for serum albumin, serum glutamic oxaloacetic transaminase, serum γ-glutamyl transpeptidase or serum alkaline phosphatase. Bilirubin added *in vitro* displaced both phenprocoumon (the binding of which correlated closely with azapropazone) and azapropazone from their plasma binding sites; however, this displacement was much smaller than the binding changes observed in patients with liver disease.

Cancer patients also have a reduced binding of azapropazone in their serum[17]. These authors using multivariate analysis of variance showed that albumin, non-esterified fatty acids and α_1-acid glycoprotein concentrations accounted for 60% of interpatient variations in the bound/free concentration ratios of azapropazone in a group of 31 cancer patients.

VI. PHARMACOKINETICS OF AZAPROPAZONE IN THE ELDERLY

Ritch *et al.*[18] have measured plasma concentrations of azapropazone in young and elderly subjects after a single oral dose (2 × 300 mg Rheumox capsules). Twelve elderly patients (aged 76 to 96 years) and six healthy volunteers (aged 19 to 37 years) took part in the study. The patients presented with either osteoarthritis ($n = 11$) or rheumatoid arthritis ($n = 1$); they were all symptom free and none were recieving azapropazone chronically. Although all drugs were witheld for 24 hours before the start of the study, five patients had received one drug each within the two weeks prior to the study (co-trimoxazole, flavoxate, benorylate, danthron with poloxamer and dextropropoxyphene with paracetamol). All subjects fasted for 10 hours prior to and for two hours post administration of the azapropazone (with 200 ml of water). Plasma samples were collected over 72 hours and the azapropazone content measured colorimetrically. Creatinine clearance and serum urea were significantly altered reflecting impaired renal function in the elderly. There were also significant differences between the two groups in terms of AUC (2368 ± 1010 mean ± SD *vs* 1144 ± 291 μg.h/ml; $p < 0.02$) and plasma clearance (0.292 ± 0.11 *vs* 0.551 ± 0.15 L/h; $p < 0.001$), the elderly patients, as expected, having an increased AUC and decreased clearance. Although there were marked differences in the half-lives (31 ± 15 *vs* 18 ± 5 h) and Cp_{max} values (51.5 ± 19 *vs* 43.4 ± 9 μg/ml) between the two groups, due to large intersubject variations, particularly in the elderly patients, the differences did not reach statistical significance. There was a significant correlation between creatinine clearance and azapropazone clearance for all the subjects studied ($r = 0.75$; $p < 0.001$) and for the younger subjects alone ($r = 0.80$; $p < 0.05$). The relationship was, however, poor in the elderly group alone ($r = 0.30$, $p > 0.05$). Using multiple regression analysis azapropazone clearance could be predicted by the equation:

$Cl_{az} = 0.206 + 0.0065\ Cl_{cr} - 0.0129 \times$ fat mass

(Cl_{az} = azapropazone clearance; Cl_{cr} = creatinine clearance)

Interestingly Vd values were the same in the elderly (0.21 ± 0.08 L/kg) and the young (0.22 ± 0.09 L/kg). The authors suggested that therapeutic plasma azapropazone concentrations may be achieved in the elderly with a dose of 600 mg daily.

VII. DISTRIBUTION OF AZAPROPAZONE INTO SYNOVIAL FLUID

Two studies have examined the distribution of azapropazone into synovial fluid. These studies have particular relevance to the pharmacodynamics of azapropazone since synovial fluid will represent a major pharmacological effect compartment in the treatment of both rheumatoid and osteoarthritis. In the first study Aylward et al.[19] investigated synovial fluid concentrations of azapropazone in five outpatients with active rheumatoid disease. None of the patients exhibited clinical or laboratory evidence of renal or hepatic dysfunction. All subjects (two of which were receiving D-penicillamine, 125 mg/day and 375 mg/day respectively) received 300 mg or 600 mg of azapropazone administered orally on two separate study days, at least 14 days apart. The patients fasted for 10 hours prior to and three hours post drug administration. Plasma samples were collected for 24 hours post dosing. Synovial fluid samples were drawn from a knee joint effusion via an indwelling cannula, only after administration of the 300 mg dose, again over a 24 hour period. Azapropazone was quantified in both plasma and synovial fluid by HPLC. Mean peak plasma concentrations of azapropazone were 22.8 ± 7.2 (SD) μg/ml and $53.4 \pm 15.3\ \mu$g/ml for the 300 and 600 mg doses respectively. The corresponding t_{max} values were three and four hours. The mean peak drug concentration in synovial fluid was $14.1 \pm 3.7\ \mu$g/ml (following a 300 mg dose) and was not achieved until 24 hours post dosing, meaning that synovial fluid concentrations were decidedly greater than those in plasma at this sampling time.

A more recent study[20] investigated azapropazone transfer into synovial fluid in 32 patients (5 males; 27 females; age range 16 ± 73 years) with rheumatoid arthritis which necessitated synovectomy of the knee joint. The investigation was carried out in two parts. In the first part 24 patients received 600 mg azapropazone i.v. as a single dose at various times (45 minutes to 60 h) prior to the operation. In the second part 13 patients received 600 mg b.i.d. for five days (steady-state) and samples were taken two, six and twelve hours after the last dose. During each operation approximately 1 ml of synovial fluid and three samples of synovium were taken from each patient. One synovial sample was taken from the cartilage/bone margin, a second from the middle of the synovial membrane (where most pathological changes were likely to be found) and the third from tissue which was more or less macroscopically normal. Plasma samples were taken at random from several patients together with tissue samples.

75

Detectable concentrations of azapropazone (9 to 55 μg/ml; direct measurement of UV absorption on TLC plate) were found in synovial tissue and fluid from all patients in samples taken approximately one hour post drug administration. Peak concentrations of azapropazone (after i.v. administration) in synovial fluid of 57 and 66 μg/ml were found 1.2 and 12 h after injection, and 36 h after medication the mean concentration was 17 μg/ml. No difference was found in the azapropazone concentrations between tissues samples taken from the various sites. The highest tissue concentration found was 25.6 μg/ml at four hours and azapropazone could still be detected 60 h after drug administration. There was good correlation between tissue and synovial fluid concentrations ($r = 0.92$) and for plasma and synovial tissue concentrations ($r = 0.91$). In some patients synovial fluid and tissue concentrations were high but they were mostly below or in the range of corresponding plasma concentrations.

Synovial fluid azapropazone concentrations after multiple dosing averaged 64, 35 and 28 μg/ml, two, six and 12 hours respectively after the last dose. The average synovial tissue and fluid concentrations at the corresponding times of removal did not indicate accumulation of azapropazone in the tissues after treatment for five days.

VIII. MAJOR PHARMACOKINETIC INTERACTIONS INVOLVING AZAPROPAZONE

Since azapropazone is highly bound to plasma proteins and since metabolism is involved in its clearance, there is the potential for pharmacokinetic interactions involving azapropazone. The pharmacokinetics of azapropazone are unlikely to be changed to a clinically significant degree but azapropazone can influence the disposition of other drugs with a narrow therapeutic index to an extent that is clinically significant. The prime example of this is the interaction been azapropazone and warfarin[21]. Azapropazone is a potent displacer of warfarin from its plasma protein binding sites[22,23] and leads to dramatic increases in prothrombin time if taken by patients receiving warfarin. It has as yet not been determined whether the underlying mechanism of the interaction involves a selective inhibition by azapropazone of the metabolism of warfarin isomers, a mechanism which has been shown to take place with phenylbutazone[24]. Other pharmacokinetic interactions of azapropazone involve phenytoin[25,26] and tolbutamide[27,28]. The underlying mechanism, although involving plasma binding displacement, is likely to be decreased hepatic clearance of both phenytoin and tolbutamide. Daly et al.[29] have suggested that the clearance of methotrexate may be impaired by azapropazone, either by inhibition of hepatic enzymes or by competition for renal tubular secretion.

References

1. Walker, FS (1985). Azapropazone and related benzotriazones. In: Rainsford, KD, (ed) *Anti-inflamatory and Anti-rheumatic Drugs*, Vol. II, *Newer Anti-inflamatory Drugs*. (Boca Raton: CRC Press) pp. 1–32
2. Mixich, G (1968). Zum chemischen Verhalten des Antiphogistikums Azapropazon (Mi85) = 3-Dimethylamino-7-methyl-1,2-(n-propylmalonyl)-1,2-dihydro-1.2.4-benzotriazin. *Helv. Chim. Acta*, **51**, 532
3. Fenner, H and Mixich, G (1973) NMR-Untersuchungen zur Molekülstruktur von Azapropazon und Deutung seiner Pharmakokinetic und Biotransformation. *Azneim. Forsch.*, **23**, 667
4. Albengres, E, Urien, S, Riant, P, Marcel, GA and Tillement, JP (1987). Binding of two anthranilic acid derivatives to human albumin, erythrocytes and lipoproteins: evidence for glafenic acid high affinity binding. *Mol. Pharmacol.*, **31**, 294–300
5. Klatt, VL and Koss, FW (1973). Pharmkokinetische Untersuchungen mit ^{14}C-Azapropazon-Dihydrat an der Ratte. *Arzneim. Forsch.*, **23**, 913
6. Jahn, V, Reller, J and Schatz, F (1973). Pharmakokinetische Untersuchungen mit Azapropazon bei Tieren. *Arzneim. Forsch.*, **23**, 660–666
7. Jones, CJ (1976). The pharmacology and pharmacokinetics of azapropazone – a review. *Curr. Med. Res. Opin.*, **4**, 3–16
8. Sturman, JA and Smith, MJH (1967). The binding of salicylate to plasma proteins in different species. *J. Pharm. Pharmacol.*, **19**, 621–623
9. Schatz, F, Adrian, RW, Mixich, G, Molnarova, M, Reller, J and Jahn, U (1970). Pharmakokinetische Untersuchungen mid dem Antiphlogistikum Azapropazon (Prolixan 300) am Menschen. *Therapiewoche*, **20**, 39
10. Klatt, VL and Koss, FW (1973). Human pharmakokinetische Untersuchungen mit ^{14}C-Azapropazon-Dihydrat. *Arzneim. Forsch.*, **23**, 920–921
11. Evans, EF (1974). Data on file, AH Robins Co.
12. Leach, H (1976). The determination of azapropazone in blood plasma. *Curr. Med. Res. Opin.*, **4**, 35
13. Breuing, K-H, Gilfrich, H-J, Meinertz, T, Weigand, V-W and Jähnchen, E (1981). Disposition of Azapropazone in chronic renal and hepatic failure. *Eur. J. Clin. Pharmacol.*, **20**, 147–155
14. Rainsford, KD (1985). Distribution of azapropazone and its principal 8-hydroxy metabolite in plasma, urine and the gastrointestinal mucosa determined by HPLC. *J. Pharm. Pharmacol.*, **37**, 341–345.
15. Kline, BJ, Wood, JH and Beightol, LA (1983). The determination of azapropazone and its 6-hydroxy metabolite in plasma and urine by HPLC. *Arzneim. Forsche.*, **33**, 504–506
16. Jähnchen, E, Blanck, KJ, Breuing, K-H, Gilfrich, H-J, Meinertz, T and Trenk, D (1981). Plasma protein binding of azapropazone in patients with kidney and liver disease. *Br. J. Clin. Pharmacol.*, **11**, 361–367
17. Urien, S, Albengres, E, Pinquier, JL and Tillement, JP (1986). Role of alpha-1 acid glycoprotein, albumin and non-esterified fatty acids in serum binding of apazone and warfarin. *Clin. Pharmacol. Ther.*, **39**, 683–689
18. Ritch, AES, Perera, WNR and Jones, CJ (1982). Pharmakokinetics of azapropazone in the elderly. *Br. J. Clin. Pharmacol.*, **14**, 116–119
19. Aylward, M, Baker, PA, Davies, DE, Hutchings, L, Lewis, PA, Maddock, J and Protheroe, DA (1977). Data on file, AH Robins Co. (Simbec Research Laboratories, Merthyr Tydfil, Wales, UK)
20. Spahn, H, Thabe, K, Mutschler, E, Tillmann, K and Gikalov, I (1987). Concentration of azapropazone in synovial tissues and fluid. *Eur. J. Clin. Pharmacol.*, **32**, 303–307

21.   Powell-Jackson, PR (1977). Interaction between azapropazone and warfarin. *Br. Med. J.*, **1**, 1193–1194

22.   McElnay, JC and D'Arcy, PF (1980). Displacement of albumin-bound warfarin by anti-inflammatory agents in vitro. *J. Pharm. Pharmacol.*, **32**, 709–711

23.   Diana, FJ, Veronich, K and Kapoor, AL (1989). Binding of nonsteroidal anti-inflammatory agents and their effect on binding of racemic warfarin and its enantiomers to human serum albumin. *J. Pharm. Sci.*, **78**, 195–199

24.   Lewis, RJ, Trager, WF, Chan, KK, Breckenridge, A, Orme, M, Roland, M and Schary, W (1974). Warfarin; stereochemical aspects of its metabolism and the interaction with phenylbutzone. *J. Clin. Invest.*, **53**, 1607–1617

25.   Roberts, CJC, Daneschmend, TK, Macfarlane, D and Dieppe, PA (1981). Anticonvulsant intoxication precipitated by azapropazone. *Postgrad. Med. J.*, **57**, 191–192

26.   Geaney, DP, Carver, JG, Davis, CL and Aronson, JK (183). Pharmacokinetic investigation of the interaction of azapropazone with phenytoin. *Br. J. Clin. Pharmcol.*, **15**, 727–734

27.   Andreasen, PB, Simonsen, K, Brocks, K, Dimo, B and Bouchelouche, P (1981). Hypoglycaemia induced by azapropazone-tolbutamide interaction. *Br. J. Clin. Pharmacol.*, **12**, 581–583

28.   Waller, DG and Waller, D (1984). Hypoglycaemia due to azapropazone-tolbutamide interaction. *Br. J. Rheumatol.*, **23**, 24–25

29.   Daly, H, Boyle, J, Roberts, C and Scott, G (1986). Interaction between methotrexate and non-steroidal anti-inflammatory drugs. *Lancet*, **1**, 557.

Summary

The pharmacokinetic properties of the 1,2,4-benzotriazine non-steroidal anti-inflammatory drug azapropazone are reviewed. Azapropazone (pKa value 6.3 at 25°C) has low aqueous solubility at low pH which leads to poor dissolution in, and therefore absorption from, the stomach. Absorption is, however, rapid when the drug reaches the small intestine in both animal species and in human subjects. Early definitive pharmacokinetic studies in animal species showed that distribution of the drug out of the plasma compartment was very limited due to extensive plasma protein binding; this binding varied greatly between species. In the rat, which has been the most widely studied species, the kidney was found to be the major organ of elimination and it was also shown that excretion took place by glomerular filtration rather than by active mechanisms. The half-life was approximately 9 h. Although some metabolites were isolated in the urine they were not conclusively identified at that time. Most of the absorbed dose was eliminated unchanged in the urine. The dog, which exhibits a particularly low plasma protein binding of azapropazone, is unsuitable to model the disposition of azapropazone in man. A range of studies have been carried out in man involving healthy subjects, patients with arthritic illnesses and in patients with compromised kidney and liver functions, after both oral and intravenous administration of azapropazone. Pharmacokinetic parameters in healthy subjects are linear. The GI absorption in man is high (F = 83%) with maximal serum concentrations occurring by six hours. Again distribution is limited due to extensive plasma protein binding (in excess of 99%) and indeed the volume of distribution approximates to only twice the blood volume. The main metabolite of azapropazone is the 8-hydroxy derivative. It can readily be extracted from urine; small amounts have also been found in plasma. The elimination half-life in subjects with good kidney and hepatic function is in the order of 12 hours. In patients with severe hepatic or renal impairment the clearance of azapropazone is very much reduced, due to reductions in serum protein binding and glomerular filtration. Plasma half-lives in excess of 50 hours have been reported in patients with severe impairment of liver function. Clearance is also reduced in the elderly due to decreased glomerular filtration.

Azapropazone distributes well into synovial fluid, a major pharmacological effect compartment. Synovial fluid and tissue concentrations of azapropazone are normally lower than in serum. Due to azapropazone's pharmacokinetic profile it can enter into drug interactions with other agents which are highly protein bound, such as warfarin.

Zusammenfassung

Die pharmakokinetischen Eigenschaften der nicht steroidalen, entzündungshemmenden Substanz Azapropazon (1,2,4-Benzotriazin) sollen kurz im Überblick dargestellt werden.
Azapropazon (pKs 6,3 bei 25°C) ist schlecht wasserlöslich und hat einen niedrigen pH-Wert. Die Substanz geht daher nur schlecht in Lösung und die Resorption aus dem Magen ist gering. Wenn die Substanz jedoch in den Dünndarm gelangt, erfolgt sowohl beim Tier als auch beim Menschen eine schnelle Resorption. Die ersten pharmakokinetischen Studien an Tieren haben gezeigt, daß die Verteilung der Substanz aus dem Plasma-Kompartiment aufgrund der starken Plasmaproteinbindung sehr gering ist. Die Plasmaproteinbindung zeigte starke Schwankungen zwischen den einzelnen Spezies.

Bei der Ratte, das für die Experimente am häufigsten verwendete Modell, war die Niere ein Hauptausscheidungsorgan, und die Ausscheidung erfolgte hauptsächlich über den glomerulären Filtrationsmechanismus und weniger über aktive Mechanismen. Die Halbwertszeit betrug ungefähr 9 Stunden. Einige Metaboliten konnten aus dem Urin isoliert werden, aber ihre Identität ist bisher noch ungeklärt. Der größte Teil der resorbierten Dosis wurde unverändert im Urin wieder ausgeschieden. Das Hunde-Modell, bei dem Azapropazon eine besonders niedrige Plasmaproteinbindung aufweist, ist für die Untersuchung des Verhaltens von Azapropazon beim Menschen nicht geeignet. Es wurden Humanstudien an gesunden Probanden, Arthritis-Patienten und Patienten mit gestörter Nieren- und Leberfunktion mit oraler und intravenöser Verabreichung von Azapropazon durchgeführt.

Die pharmakokinetischen Parameter verlaufen bei gesunden Probanden linear. Die Resorption der Substanz aus dem Magen-Darm-Trakt beträgt beim Menschen 83%, wobei die maximale Serumkonzentration nach 6 Stunden erreicht ist. Wiederum wird die Verteilung durch die hohe Plasmaproteinbindung (über 99%) eingeschränkt; die Volumenverteilung beträgt in der Tat nur ungefähr das zweifache des Blutvolumens. Der Hauptmetabolit des Azapropazons ist das 8-Hydroxy-Derivat; er läßt sich leicht aus dem Urin extrahieren. Der Metabolit wurde auch in kleinen Mengen im Plasma vorgefunden. Die Halbwertszeit für die Elimination beträgt bei Versuchspersonen mit gesunder Nieren- und Leberfunktion ungefähr 12 Stunden. Bei Patienten mit schweren Leber- oder Nierenfunktionsstörungen ist die Clearance von Azapropazon aus dem Plasma aufgrund der Plasmaproteinbindung und der glomerulären Filtration stark herabgesetzt.

Patienten mit schweren Leberfunktionsstörungen weisen im Plasma Halbwertszeiten von über 50 Stunden auf. Auch bei älteren Personen ist die Clearance aufgrund der niedrigeren glomerulären Filtrationsrate herabgesetzt. Azapropazon verteilt sich gut in der Synovia, dem wichtigsten Kompartiment für pharmakologische Wirkungen.

Die Konzentration von Azapropazon in Synovia und Gewebe ist normalerweise niedriger als im Plasma. Aufgrund seines pharmakokinetischen Profils kann Azapropazon mit anderen Arzneimitteln mit ebenfalls hoher Eiweißbindung, wie z.B. Warfarin, in Wechselwirkung treten.

Resumé

On a réexaminé les propriétés pharmacocinétiques du médicament anti-inflammatoire non stéroïdien à base de 1,2,4-benzotriazine appelé azapropazone. L'azapropazone (valeur pKa 6,3 à 25 Degrés C) a une faible solubilité aqueuse à pH bas d'où une dissolution médiocre et une faible absorption à partir de l'estomac. L'absorption est toutefois rapide lorsque le médicament arrive au niveau du petit intestin chez les espèces animales comme chez l'homme. Les premières études pharmacocinétiques effectuées sur des animaux ont montré que la distribution du médicament en-dehors du compartiment plasmatique était très limitée à cause de l'extensive fixation aux protéines plasmatiques; cette fixation variait énormément d'une espèce à l'autre.

Chez le rat, l'espèce étudiée le plus couramment, on a découvert que le rein était l'organe d'élimination le plus important et que l'excrétion s'effectuait par filtration glomérulaire plutôt que par des mécanismes actifs. La demi-vie était d'environ 9 heures. Bien que l'on ait réussi à isoler certains métabolites dans l'urine, on n'a pas pu les identifier de manière conclusive. Presque toute la dose absorbée a montré que l'élimination était restée inchangée dans l'urine. Le chien, chez qui on a observé une fixation aux protéines plasmatiques de l'azapropazone particulièrement limitée, ne convient pas pour modeler la disposition de l'azapropazone chez l'homme. On a effectué une série d'études chez l'homme avec des sujets en bonne santé, des malades atteints d'une maladie arthritique et chez des malades avec des fonctions rénales et hépatiques altérées, après administration d'azapropazone tout à la fois par voie orale et par voie intraveineuse.

Chez les sujets en bonne santé, les paramètres pharmacocinétiques sont linéaires. Chez l'homme, l'absorption gastro-intestinale est très élevée (83%), la concentration aérique maximum étant obtenue en 6 heures. A nouveau, la distribution est limitée à cause de l'extensive fixation aux protéines plasmatiques (qui est de plus de 99%): en effet, le volume de distribution ne se rapproche que de deux fois le volume du sang. Le principal métabolite de l'azapropazone est le 8-hydroxy dérivé. On peut facilement l'extraire de l'urine et on en a trouvé de petites quantités dans le plasma. Le demi-vie d'élimination chez des sujets dont les fonctions rénales et hépatiques sont normales est de l'ordre de 12 heures. Chez des malades souffrant d'une grave insuffisance hépatique ou rénale, la clairance de l'azapropazone est énormément réduite à cause de la fixation aux protéines plasmatique réduite et de la filtration glomérulaire.

On a observé des demi-vies plasmatiques d'au delà de 50 heures chez des malades avec une grave insuffisance hépatique. La clairance est également réduite chez les personnes âgées en raison de la diminution de la filtration glomérulaire. L'azapropazone se distribue bien dans le liquide synovial, le compartiment de l'effet pharmacologique principal.

Les concentrations de l'azapropazone dans le liquide synovial et dans les tissus sont normalement plus faibles que dans le plasma. A cause de son profil pharmacocinétique, l'azapropazone peut causer une interaction médicamenteuse avec d'autres agents qui sont en grande mesure liés aux protéines, comme par exemple la warfarine.

7
Mathematical model for assessing risk of gastrointestinal reactions to NSAIDs

K McCormack

I. INTRODUCTION

In vitro data indicate that all clinically useful non-steroidal anti-inflammatory drugs (NSAIDs) inhibit to a varying degree the activity of the enzyme cyclo-oxygenase. It has been argued that the failure of certain NSAIDs to significantly reduce gastric mucosal levels of prostaglandins (PG) *in vivo* may reflect pharmacokinetic differences between NSAIDs rather than tissue-specific differences in their potency as inhibitors of cyclo-oxygenase[1]. A corollary of such an argument is that accumulation of NSAID within gastric mucosal cells is a principal factor associated with the intervention of intracellular biochemical events and resultant gastric mucosal damage.

In vivo, attempts to describe NSAID-induced gastric mucosal damage have been based on simple models derived from classical absorption theory. In clinical practice, however, such models must be extended to include transfer of NSAID from plasma to gastric mucosal cells, enterohepatically circulated NSAID, and the effects of age on gastric mucosa. This brief overview examines the impact of an early hypothesis on our current thinking concerning the importance of pharmacokinetic factors on the aetiology of NSAID gastric toxicity. The limitations of this early hypothesis are examined.

II. pH-PARTITION HYPOTHESIS

In the 1950s, the quantitative experimental work of Shore *et al.*[2], Hogben *et al.*[3,4] and Schanker *et al.*[5-7] culminated in the creation of the classical pH-partition hypothesis of drug absorption. In brief, this hypothesis states that the passage of a drug across the gastrointestinal barrier is restricted to the uncharged lipid-soluble species.

It was Martin in 1963[8] who proposed that theoretical considerations (i.e. the pH partition hypothesis) suggest that after the oral administration of certain acidic drugs, appreciable quantities of drug anion ($R.COO^-$) may accumulate in the gastric mucosal cells (specifically the parietal cells). Such a phenomenon, he argued, is a consequence of the pH gradient which exists

Azapropazone – 20 years of clinical use. Rainsford, KD (ed)
© Kluwer Academic Publishers. Printed in Great Britain

between the surface of the mucosal cell, which borders the gastric lumen, and the interior of a mucosal cell. He considered that in the gastric fluid, all acidic drugs exist largely in their un-ionized form (R.COOH) which, on entering the cell interior, dissociate to exist as the anion. At pH 7.0 the ionized form will predominate, and being the lipid-insoluble form, it will accumulate. Martin speculated that this 'ion trapping' might be the basis by which certain acids such as aspirin give rise to gastric mucosal damage.

1. NSAIDs and the gastric parietal cell

In the stomach, proton-secreting parietal cells are directly surrounded by fluid at pH 1.5–6.0 and they are not covered by the protective mucus layer afforded to more superficial cells in the gastric pit. Thus, the parietal cell may be postulated to occupy a focal role in the development of NSAID-induced gastric mucosal damage. Indeed, autoradiographs of the glandular mucosa (which contains parietal cells) of the stomach in rats treated with ^{3}H-salicylic acid reveal high concentrations throughout glandular mucosa only 1 minute after drug administration[9,10]. Electron microscope studies support the speculation that the areas where accumulation is observed contain parietal cells and may well be the foci from which ulcers of the stomach mucosa develop (in the rat)[11]. Autoradiographs of rats treated with ^{3}H-salicylic acid at high magnification reveal the presence of activity in individual parietal cells[10].

2. The significance of Martin's hypothesis to modern NSAIDs

At a given temperature, the total aqueous solubility, S_T, of a univalent acidic NSAID increases with pH according to the equation:

$$S_T = S_o(1 + 10^{pH-pKa})$$

where S_o is the intrinsic solubility of the un-ionized moiety. Decreasing pH favours an increase in the ratio of un-ionized/ionized NSAID with a proportional decrease in solubility. Thus with decreasing pH, predominant hydrophobic character (as defined by the magnitude of the partition coefficient) precludes significant aqueous solubility. Whilst most acidic NSAIDs conform to analogues of aspirin or indomethacin, the degree of lipophilia is variable, and many NSAIDs contain functional groups, in addition to the carboxyl moiety, which enable adequate aqueous solvation through hydrogen bonding. It is not surprising, therefore, that some compounds reach sufficiently high concentrations in gastric juice for measurable absorption in the stomach.

With solid form under conditions of fast distintegration, the solubility of the un-ionized moiety is directly related to the dissolution rate and limits the rate of appearance of drug in the circulation. Salicylic acid released from acetylsalicylic acid (ASA) within gastric juice is absorbed from the stomach and reaches high concentrations in plasma within 1 hour after administration if given in a formulation designed for rapid disintegration and dissolution of ASA[12]. Less hydrophilic compounds do not dissolve to a sufficient degree in gastric juice at low pH and hence achieve peak plasma concentrations later than 2 hour after administration, probably due to the fact that absorption becomes pronounced only after the drug has passed the stomach and reached the upper small intestine[13].

Another salicylate, diflunisal, appears to be absorbed only distal to the stomach since the time-to-peak value is around 2–3 hours. According to time-to-peak values, other drugs like indomethacin, fenoprofen, flurbiprofen, naproxen, phenylbutazone, tolmetin and ibuprofen hold intermediate positions between ASA and diflusinal, i.e. some absorption occurs in the stomach. Clearly, Martin's hypothesis cannot be assumed to apply generally.

III. CLASSICAL ABSORPTION THEORY AND NSAID-INDUCED GASTRIC MUCOSAL DAMAGE IN VIVO

In vivo, classical absorption theory may be used to predict the proportion of prostaglandin synthesis inhibited by NSAID at any time t. Such a model presupposes that inhibition of PG synthesis is an important factor in the aetiology of NSAID-induced gastric mucosal damage and makes no allowance for a systemic component to such damage. Using this model then, we may derive the following empirical relationship:

$$PG(t) = \frac{\exp(K(conc_{IN(t)} - IC_{50}))}{1 + \exp(K(conc_{IN(t)} - IC_{50}))}$$

where:

$PG(t)$ = proportion of PG synthesis inhibited at time t
IC_{50} = concentration of NSAID required for 50% inhibition of PG synthesis
K = rate constant
$\exp$ = exporent, e

and

$$conc_{IN} = \frac{conc_S P_{2.0}}{P_{7.0}}$$

where $P_{2.0}$ and $P_{7.0}$ are the apparent partition coefficients which respectively represent NSAID in the gastric lumen and gastric mucosal cell (parietal).

The mean number of lesions produced by drug i at dose D will be given by an equation of the following form:

mean number of lesions = constant $\times g(PG^i(t_o)) \times f(D)$

where $f(-)$ and $g(-)$ are monotonically increasing functions and t_0 is the time the drug is in the stomach.

Given suitable data, it should be possible to determine the shape of $f(-)$

and $g(-)$ and subsequently determine the influence of partition coefficient, partition rate constant (Kp), solubility and IC_{50} on gastric damage. For a series of NSAIDs such data is now available and we hope to shortly publish our findings. These findings provide a means whereby the topical component of gastric mucosal damage may be calculated for an individual NSAID based on our model described herein.

IV. GASTRIC MUCOSAL DAMAGE ASSOCIATED WITH NSAIDs IN CLINICAL USE

The above model, however, does not explain why in clinical practice it is the antral region which is apparently the preferred site for NSAID-associated gastric mucosal damage. Nor does the above model explain why some orally ingested non-acidic compounds (which, following absorption, are subsequently converted to weak organic acids capable of inhibiting PG synthesis) and parenterally administered NSAIDs cause gastric damage. Clearly, the above model needs to be extended to include the transfer of NSAID from plasma to gastric mucosal cell.

Presently, the systemic transfer of NSAID cannot be adequately explained. The following hypothesis, however, is presented which does provide a working model as a basis for further studies. Once again, such a model presupposes that intracellular accumulation of NSAID is an important factor in the aetiology of gastric mucosal damage.

In man, the antral mucosa is especially vulnerable to the deleterious effects of various micro- and macroenvironmental factors such as bile reflux, alcohol, tobacco, drugs, infection (*Campylobacter pylori*)[14-23], etc. In genetically pre-disposed individuals, collectively such factors may be important in the development of chronic atrophic antral gastritis[24] — a condition characterized by a marked reduction or even disappearance of the parenchyma. Both the severity and frequency of chronic atrophic gastritis increase significantly with age. At about age 50, the prevalence of chronic atrophic antral gastritis is about 1 in 2^{25-28}. Indeed, Cheli *et al.*[29] recorded a prevalance of about 80% in the 70–79 age group of an asymptomatic Hungarian population which was free of radiological and endoscopic evidence of gastric pathology.

Experimentally, intact atrophic gastritic tissue in the human presents less of a resistant barrier to the back-diffusion of hydrogen ions[30,31]. Under experimental conditions in the dog, atrophic gastritic tissue is demonstrated to be very prone to ulceration[32,33]. Whilst the reasons for such vulnerability are documented, it is not the intention to discuss them here; rather it is important to acknowledge that in certain ididivuals, the antral mucosa is especially vulnerable to back-diffusion of hydrogen ions, especially in the presence of a 'barrier-breaker' (e.g. bile, alcohol, aspirin). Such a back-diffusion may be expected to reduce the intramural pH in the lamina propria of the gastric mucosa[34,35]. With this insult, one may further postulate that circulating NSAID will accumulate intramurally following an increase in capillary 'leakiness' mediated, for example, by histamine release. Given the reduced intramural pH relative to the interior of the gastric mucosal cell then passive diffusion of un-ionized NSAID down a concentration gradient will lead to 'ion-trapping'.

V. 'GASTRIC-SPARING' NSAIDs IN CLINICAL PRACTICE

Attempts to reduce the problem of NSAID-associated gastric toxicity in clinical practice have been concentrated on minimizing direct contact of drug with gastric mucosa. These efforts reflect the use of a simple model which almost certainly has limited clinical relevance. In the light of this article, some examples of 'gastric-sparing' NSAIDs are now considered.

1. Prodrugs

Prodrugs commercially available in the UK can be divided into two groups, acidic and non-acidic:

    1. Acidic drugs; fenbufen, sulindac, salsalate.
    2. Non-acidic drugs: benorylate, nabumetone.

Table 1   The minimum aqueous solubility of some common NSAIDs together with time-to-peak plasma concentration

	Minimum aqueous solubility		Time-to-peak plasma concentration	
	S_o (μmol/L)	Log S_o	T_m (h)	Log T_m
Azapropazone (AZA)	205.1	2.312	4.0–4.5	0.602–0.653
Fenbufen (FEN)	7.9	0.898	2.0	0.301
Fenoprofen Ca (FENO)	32.2	1.508	1.0–2.0	0–0.301
Flufenamic acid (FLU)	9.2	0.964	6.0	0.778
Flurbiprofen (FLUR)	32.7	1.515	1.5–3.0	0.176–0.477
Ibuprofen (IBU)	101.8	2.008	0.5–1.5	(−0.301)*–0.176
Indomethacin (IND)	25.2	1.401	1.0–2.0	0–0.301
Ketoprofen (KETO)	192.7	2.285	0.3	(−0.523)*
Naproxen (NAP)	56.4	1.751	1.0–2.0	0–0.301
Phenylbutazone (PHE)	25.9	1.413	2.0	0.301
Piroxicam (PIR)	48.3	1.684	2.0	0.301
Tolmetin (TOL)	72.9	1.863	0.5–1.0	(−0.301)*–0

*Parentheses denote negative quantity.
Solubility data is from Herzfeldt et al.[41]. Lowest solubility (s_o) for each NSAID was determined in HCl buffer at several pH units below the pK_a. This value is considered to represent the inherent solubility of the un-ionized moiety. Solubility data for flufenamic acid is not available below the pK_a values for this drug, so was estimated from available data using the relationship $S_T = S_o(1 + 10^{pH-pK_a})$, where S_T is the total solubility at a given pH (Krebs and Speakman[42]). Time-to-peak plasma concentration values (T_m) are those reported in the literature following the oral administration of drug in the solid form in apparently healthy individuals. For reference purposes, these data have been comprehensively reviewed by Verbeeck et al.[43]; Brune and Lanz[13]; Grennan and Higham[44]; Marsh et al.[45].

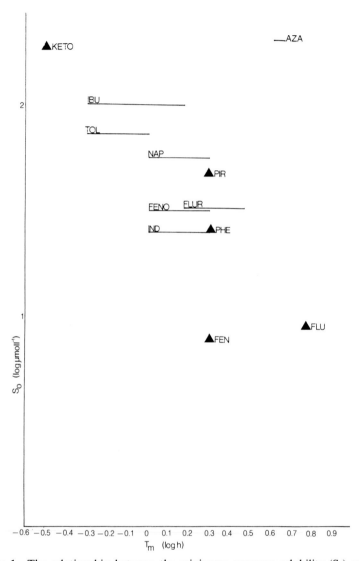

Figure 1 The relationship between the minimum aqueous solubility (S$_o$) and the time-to-peak plasma concentration (T$_m$) for some common NSAIDs (for details see Table 1). For a given range of T$_m$ (Table 1), the earliest value is used for regression analysis, since later peaks may include enterohepatically circulated drug. AZA = azapropazone, which appears to fall outside the trend shown by other NSAIDs and which contributes to the weak correlation r = −0.5 (not significant). The correlation is improved considerably by excluding AZA; r = −0.84 (p < 0.01). However, even with the weaker correlation, AZA falls outside the 99% confidence limit calculated as three standard errors (S$_x$) of the estimate of T$_m$ (r = −0.5 S$_x$ = 0.314; r = −0.84 S$_x$ = 0.189).

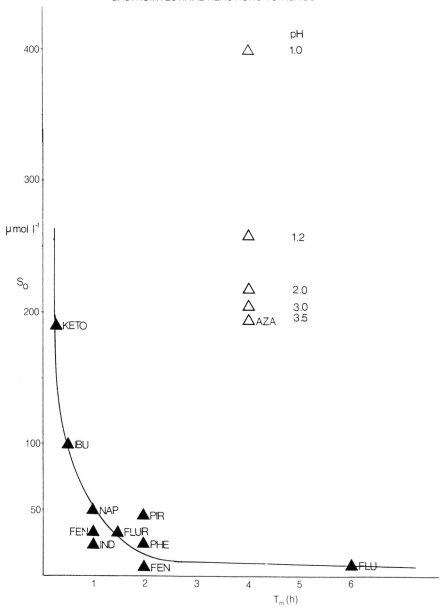

Figure 2 The relationship between the minimum aqueous solubility (S_o) and the time-to-peak plasma concentration (T_m) for some common NSAIDs (for details see Table 1). The S_o value for azapropazone occurs at pH 3.5 and accordingly is the value used in the statistical methods described in Figure 1. The additional solubility values illustrated at pH 3.0 and below are added merely to demonstrate the unique dissolution behaviour of azapropazone with decreasing pH within the above series of NSAIDs tested.

Whilst significant absorption of these prodrugs occurs distal to the stomach, i.e. in the upper small intestine, solubility and pharmacokinetic data for these drugs suggest that, to a variable degree, *some* absorption does occur in the stomach. In the case of the *acidic* prodrugs, according to basic principles of chemistry, these drugs are able to accumulate within the cells of the stomach wall. Such phenomena may be important for sulindac, which in its prodrug form is demonstrated to be a moderate inhibitor of PG synthesis[36], i.e. *before* being converted to the more potent active metabolite.

The principal metabolite, i.e. the 'active' form, of both fenbufen and sulindac is a potent inhibitor of PG synthesis. Thus, for these drugs, damage to the gastric mucosa via the circulation may be more important.

2. Sustained/controlled release and enteric-coated forms

The theoretical advantage of these formulations is that the amount of drug available for direct contact with the gastric mucosa is reduced. Indomethacin, formulated as slow-release polymer-coated pellets, has been available for some time. A characteristic of this formulation is that a third of the dose exists as uncoated indomethacin and undergoes a 'burst' release upon swallowing and this may result in greater direct gastric exposure to indomethacin than other formulations.

Attempts to solve the problem of 'dumping' include controlled release pellets in an enteric coat, and the use of a special cellulose/alcohol granular matrix which, it is claimed, provides controlled release of indomethacin regardless of whether the tablet is whole or disintegrated. Any clinical superiority of these new systems remains to be proven.

3. 'Chemical' approach

Chemical modification of an NSAID's molecular structure has been used as a means to influence solubility in gastric juice and hence gastric absorption. For example, removal of the 'acetyl' moiety of aspirin together with the incorporation of two fluorine atoms results in the salicylate analogue — diflunisal, which by comparison with plain aspirin is virtually insoluble in gastric juice. Since this 'fluorinated' salicylate molecule is a considerably more potent inhibitor of PG synthesis than plain aspirin, then once again the systemic effect on the gastric mucosa cannot be ignored.

Perhaps the most interesting NSAID in the so-called 'chemical' category is azapropazone. Many workers however prefer to class azapropazone separately as an 'amphiprotic' NSAID[37]. This description aptly describes the ability of un-ionized azapropazone to protonate with decreasing pH. The aqueous solubility curve for azapropazone is clearly suggestive of amphiprotic character[37].

The minimum aqueous solubility of selected acidic NSAIDs (Table 1), determined in aqueous buffer at several pH units below the pK_a value, correlates closely with the time-to-peak plasma concentrations as shown in Figure 1. Within the realms of the simple equation,

$$S_T = S_o(1 + 10^{pH-pKa})$$

then such behaviour accords with theoretical expectation.

Figure 1 illustrates that azapropazone is clearly the exception. In spite of relatively high aqueous solubility in an acid environment (the minimum aqueous solubility of azapropazone occurs at pH 3.0–4.0 and is approximately 8 times that of indomethacin, 26 times that of fenbufen, 16 times that of diclofenac, for example), the time-to-peak plasma concentration of 4.0–4.5 hours for azapropazone in man is highly suggestive of pronounced absorption distal to the stomach. *A priori*, this may be explained by the proportional increase in the amount of lipid insoluble cationic moiety relative to the lipid soluble un-ionized moiety calculated to occur with decreasing pH below about pH 5.0 (see chapter by FM Dean). Indeed, this view is supported by the observation that the aqueous solubility of azapropazone at pH 1.0 is approximately double that observed at pH 3.0–4.0 (Figure 2).

Experimentally, Klatt and Koss[38] and Jahn et al.[39] conclude that in the rat, orally administered azapropazone is insignificantly absorbed in the stomach, with maximal rates of absorption occurring in the upper small intestine.

More recently, Upadhyay et al.[40] investigated the site of absorption of azapropazone in apparently healthy human volunteers using a multiple tube oro-gastric catheter positioned to allow the selective release of drug in either the stomach or duodenum. Balloons inflated immediately distal and proximal to the pylorus provided an effective fluid seal (confirmed in a separate study using ^{14}C-glycerol).

Following the intragastric administration of an aqueous suspension of 600 mg azapropazone, during a 4 hour period plasma levels of the drug were below the limits of confidence for detection. However, the drug rapidly appeared in plasma following intraduodenal administration.

Whilst exercising caution in extrapolating results obtained from the pylorus-occluded stomach, these observations are in accordance with the physical data which suggests that at low pH values, azapropazone exists as a positively charged lipid-insoluble species. With distally rising pH in the gastrointestinal tract, appearance of azapropazone in plasma parallels the increasing amounts of the lipid soluble un-ionized moiety.

Since azapropazone is a weak inhibitor of PG synthesis[36] then systemic transfer of azapropazone to gastric mucosal cells may be of less importance by comparison with stronger inhibitors. The significance of this feature in clinical practice, however, remains conjecture.

References

1. McCormack, K and Brune, K (1987). Classical absorption theory and the development of gastric mucosal damage associated with the non-steroidal anti-

inflammatory drugs. *Arch Toxicol*, **60**, 261–9

2. Shore, PA, Brodie, BB and Hogben, CAM (1950). The gastric secretion of drugs. A pH partition hypothesis. *J Pharmacol*, **119**, 361–9

3. Hogben, CAM, Schanker, LS, Tocco, DJ and Brodie, BB (1957). Absorption of drugs from the stomach. II. The human. *J Pharmacol*, **120**, 540–5

4. Hogben, CAM, Tocco, DJ, Brodie, BB and Schanker, LS (1959). On the mechanism of intestinal absorption of drugs. *J Pharmacol*, **125**, 275–82

5. Schanker, LS (1959). Absorption of drugs from the rat colon. *J Pharmacol*, **126**, 81–8

6. Schanker, LS, Shore, PA, Brodie, BB and Hogben, CAM (1957). Absorption of drugs from the stomach. The rat. *J Pharmacol*, **123**, 81–8

7. Schanker, LS, Tocco, DJ, Brodie, BB and Hogben, CAM (1958). Absorption of drugs from the rat small intestine. *J Pharmacol*, **123**, 81–8

8. Martin, BK (1963). Accumulation of drug anions in gastric mucosal cells. *Nature*, **198**, 896–7

9. Brune, K, Schweitzer, A and Eckert, H (1977). Parietal cells of the stomach trap salicylates during absorption. *Biochem Pharmacol*, **26**, 1735–40

10. Brune, K, Gubler, H and Schweitzer, A (1979). Autoradiographic methods for the evaluation of ulcerogenic effects of anti-inflammatory drugs. *Pharmacol Ther*, **5**, 199–207

11. Rainsford, KD and Brune, K (1978). Selective cytotoxic actions of aspirin on parietal cells: a principal factor in the early stages of aspirin-induced gastric damage. *Arch Toxicol*, **40**, 143–50

12. Leonards, JR (1963). The influence of solubility on the rate of gastrointestinal absorption of aspirin. *Clin Pharmacol Ther*, **4**, 476–81

13. Brune, K and Lanze, R (1985). Pharmacokinetics of non-steroidal anti-inflammatory drugs. *Handbook of Inflammation*, **5**, 413–49

14. Edwards, FC and Coghill, NF (1966). Aetiological factors in chronic atrophic gastritis. *Brit Med J*, **2**, 1409–15

15. Mukawa, K, Nakamura, T, Nakano, G and Magamachi, Y (1987). Histopathogenesis of intestinal metaplasia: minute lesions of intestinal metaplasia in ulcerated stomachs. *J Clin Pathol*, **40**, 13–8

16. Tatsuta, M, Iishi, H and Okada, S. (1988). *Dig Dis Sci*, **33**, 23–9

17. Upadhyay, R, Howatson, A, McKinlay, A, Danesh, BJZ, Sturrock, RD and Russell, RI (1988). *Campylobacter pylori* associated gastritis in patients with rheumatoid arthritis taking non-steroidal anti-inflammatory drugs. *Brit J Rheum*, **27**, 113–6

18. Doube, A and Morris, A (1988). Non-steroidal anti-inflammatory drug-induced dyspepsia — is *Campylobacter pyloridis* implicated? *Brit J Rheum*, **27**, 110–2

19. Kohli, Y, Kato, T, Suzuki, K, Tada, T and Fujiki, N (1987). Incidence of atrophic gastritis with age in Japan and Canada. *Jpn J Med*, **26**, 158–61

20. Tsuneoka, K, Hirakawa, T, Matsushita, K *et al.* (1977). The digestive tract in aging. *Stomach Intest*, **12**, 577–90

21. Roberts, DM (1972). Chronic gastritis, alcohol and non-ulcer dyspepsia. *Gut*, **13**, 768–74

22. Delaney, JP, Broadie, TA and Robbins, PL (1975). Pyloric reflux gastritis: the offending agent. *Surgery*, **6**, 764–72

23. Strickland, RG and Mackay, IR (1973). A reappraisal of the nature and significance of chronic atrophic gastritis. *Am J Dig Dis*, **18**, 426–40

24. Kekki, M, Siurala, M, Varis, K, Sipponen, P, Sistonen, P and Nevanlinna, HR (1987). Classification principles and genetics of chronic gastritis. *Scand J Gastroent*, **22**, (Suppl. 141), 1–28

25. Siurala, M, Isokoski, M, Varis, K and Kekki, M (1968). Prevalence of gastritis in a rural population. *Scand J Gastroent*, **3**, 211–23

26. Siurala, M, Varis, K and Kekki, M (1980). New aspects on epidemiology, genetics and dynamics of chronic gastritis. *Front Gastrointest Res*, **6**, 148–66

27. Ihamaki, T, Saukkonen, M and Siurala, M (1978). Long-term observation of subjects with normal mucosa and with superficial gastritis: results of 23–27 years follow-up examinations. *Scand J Gastroent*, **13**, 771–5

28. Villako, K, Kekki, M, Tamm, A and Savisaar, E (1986). Development and progression of chronic gastritis in the antrum and body mucosa: results of long-term follow-up examinations. *Ann Clin Res*, **18**, 121–3

29. Cheli, R, Simon, L, Aste, H *et al.* (1980). Atrophic gastritis and intestinal metaplasia in asymptomatic Hungarian and Italian populations. *Endoscopy*, **12**, 105–8

30. Winawer, SJ, Bejar, J, McCray, RS and Zamcheck, N (1971). Hemorrhagic gastritis. *Arch Intern Med*, **127**, 129–31

31. Chapman, MA, Werther, JL and Janowitz, HD (1968). Response of the normal and pathological human gastic mucosa to an instilled acid load. *Gastroenterology*, **55**, 344–53

32. Ritchie, WP and Delaney, JP (1971). Susceptibility of experimental atrophic gastritis to ulceration. *Gastroenterology*, **60**, 554–9

33. Ritchie, WP, Butler, BA and Delaney, JP (1972). Studies on the pathogenesis of benign gastric ulcer: increased back diffusion of hydrogen ion in experimental atrophic gastritis. *Ann Surg*, **175**, 594–600

34. Kivilaakso, E, Fromm, D and Silen, W (1978). Effect of the acid secretory state on intramural pH of rabbit gastric mucosa. *Gastroenterology*, **75**, 641–8

35. Fromm, D and Kolois, M (1982). Effects of sodium salicylate and acetylsalicylic acid on intramural pH and ulceration of rabbit antral mucosa. *Surgery*, **91**, 438–47

36. Brune, K, Rainsford, KD, Wagner, K and Peskar, BA (1981). Inhibition by anti-inflammatory drugs of prostaglandin production in cultured macrophages. *Arch Pharmacol*, **315**, 269–76

37. McCormack, K and Brune, K (1989). The amphiprotic character of azapropazone and its relevance to the gastric mucosa. Article in press — *Arch Toxicol.*

38. Klatt, L, and Koss, FW (1973). Pharmacokinetic studies with azapropazone dihydrate, labelled with carbon-14, in the rat. *Arzneim Forsch*, **23**(7), 913–9

39. Jahn, V, Reller, J and Schatz, F (1973). Pharmacokinetic experiments with azapropazone in animals. *Arzneim Forsch*, **13**(5), 660–6

40. Upadhyay, R, Duncan, A, Walker, FS and Russell, RI (1989). A new method for studying gastric and intestinal absorption of drugs and its application to azapropazone. *Eur J Clin Pharmacol* (In press)

41. Herzfeldt, CD and Kummel, R (1983). Dissociation constants, solubilities and dissolution rates of some selected non-steroidal anti-inflammatories. *Drug Dev Ind Pharm*, **9**(5), 767–93

42. Krebs, HA and Speakman, JC (1945). The effect of pH on the solubility of sulphanamides. *Biochem J*, **39**, xlii

43. Verbeeck, RK, Blackburn, JL and Loewen, GR (1983). Clinical pharmacokinetics of non-steroidal anti-inflammatory drugs. *Clin Pharmacokinet*, **8**, 297–331

44. Grennan, DM and Higham, C (1986). Non-steroidal anti-inflammatory drugs. In: Mol, JMH *et al.* (eds), *Therapeutics in Rheumatology* (Cambridge: Cambridge University Press)

45. Marsh, CC, Schuna, AA and Sundstrom, MD (1986). A review of selected investigational non-steroidal anti-inflammatory drugs of the 1980s. *Pharmacotherapy*, **6**(1), 10–25

Summary

It has been argued that the failure of certain non-steroidal anti-inflammatory drugs (NSAIDs) to reduce gastric mucosal levels of prostaglandins (PG) *in vivo* may reflect pharmacokinetic differences between NSAIDs rather than tissue-specific differences in their potency as inhibitors of the enzyme cyclo-oxygenase. A corollary of such an argument is that accumulation of NSAIDs within gastric mucosal cells is a principal factor associated with the intervention of intracellular biochemical events, and resultant gastric mucosal damage. *In vivo*, attempts to describe NSAID-induced gastric mucosal damage have been based on simple models derived from classical absorption theory in which the parietal cell is generally postulated to occupy a focal role. Such models, however, do not explain why in clinical practice it is the antral region which is apparently the preferred site for NSAID-associated gastric mucosal damage. Neither do such models adequately explain why some orally ingested non-acidic compounds (which, following absorption, are subsequently converted to weak organic acids capable of inhibiting PG synthesis) and parentally administered NSAIDs are damaging.

This brief overview examines the impact of hypotheses on our current thinking concerning the importance of pharmacokinetic factors on the aetiology of NSAID-associated gastric toxicity. The limitations of previous hypotheses are examined together with the limitations of models subsequently derived.

Zusammenfassung

Es wurde argumentiert, dass die fehlende *in vivo*-Senkung der Konzentrationen von Prostaglandinen (PG) in der Magenschleimhaut nach Verabreichung gewisser nichtsteroidaler Antirheumatika (NSAID) eher auf pharmakokinetische Unterschiede zwischen verschiedenen NSAID als auf gewebespezifische Unterschiede ihrer hemmenden Potenz des Enzyms Cyclooxygenase hinweist. Eine logische Folge dieser Argumentation wäre, dass die Ansammlung von NSAID in den Zellen der Magenschleimhaut den Hauptfaktor darstellt bei der Entstehung biochemischer Vorgänge in der Zelle, welche letztlich zur Schädigung der Magenschleimhaut führen. Versuche zur Beschreibung der NSAID-induzierten Magenschleimhautschädigung *in vivo* stützten sich auf einfache Modelle, die von der klassischen Resorptionstheorie abgeleitet waren, bei welcher der Parietalzelle im allgemeinen eine zentrale Rolle beigemessen wird. Solche Modelle vermögen aber die klinische Beobachtung nicht zu erklären, dass die NSAID-induzierte Schädigung der Magenschleimhaut anscheinend bevorzugt in der Antrumgegend lokalisiert ist. Ebensowenig liefern die Modelle eine adäquate Erklärung dafür, wieso sich einige oral verabreichte, nicht säurebildende Substanzen (die nach erfolgter Resorption in schwache organische Säuren umgewandelt werden, welche die Prostaglandinsynthese hemmen) sowie parenteral verabreichte NSAID schädigend auswirken.

Diese kurze Übersichtsarbeit untersucht die Auswirkungen einer früh formulierten Hypothese auf unsere heutige Einschätzung der Bedeutung pharmakokinetischer Aspekte bei der Entstehung der NSAID-assoziierten Magentoxizität. Auf die Grenzen dieser frühen Hypothese wird ebenso eingegangen wie auf die Grenzen der später abgeleiteten Modelle.

Resumé

On a prétendu que le fait que certains anti-inflammatoires non stéroïdiens (AINS) faisaient diminuer les taux de prostaglandines (PG) au niveau de la muqueuse gastrique *in vivo*, pouvait être le reflet de différences pharmacocinétiques entre AINS plutôt que de différences tissulaires spécifiques, dans leur puissance inhibitrice de l'enzyme cyclo-oxygénase. L'un des corollaires d'un tel argument est que l'accumulation d'AINS à l'intérieur des cellules de la muqueuse gastrique est un facteur important dans la mise en jeu de phénomènes biochimiques intracellulaires, et de la lésion de la muqueuse gastrique qui en résulte. *In vivo*, les tentatives de décrire la lésion de la muqueuse gastrique se sont basées sur des modèles simples, dérivés de la théorie classique de la résorption, dans laquelle on suppose généralement que la cellule pariétale occupe un position centrale. Mais de tels modèles n'expliquent pas pourquoi, en clinique, c'est la région antrale qui semble être le site de prédilection de la lésion de la muqueuse gastrique induite par les AINS. De tels modéle n'expliquent pas non plus de manière satisfaisante pourquoi certaines substances non acidifiantes prises par voie orale (converties suite à leur absorption en acides faibles organiques capables d'inhiber la synthèse de PG), et les AINS administrés par voie parentérale, sont nocifs.

Ce bref aperçu examine l'impact d'une ancienne hypothèse sur notre raisonnement actuel, quant à l'importance des facteurs pharmacocinétiques sur l'étiologie de la toxicité gastrique des

AINS. Les limites de cette ancienne hypothèse sont examinées en même temps que les limites des modèles qui en sont dérivés par la suite.

8
Reduction of irreversible injury in animal models of myocardial ischaemia by treatment with azapropazone

RM Knabb, MJMC Thoolen, SA Mousa and PBMWM Timmermans

I. BACKGROUND

Despite considerable advances in the last twenty years, myocardial infarction remains one of the leading causes of morbidity and mortality in industrialized countries. Myocardial infarction is precipitated by occlusion of one of the coronary arteries, which supply blood to the muscular tissue of the heart itself. The coronary arteries are frequently sites of advanced atherosclerotic lesions, and damage at these sites can result in the formation of an occlusive thrombus. The resultant ischaemia leads to depletion of high energy phosphates (ATP, CP) and tissue damage which progresses from reversible to irreversible injury[1]. Although this progression can be interrupted by timely restoration of perfusion by thrombolysis or angioplasty, it is believed that reperfusion exacerbates an inflammatory process which begins during ischaemia, and is characterized by the generation of cytotoxic oxygen free radicals[2,3] and an influx of activated neutrophils[4-7], leading to additional irreversible injury. Thus, to maximize the benefits of reperfusion and minimize the area which is irreversibly injured, it may be necessary to accompany therapies which restore perfusion by interventions which reduce reperfusion injury.

Numerous investigators have attempted to reduce the extent of reperfusion injury to experimental animals by enhancing the elimination of oxygen free radicals with free radical scavengers such as superoxide dismutase[8-13]. Superoxide dismutase is involved in manifesting natural defences against free radicals, which are produced in small amounts under normal circumstances. Endogenous superoxide dismutase and other radical scavengers are presumably overwhelmed by the burst of free radicals which follows reoxygenation of ischaemic tissue. Exogenous administration of native or recombinant superoxide dismutase has been found, in some laboratories, to dramatically reduce infarct size but has been without effect in others.

Azapropazone – 20 years of clinical use. Rainsford, KD (ed)
© Kluwer Academic Publishers. Printed in Great Britain

Another approach considered here is to block the sources of oxygen free radicals in ischaemic and reperfused tissue. Studies by McCord and others have demonstrated that the enzyme xanthine oxidase is a potential source of oxygen free radicals in reperfused tissue[2,3,14]. Under normal conditions, this enzyme is present as a dehydrogenase. Limited proteolysis under conditions present in ischaemic tissue converts the dehydrogenase form to the active oxidase, which then releases superoxide anion in the process of converting hypoxanthine to xanthine, and xanthine to uric acid. Reduction of high energy phosphates with concomitant formation of AMP during ischaemia provides a substrate to the enzyme from the further breakdown of AMP to hypoxanthine. Thus ischaemia converts xanthine dehydrogenase to a superoxide producing oxidase form, and provides increased levels of hypoxanthine. With reperfusion, the abrupt reintroduction of oxygen allows this enzyme to produce large amounts of superoxide anion, which is converted to hydrogen peroxide and the highly toxic hydroxyl radical.

Based on the hypothesis that xanthine oxidase is the major source of free radicals, various investigators have tested allopurinol, or its active metabolite oxypurinol in animal models of ischaemia and reperfusion[15-17]. As with the results from superoxide dismutase, the results have varied greatly.

In addition to the direct damage caused by reactive oxygen species, they also produce chemoattractant substances which result in the invasion of reperfused tissue by large numbers of activated neutrophils[5-7]. Neutrophils are also capable of producing large amounts of free radicals[18,19] and upon activation release lysosomal enzymes which produce additional tissue damage. Although the cytotoxic actions of neutrophils normally play a beneficial role in the organism, by killing bacteria or aiding in the degradation of necrotic tissue, in the setting of reperfusion they can cause irreversible damage to ischaemic tissue which could otherwise recover from the ischaemic insult.

The importance of neutrophils in reperfusion injury has been shown by studies in which dogs were rendered neutropenic prior to induction of ischaemia and reperfusion[20]. Reduction in leukocyte count by 77% with rabbit antiserum to dog neutrophils was shown to significantly reduce infarction by 43% following reperfusion, as compared to control animals which received nonimmune serum or saline. Other approaches to inhibition of neutrophils which may be more readily applicable to man include use of nonsteroidal anti-inflammatory agents, such as ibuprofen[4], or nafazatrom[21], eicosanoids such as prostacyclin[22-24], or perfluorochemicals[25].

II. EFFECTS OF AZAPROPAZONE ON REPERFUSION INJURY

The ability of azapropazone to inhibit xanthine oxidase[26,27] would afford one possible basis for determining the influence of azapropazone in animal models of ischaemia and reperfusion. The drug was also found by Mackin *et al.*[28] to inhibit various functions of activated neutrophils, including their migration, superoxide production, aggregation, and degranulation. Thus, with one molecule there are multiple activities which should not only reduce free radical production, but also the tissue damage caused by activated neutrophils.

III. EXPERIMENTAL STUDIES

1. Studies in rats

Montor *et al.*[29] tested the effects of azapropazone and the xanthine oxidase inhibitor allopurinol on myocardial infarction in rats. For these studies, occlusion of the left anterior descending coronary artery (LAD) was performed under diethyl ether anaesthesia. The chest was opened, the LAD ligated, and the chest wall closed during a very brief (20 second) period without ventilation. The extent of infarction was determined 48 hours after LAD occlusion by gross staining of the hearts with triphenyltetrazolium chloride (TTC), in which viable tissue appears dark red, whereas infarcted tissue remains pale[30].

Rats treated with either azapropazone (100mg/kg b.i.d., i.p.) or allopurinol (50 mg/kg b.i.d., i.p.) from 24 hours before LAD occlusion to 48 hours after occlusion had significantly smaller infarcts than saline-treated rats. In contrast, no beneficial effect was observed in rats which received azapropazone or allopurinol beginning one hour before LAD occlusion.

Although in these studies occlusion of the coronary artery was not followed by reperfusion, it is likely that sufficient oxygen to produce free radicals reaches the ischaemic myocardium by collateral blood flow and by diffusion from the left ventricular chamber across the relatively thin myocardial wall. Furthermore, neutrophils have been shown to accumulate in ischaemic myocardium without reperfusion[31].

2. Reperfusion in open chest dogs

Initial experiments to explore the effects of azapropazone on myocardial injury after ischaemia followed by reperfusion were performed in open chest dogs, anaesthetized with pentobarbitone/barbitone[32]. Myocardial ischaemia was induced by ligating the left anterior descending coronary artery. After 90 minutes of complete occlusion, the ligature was released to restore perfusion. Animals were sacrificed after 5 hours of reperfusion, and their hearts were removed for *ex vivo* analysis. The LAD was cannulated at the site of the previous occlusion, and perfused with TTC, while the remainder of the heart was perfused with Monastral blue dye via the aorta. This permitted identification of both the area at risk of infarction as well as the infarcted tissue within the area at risk. After fixation in formalin for 48 hours, the hearts were sectioned into six slices pendicular to the long axis of the heart, and the area at risk and infarction were quantified by planimetry.

Four groups of dogs were studied. Control animals (group I) received the vehicle for azapropazone, 1 ml/kg one hour before LAD occlusion, and 0.5 ml/kg 5 minutes before and 2.5 hours after reperfusion. Group II was treated with 100 mg/kg azapropazone one hour before LAD occlusion, and 50 mg/kg 5 minutes before and 2.5 hours after reperfusion. Group III received a single dose of 50 mg/kg azapropazone 5 minutes before reperfusion. Group IV received a single dose of 15 mg/kg azapropazone 5 minutes before reperfusion.

There were no significant differences in mean arterial pressure or heart rate among the four groups before, during and after LAD occlusion. Treatment with azapropazone did not alter these parameters. In addition, the area at risk was similar in the four groups. Despite the fact that haemodynamics and area at risk were similar in the four groups, the portion of the area at risk which was infarcted was greatly reduced in azapropazone-treated animals from groups II and III. Infarction averaged $34.7 \pm 4.8\%$ in 11 control dogs. Treatment with azapropazone before LAD occlusion resulted in only $7.6 \pm 1.8\%$ of the area at risk becoming infarcted. A smaller, but significant protective effect was also observed when azapropazone treatment was started 5 minutes before reperfusion ($14.8 \pm 4.4\%$ of area at risk), but not with a single dose of 15 mg/kg ($40.4 \pm 4.9\%$).

Histological examination of tissue from groups I and II also demonstrated beneficial effects of azapropazone. The extent of neutrophil infiltration was significantly reduced in both infarcted and noninfarcted portions of the area at risk. Similarly, myocardial oedema and haemorrhage were reduced in azapropazone-treated dogs.

Mousa et al.[33] studied further the factors which influence the protective effects of azapropazone in open chest dogs subjected to 2 hours of LAD occlusion followed by 5 hours of reperfusion. They utilized ^{14}C-labelled deoxy-2-D-glucose to assess the degree of ischaemia, and ^{111}Indium-labelled antimyosin to detect infarction. Azapropazone decreased the degree and extent of ischaemia, and reduced infarction in mild and moderately ischaemic tissue, but had no effect on myocardium, in which flow was severely decreased ($< 30\%$ of normal myocardial blood flow). Thus, the protective effects of azapropazone occur predominantly in the border zones, rather than in the centre of the ischaemic area.

3. Coronary thrombosis/thrombolysis in dogs

Since myocardial infarction in man is precipitated by the thrombotic occlusion of a coronary artery, it was desirable to test the effects of azapropazone in a model which closely mimics these conditions. For these studies[34,35], we utilized a model in which coronary thrombosis is induced in anaesthetized dogs by insertion of a small copper coil within the lumen of the left anterior descending coronary artery under fluoroscopic guidance. Thrombosis occurs within about 10 minutes after insertion of the copper coil, and is verified by angiography.

One hour after coronary occlusion, the animals were treated with intracoronary streptokinase to dissolve the thrombus and restore perfusion. Animals were treated with azapropazone either beginning prior to induction of coronary occlusion, or just prior to beginning thrombolytic therapy. Control dogs received injections of the vehicle for azapropazone.

Regional myocardial blood flow was determined with radiolabelled microspheres[36] during coronary artery occlusion, and again one hour and approximately 24 hours after reperfusion. Animals were euthanazed after the 24 hour flow measurement, and the hearts were perfused with TTC to delineate infarction. Area at risk was determined by measuring the blood flow throughout the heart during LAD occlusion and calculating the amount of tissue with less than 50% of normal blood flow.

We observed no differences in mean arterial blood pressure, heart rate, or the rate pressure product (an index of cardiac work) among the three groups. In addition, the time required for lysis of the occlusive thrombus was similar in the three groups, so that the total duration of ischaemia was not significantly different in azapropazone-treated animals. Importantly, the three groups had a similar amount of collateral blood flow to the ischaemic zone. Myocardial blood flow to normal tissue, or within the region at risk was not different among the three groups at any of the three times at which flow was assessed. The portion of the left ventricle which was at risk of infarction was similar in the three groups. As compared with control animals, the extent of the ischaemic tissue which became infarcted was reduced by 72% after treatment with azapropazone prior to induction of ischaemia. Delaying treatment with azapropazone until just prior to initiation of thrombolytic therapy still resulted in a 66% reduction in infarct size as compared to control animals.

Since, in these studies, treatment with azapropazone was maintained throughout the period of reperfusion until the animals were euthanazed, it is possible that the observed protection was due to postponement of reperfusion damage rather than true protection. To determine if the protective effects of azapropazone would be maintained after stopping treatment, another series of dogs were studied in which the extent of infarction was determined 4 days after induction of ischaemia and reperfusion[37]. Azapropazone (100 mg/kg i.v.) was administered to one group of dogs beginning just prior to thrombolytic treatment, and continuing by intravenous infusion (10 mg $kg^{-1}h^{-1}$) for 24 hours using a portable infusion pump carried in a pack on the animals. Control dogs received an equivalent volume of the vehicle for azapropazone solution.

Infarction was again determined by staining with TTC, and regional myocardial blood flow and area at risk were measured with radiolabelled microspheres. Serial blood samples taken during and after administration of azapropazone showed that plasma levels of azapropazone were relatively steady throughout azapropazone infusion (mean 140–160 μg/ml), but fell rapidly afterwards. Although the extent of infarction was larger in both groups of dogs which were sacrificed after 4 days as compared to earlier studies, the protective effects of azapropazone were maintained, with an approximately 50% reduction in the percentage of the area at risk which became infarcted, attributable to azapropazone. As in previous studies, there were no significant differences in haemodynamic parameters which determine cardiac work or in blood flow to ischaemic tissue during ischaemia or reperfusion.

Additional studies were performed to characterize a dose response relationship between azapropazone and the extent of infarction. These studies employed the same model, with the exception that thrombolysis was induced with intravenous tissue plasminogen activator (tPA) instead of intracoronary streptokinase. Animals were randomized to receive the vehicle for azapropazone, or one of three doses: 75 mg/kg just prior to treatment with tPA followed by an infusion of 7.5 mg kg^{-1} h^{-1} for 24 hours, 35 mg/kg plus infusion of 3.5 mg kg^{-1} h^{-1} for 24 hours, or 25 mg/kg plus 2.5 mg kg^{-1} h^{-1} for 24 hours. Animals were sacrificed 24 hours after discontinuing treatment with vehicle or azapropazone. A significant reduction in infarct size as compared to control dogs was observed in animals treated with azapropazone at a dose of 75 mg/kg followed by infusion with 7.5 mg kg^{-1} h^{-1} over 24 hours, but no significant effect was observed with the two lower doses. The four groups had similar baseline haemodynamic characteristics, and there were no differences in duration of occlusion or collateral blood flow.

4. Myocardial infarction in rabbits

Recent studies have examined McCord's hypothesis that xanthine oxidase is a major source of superoxide anion in reperfused tissues[14,38]. Specifically, studies from several laboratories have documented a marked variation in the levels of xanthine dehydrogenase and xanthine oxidase in myocardium from different species. Whereas the rat and the dog have easily detectable levels of xanthine oxidase in the heart, it has been found that rabbit, pig, and man have undetectable levels. If large amounts of free radicals are produced by xanthine oxidase in dogs and rats, the protective effects of allopurinol or azapropazone in these species could be misleading in regard to the efficacy of these agents in man.

For this reason, studies were performed in anaesthetized, open chest rabbits. Since collateral blood flow is minimal in rabbit hearts, ischaemic damage develops more rapidly than in dogs. Thus shorter periods of ischaemia must be employed in order to demonstrate reperfusion-induced damage. For these studies, a coronary artery was ligated for 30 minutes, and reperfused for 5 hours. The extent of infarction was quantified at the end of reperfusion using TTC. In control rabbits, infarction comprised $29 \pm 4\%$ of the left ventricle. Treatment with azapropazone reduced infarction significantly to

$20 \pm 1\%$ of the left ventricle. Thus myocardial salvage by azapropazone occurs not only in species with high levels of xanthine oxidase, and as well in animals in which this enzyme is lacking.

5. Swine studies

The effects of azapropazone on regional myocardial function were assessed in open chest swine subjected to 30 minutes of LAD occlusion followed by 2 hours of reperfusion. Swine also have limited collateral blood flow in comparison with dogs, and even short periods of ischaemia result in some irreversible ischaemic damage. Azapropazone or saline were given 15 minutes prior to reperfusion, and regional myocardial function was assessed by measuring segmental shortening with Doppler ultrasound crystals sutured to the epicardial surface of the heart. During ischaemia, normal contraction is impaired, and ischaemic areas may actually lengthen due to the pressure in the ventricle. Recovery of shortening is dependent on the severity of myocardial damage.

Azapropazone-treated animals had significantly better recovery of segmental shortening in border zones of the ischaemic area. Shortening was depressed in the central ischaemic area to a similar extent in azapropazone and control animals. There were no differences in heart rate, mean arterial blood pressure, or left ventricular pressure development between the two groups. Analysis of tissue samples for myeloperoxidase, a marker enzyme for neutrophils, revealed that azapropazone significantly reduced the extent of neutrophil accumulation in ischaemic/reperfused tissue.

IV. DISCUSSION

Numerous studies in patients have demonstrated the therapeutic value of early reperfusion during acute myocardial infarction[39-42]. However, considerable evidence in animal models of ischaemia followed by reperfusion supports the need for adjunctive therapy to reduce reperfusion-induced damage and thereby maximize the potential benefits of reperfusion. These studies show that azapropazone is highly effective in reducing the extent of infarction that occurs with coronary artery occlusion followed by reperfusion.

In each of the above studies, differences in the extent of infarction could not be attributed to differences in baseline variables which have been shown to influence infarction. Thus, the reductions in infarct size observed can be attributed to a protective effect of azapropazone. Furthermore, the effects of azapropazone are not due to modulation of the balance between myocardial oxygen supply and demand. Although interventions which reduce oxygen demand or increase oxygen supply may result in temporary improvement in cardiac function, these interventions do not appear to positively alter final infarct size. In contrast, treatment with azapropazone results in a persistent protecton of jeopardized myocardium, as shown by the reduced infarct size observed 24–72 hours after discontinuation of azapropazone treatment.

The protective effects of azapropazone could be due to inhibition of xanthine oxidase[26,27], inhibition of neutrophil functions[28], or a combination of these actions. The observations that azapropazone reduced the extent of infarction in rabbits and improved cardiac function during ischaemia and reperfusion in swine (both species without detectable xanthine oxidase) indicate that high levels of xanthine oxidase are not alone, required for the beneficial effects of azapropazone. This is important since it has been reported that xanthine oxidase is not present in human hearts[29]. The protective effects of azapropazone in species which lack myocardial xanthine oxidase may indicate that the action of azapropazone on neutrophils is of some importance to its efficacy.

Although other agents have been reported to reduce infarct size through inhibition of neutrophils, the use of these agents during evolving myocardial infarction in man may be difficult. Prostacyclin and related compounds result in hypotension, and therefore may not be safe during ischaemia and reperfusion. Other anti-inflammatory agents such as ibuprofen have been found to reduce infarct size, but also interfere with healing and scar formation after infarction[43,44]. This may be similar to the situation in which patients treated with steroids during myocardial infarction had a higher rate of ventricular aneurysm presumably due to impaired healing[45].

Beneficial effects of azapropazone did not require treatment prior to induction of ischaemia, but rather were observed when treatment was begun just prior to reperfusion. Thus azapropazone could easily be administered to patients after the onset of symptoms of acute myocardial infarction. For this use it is important to note that the time to lysis after administration of streptokinase or tissue plasminogen activator were not significantly different in the azapropazone-treated groups than in control animals. Thus azapropazone does not appear to interfere with or potentiate the fibrinolytic activation produced by plasminogen activators.

In summary, our studies with azapropazone in animal models of myocardial ischaemia and reperfusion show that the ability of azapropazone to inhibit both xanthine oxidase and the functional responses of neutrophils results in a reduction of irreversible injury to the heart as compared to that which would occur with reperfusion alone. The testing of this principle in clinical studies is underway, and other uses for azapropazone in diseases related to activated neutrophils and/or ischaemia followed by reperfusion should be considered.

Acknowledgements

The authors wish to thank Stephanie Montor, Andrew Leamy, Denver Fernando, Dolores Rasbach, Thomas Powers, and Martin Hulse for their contributions to these studies.

References

1. Reimer, KA, Lowe, JE, Rasmussen, MM and Jennings, RB (1977). The wavefront phenomenon of ischemic cell death. I. Myocardial infarct size vs. duration of coronary occlusion in dogs. *Circulation*, **56**, 786–94

2. McCord, JM (1985). Oxygen-derived free radicals in postischemic tissue injury. *New Engl J Med*, **312**, 159–63

3. McCord, JM (1986). Superoxide radical: a likely link between reperfusion injury and inflammation *Adv Free Radical Biol Med*, **2**, 325–45

4. Mullane, KM, Read, N, Salmon, JA and Moncada, S (1984). Role of leukocytes in acute myocardial infarction in anesthetized dogs: relationship to myocardial salvage by anti-inflammatory drugs. *J Pharmacol Exp Ther*, **228**, 510–22

5. Engler, RL, Dahlgren, MD, Morris, D, Peterson, M, Schmid–Schoenbein, GW (1986). Role of leukocytes in response to acute myocardial ischemia and reflow in dogs. *Am J Physiol*, **252**, H314–H322

6. Mehta, JL, Nichols, WW and Mehta, P (1988). Neutrophils as potential participants in acute myocardial ischemia: relevance to reperfusion. *J Am Col Cardiol*, **11**, 1309–16

7. Engler, RL (1989). Free radical and granulocyte-mediated injury during myocardial ischemia and reperfusion. *Am J Cardiol*, **63**, 19E–23E

8. Jolly, SR, Kane, WJ, Bailie, MB, Abrams, GD and Lucchesi, BR (1984). Canine myocardial reperfusion injury: its reduction by the combined administration of superoxide dismutase and catalase. *Circ Res*, **54**, 277–84

9. Werns, SW, Shea, MJ, Driscoll, EM *et al.* (1985). The independent effects of oxygen radical scavengers on canine infarct size. Reduction by superoxide dismutase but not catalase. *Circ Res*, **56**, 895–8

10. Ambrosio, G, Becker, LC, Hutchins, GM, Weisman, HF and Weisfeldt, ML (1986). Reduction in experimental infarct size by recombinant human superoxide dismutase: insights into the pathophysiology of reperfusion injury. *Circulation*, 74, 1424–33

11. Gallagher, KP, Buda, AJ, Pace, D, Gerren, RA and Schlafer, M (1986). Failure of superoxide dismutase and catalase to alter size of infarction in conscious dogs after 3 hours of occlusion followed by reperfusion. *Circulation*, **73**, 1065–76

12. Uraizee, A, Reimer, KA, Murray, CE and Jennings, RB (1987). Failure of superoxide dismutase to limit size of myocardial infarction after 40 minutes of ischemia and 4 days of reperfusion in dogs. *Circulation*, **75**, 1237–48

13. Werns, SW, Simpson, PJ, Mickelson, JK, Shea, MJ, Pitt, B and Lucchesi, BR (1988). Sustained limitation by superoxide dismutase of canine myocardial injury due to regional ischemia followed by reperfusion. *J Cardiovasc Pharmacol*, **11**, 36–44

14. Roy, RS and McCord, J (1983). Superoxide and ischemia: conversion of xanthine dehydrogenase to xanthine oxidase. In: Greenwald, RA and Cohen J (ed), *Oxy Radicals and Their Scavenger Systems*, Vol. 2. (New York: Elsevier Science), pp.145–53

15. Akizuki, S, Yoshida, S, Chambers, DE *et al.* (1985). Infarct size limitation by the xanthine oxidase inhibitor, allopurinol, in closed chest dogs with small infarcts. *Cardiovasc Res*, **19**, 686–92

16. Reimer, KA and Jennings, RB (1985). Failure of the xanthine oxidase inhibitor allopurinol to limit infarct size after ischemia and reperfusion in dogs. *Circulation*, **71**, 1069–75

17. Werns, SW, Shea, MJ, Mitsos, SE *et al.* (1986). Reduction of the size of infarction by allopurinol in the ischemic-reperfused canine heart. *Circulation*, **73**, 518–22

18. Babior, BM (1978). Oxygen dependent microbial killing by phagocytes. *N Engl J Med*, **298**, 659–68, 721–5

19. Fantone, JC and Ward, PA (1982). Role of oxygen-derived free radicals and metabolites in leukocyte-dependent inflammatory reactions. *Am J Pathol*, **107**, 397–418

20. Romson, JL, Hook, BG, Kunkel, SL, Abrams, GD, Schork, MA and Lucchesi, BR (1983). Reduction of the extent of ischemic myocardial injury by neutrophil depletion in the dog. *Circulation*, **67**, 1016–23

21. Bednar, M, Smith, B, Pinto, A and Mullane, KM (1985). Nafazatrom-induced salvage of ischemic myocardium in anesthetized dogs is mediated through inhibition of neutrophil function. *Circ Res*, **57**, 131–41

22. Ogletree, ML, Lefer, AM, Smith, JB and Nicolaou, KC (1979). Studies on the protective effects of prostacyclin in acute myocardial ischemia. *Eur J Pharmacol*, **56**, 95–103

23. Simpson, PJ, Mitsos, SE, Ventura, A *et al.* (1987). Prostacyclin protects ischemic reperfused myocardium in the dog by inhibition of neutrophil activation. *Am Heart J*, **113**, 129–37

24. Simpson, PJ, Mickelson, JK, Fantone, JC, Gallagher, KP and Lucchesi, BR (1987). Iloprost inhibits neutrophil function *in vitro* and *in vivo* and limits experimental infarct size in canine heart. *Circ Res*, **60**, 666–73

25. Bajaj, AK, Cobb, MA, Virmani, R, Gay, JC, Light, RT and Forman, MB (1989). Limitation of myocardial reperfusion injury by intravenous perfluorochemicals: role of neutrophil activation. *Circulation*, **79**, 645–56

26. Thiele, K, Cox, JSG, Fischer, J and Jahn, U (1981). Xanthine oxidase inhibitor and therapeutic treatment using same. *United States Patent* 4,305,942

27. Jahn, U and Thiele, K (1988). *In vitro* inhibition of xanthine oxidase by azapropazone and 8-hydroxy-azapropazone. *Arzneim-Forsch / Drug Res*, **38**, 507–8

28. Mackin, WM, Rakich, SM and Marshal, CL (1986). Inhibition of rat neutrophil functional responses by azapropazone, an anti-gout drug. *Biochem Pharmacol*, **35**, 917–24

29. Montor, SG, Thoolen, MJMC, Mackin, WM and Timmermans, PBMWM (1987). Effect of azapropazone and allopurinol on myocardial infarct size in rats. *Eur J Pharmacol*, **140**, 203–7

30. Fishbein, M, Meerbaum, S, Rit, J *et al.* (1981). Early phase acute myocardial infarct size quantification: validation of the triphenyl tetrazolium chloride tissue enzyme staining technique. *Am Heart J* **101**, 593–600

31. Engler, RL, Dahlgren, MD, Peterson, M, Dobbs, A and Schmid–Schoenbein, GW (1986). Accumulation of polymorphonuclear leukocytes during 3-hour experimental myocardial ischemia. *Am J Physiol*, **251**, H93–100

32. Thoolen, MJMC, Mackin, WM and Timmermans, PBMWM (1987). Effect of azapropazone on ischemia/reperfusion induced myocardial infarction in dogs (abstract). *Fed Proc*, **46**, 56

33. Mousa, SA, Cooney, JM, Thoolen, MJMC and Timmermans, PBMWM (1989). Myocardial cytoprotective efficacy of azapropazone in a canine heart model of regional ischemia and reperfusion. *J Cardiovasc Pharmacol* (in press)

34. Knabb, RM, Leamy, AW, Thoolen, MJMC and Timmermans, PBMWM (1987). Salvage of ischemic myocardium by azapropazone in a canine model of coronary thrombosis and reperfusion (abstract). *Fed Proc*, **46**, 557

35. Knabb, RM, Leamy, AW, Thoolen, MJ and Timmermans, PB (1988). Reduced infarction in dogs given azapropazone prior to coronary thrombolysis (abstract). *J Am Coll Cardiol*, **11**, 208A

36. Heymann, MA, Payne, DB, Hoffman, JIE and Rudolph, AM (1977). Blood flow measurements with radionuclide-labeled particles. *Prog Cardiovasc Dis*,

20, 55–79

37. Thoolen, MJMC, Rasbach, DE, Leamy, AW, Fernando, D, Timmermans, PBMWM and Knabb, RM (1987). Persistent cardioprotection by azapropazone in a canine model of coronary thrombosis and thrombolysis (abstract). *Circulation*, **76**, (Suppl. IV), 201

38. Eddy, LJ, Stewart, JR, Jones, HP, Engerson, TD, McCord, JM and Downey, JM (1987). Free radical-producing enzyme, xanthine oxidase, is undetectable in human hearts. *Am J Physiol*, **253**, H709–11

39. Gruppo Italiano per lo studio della streptochinasi nell'infarcto miocardico (1987). Long-term effects of intravenous thrombolysis in acute myocardial infarction: final report of the GISSI study. *Lancet*, **2**, 871–4

40. The AIMS Study Group (1988). Effect of intravenous APSAC on mortality after acute myocardial infarction: preliminary report of a placebo-controlled trial. *Lancet*, **1**, 545–9

41. ISIS 2 Collaborative Group (1988). Randomized trial of intravenous streptokinase, oral aspirin, both, or neither among 17187 cases of suspected acute myocardial infarction: ISIS 2. *Lancet*, **2**, 349–60

42. Wilcox, RG, Olsson, CB, Skene, AM, von der Lippe, G, Jensen, G and Hampton, JR (1988). Trial of tissue plasminogen activator for mortality reduction in acute myocardial infarction: Anglo-Scandinavian Study of Early Thrombolysis (ASSET). *Lancet*, **2**, 525–30

43. Brown, EJ, Kloner, RA, Schoen, FJ, Hammerman, H, Hale, S and Braunwald, E (1983). Scar thinning due to ibuprofen administration after experimental myocardial infarction. *Am J Cardiol*, **51**, 877–83

44. Jugdutt, BI (1985). Delayed effects of early infarct-limiting therapies on healing after myocardial infarction. *Circulation*, **72**, 907–14

45. Bulkley, BH and Roberts, WC (1974). Steroid therapy during acute myocardial infarction. A cause of delayed healing and of ventricular aneurysm. *Am J Med*, **56**, 244–50

Summary

Reperfusion of an occluded coronary artery reduces the extent of myocardial infarction, but is associated with an inflammatory process which results in additional irreversible injury. Manifestations of this 'reperfusion injury' include oxygen free radicals and the cytotoxic actions of activated neutrophils. Azapropazone has been shown to inhibit xanthine oxidase, a source of oxygen free radicals, as well as the functional responses of neutrophils, including migration, free radical production, and degranulation. We tested the effects of azapropazone on the extent of myocardial infarction in various animal models of ischaemia with or without reperfusion. Treatment with azapropazone prior to ischaemia, or just prior to reperfusion reduced infarction in every model studied. Reduced accumulation of neutrophils was also demonstrated in some studies. The beneficial effects of azapropazone occurred without alterations of haemodynamics which modify infarct development, and may be attributable to inhibition of xanthine oxidase and/or the responses of activated neutrophils. Our results suggest that therapeutic administration of azapropazone together with therapies to restore perfusion may minimize the extent of irreversible injury which occurs during acute myocardial infarction.

Zusammenfassung

Die Reperfusion einer verschlossenen Koronararterie vermindert die Ausdehnung des Myokardinfarkts, führt aber einen entzündlichen Vorgang herbei, der seinerseits zusätzliche, irreversible Schäden nach sich zieht. Dieser 'Reperfusionsschaden' wird unter anderem durch freie Sauerstoffradikale und zytotoxische Wirkungen von aktivierten neutrophilen Leukozyten verursacht. Es konnte gezeigt werden, dass Azapropazon sowohl auf die Xanthinoxidase als Quelle freier Sauerstoffradikale als auch auf die Funktionen neutrophiler Leukozyten wie Migration, Bildung freier Radikale und Degranulation eine hemmende Wirkung ausübt. Wir untersuchten die Auswirkungen von Azapropazon auf die Ausdehnung des Myokardinfarkts an unterschiedlichen Ischämiemodellen beim Versuchstier, mit und ohne Reperfusion. Bei allen Ischämiemodellen verminderte die Behandlung mit Azapropazon die Infarktgrösse, wenn sie vor der Ischämie oder kurz vor der Reperfusion erfolgte. In einigen Arbeiten konnte zudem eine geringere Ansammlung von Neutrophilen nachgewiesen werden. Die günstige Wirkung von Azapropazon stellte sich ohne hämodynamische Veränderungen ein, welche die Infarktentwicklung beeinflusst hätten; sie ist auf die Hemmung der Xanthinoxidase und/oder der Funktion aktivierter Neutrophiler zurückzuführen. Unsere Resultate weisen darauf hin, dass bei Massnahmen zur Wiederherstellung der Perfusion die gleichzeitige therapeutische Gabe von Azapropazon das Ausmass der irreversiblen Gewebeschädigung beim akuten Myokardinfarkt auf ein Minimum senken kann.

Resumé

La reperméabilisation d'une artère coronaire obstruée limite l'extension de l'infarctus du myocarde, mais cela va de pair avec un phénomène inflammatoire ayant pour conséquence une lésion supplémentaire irréversible. Parmi les témoins de cette 'lésion de reperméabilisation', citons les radicaux oxygénes libres et les effets cytotoxiques des neutrophiles activés. Il a été prouvé que l'azapropazone inhibe la xantine-oxydase, l'une des sources de radicaux oxygènes libres, de même que les réponses fonctionnelles des neutrophiles, dont la migration, la production de radicaux libres et la dégranulation. Nous avons testé les effets de l'azapropazone sur l'étendue de l'infarctus du myocarde sur différents modèles animaux d'ischémie, avec ou sans reperméabilisation. Le traitement d'azapropazone avant l'ischémie, ou juste avant la reperméabilisation, a limité l'infarctus dans chacun des modèles examinés. Une diminution de l'accumulation des neutrophiles a également été démontrée dans certains travaux. Les effets favorables de l'azapropazone se sont manifestés sans qu'il n'y ait de répercussion sur les fonctions hémodynamiques modifiant l'évolution de l'infarctus, et ils peuvent être attribués à l'inhibition de la xanthine-oxydase et/ou aux réponses de neutrophiles activés. Nos résultats suggèrent que l'administration thérapeutique d'azapropazone, conjointement aux traitements reperméabilisateurs, peut limiter l'étendue de la lésion irréversible résultant d'un infarctus aigu du myocarde.

9

Dual inhibitory effects of azapropazone on both neutrophil migration and function: relation to cardiovascular protection

SA Mousa, R Brown, WM Mackin, P Turlapaty, RD Smith
and PBMWM Timmermans

I. INTRODUCTION

Azapropazone (AZA) is a non-steroidal anti-inflammatory drug (NSAID) and xanthine oxidase inhibitor developed by Siegfried AG[1]. It is presently marketed in Europe as Prolixan® for the treatment of gout[1,2,3]. It has been shown that AZA enhances the excretion of uric acid, leading to decreased crystal deposition[4]. Evidence also suggests that human neutrophils (hPMN) participate in the deposition of sodium urate crytals in inflammatory responses. These responses involve the release of pro-inflammatory substances such as chemotactic factors and free radicals from hPMNs which further exacerbate the inflammatory condition[5,6]. In that regard, a role for neutrophils has been implicated in different tissue destructive events including rheumatoid arthritis, myocardial reperfusion injury, adult respiratory distress syndromes (ARDs), blistering skin disorders and ulcerative colitis[7,8]. The neutrophil releases toxins normally to defend the host against invading microbes, but has little intrinsic ability to control the release of these toxins under different sets of situations. Therefore, an agent which inhibits neutrophil function may be therapeutically important.

In vitro studies have demonstrated that AZA is a xanthine oxidase inhibitor with an IC_{50} of 70–140 $\mu g/ml$ and an inhibitor of a variety of neutrophil functions (migration, aggregation, superoxide production) at 40–400 $\mu g/ml$[9,10]. The broad spectrum of actions on neutrophils suggests that AZA inhibits an early process of neutrophil activation, such as the increase in intracellular calcium or the generation of cyclic adenosine monophosphate, which precedes mediator release. Numerous reports have implicated xanthine oxidase and neutrophil-derived oxygen free radicals in reperfusion-induced myocardial damages[11,12]. For these reasons, it has been postulated that AZA should exert a beneficial effect in myocardial infarction due to ischaemia

Azapropazone – 20 years of clinical use. Rainsford, KD (ed)
© Kluwer Academic Publishers. Printed in Great Britain

and reperfusion. Subsequent studies in rats and dogs have supported these suggestions[13-15].

This study was undertaken to determine the *in vivo* inhibitory efficacy of AZA on neutrophil migration using a model of topical inflammation (multiblister suction technique) and a model of regional myocardial ischaemia /reperfusion injury in swine. Additionally, the inhibitory efficacy of AZA on neutrophil function (superoxide generation) and its potential mechanisms of action were evaluated. Furthermore, pharmacokinetic and tolerance studies were carried out in normal volunteers.

II. MATERIALS AND METHODS

Chemicals Azapropazone 100 mg/ml was solubilized in saline, bubbled with N_2 and the pH was adjusted to 9.0–9.5. Monastral blue dye, hexadecyltrimethyl ammonium bromide, O-diansidine HCl, 30% hydrogen peroxide and formyl-methionyl-leucyl-phenylalanine (FMLP) were obtained from Sigma Chemical Co. (St. Louis, MO).

1. Neutrophil migration studies

A. Topical inflammation model in swine (multiblister suction technique)

Experimental preparation Ten male Hampshire/Yorkshire swine (SPF, 10–15 kg) obtained from Bio Medical Alternatives International Inc., Raleigh, NC, were used in the study. Swine were sedated with an intramuscular injection of ketamine (10 mg/kg) and anaesthetized by intravenous administration of sodium pentobarbital (30 mg/kg). Animals were placed on a respiratory ventilator using a positive pressure pump (Harvard Instrument). The common carotid artery and the left femoral vein were exposed and cannulated for monitoring heart rate/arterial blood pressure and blood samplings, respectively. AZA was administered intravenously via the marginal ear vein.

Skin chamber device The skin suction and chamber units were obtained from Neuro probe (Neuro probe, Cabin John, MD). The suction unit has two rows of four wells in each row (Figure 1). Each well has a diameter of 7 mm, allowing blisters to form with a maximal area of 0.38 cm^2. Each row can be connected separately or together (with a Y-tube) to a vacuum pump. The second chamber unit which covers the blister lesion is very similar to the suction unit, but has bigger wells, each with a diameter of 12 mm and a volume of 1 ml. A 2 mm wide and 1 mm deep trough filled with a plastic ring surrounds the wells in order to prevent the leakage of the serum. A hole in the top of each well allows the introduction of a 20 gauge subcutaneous needle for the injection and the withdrawal of fluid.

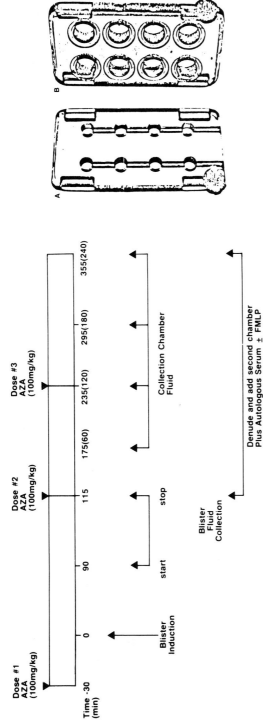

Figure 1 Diagrammatic sketch describing the protocol used in the study. AZA was given at a dose of 100 mg/kg i.v., 30 min prior to the induction of the blister. Eight blisters were induced over the swine's thigh muscle (time for induction = 90 min). Blister fluid from each blister was removed and frozen for the analysis of neutrophil migration (myeloperoxidase MPO activity). A second chamber was placed above the lesion site after the removal of the epidermal surface of the lesion. An autologous serum ± chemo-attractant (FMLP) was added to each well of the chamber. At different time intervals, the autologous serum and blood samples were withdrawn for MPO and AZA analysis. The blister chamber device used to induce the blister and the device used to cover the floor of the blister are shown.

Experimental protocol (Figure 1). The flat surface of the swine's thigh muscle was shaved and disinfected with ethanol. The suction unit was secured in place with a velcro bandage. A constant suction of ~300 mmHg was applied using a vacuum pump. The suction field was warmed up in order to increase the rate of the blister formation. After $1\frac{1}{2}$ hours, the blisters were complete. The blister fluid was removed and frozen for further analysis of myeloperoxidase (MPO) activity. The blister roofs were then gently removed with a scissors. The eight lesions (0.38 cm^2 area) were covered with the skin chamber unit and filled with 0.5 ml autologous serum with or without the chemo-attractant, FMLP (1 μg/ml). At different time intervals, the fluids from one chamber with FMLP and from another chamber without FMLP were withdrawn and frozen at $-70°$C for further analysis of neutrophil migration (MPO activity). Five swine were treated with AZA and five were given only saline. AZA 100 mg/kg, i.v., or saline was administered 30 min prior to the induction of the multiblister and every 2 hours throughout the study (Figure 1).

B. Regional myocardial ischaemia/reperfusion injury model in swine

Preparation Thirty-six male, Hampshire/Yorkshire swine (SPF, 12–16 kg) obtained from Biomedical Alternatives International Inc., Raleigh, NC, were used in the study. Swine were sedated with an intramuscular injection of ketamine (10 mg/kg) and anaesthetized by an intravenous administration of sodium pentobarbital (30 mg/kg). Animals were placed on a respiratory pump (Model 665; Harvard Apparatus, South Natick, MA). Mean arterial blood pressure was monitored by placing a catheter in the femoral artery. A midsternum thoracotomy was performed and the heart was surgically exposed and suspended in a pericardial cradle. The left anterior descending coronary artery (LAD) was dissected free from the cardiac tissues (approximately 5–10 mm) and a 2–0 silk snare was placed for subsequent occlusion with an occluder. A cathetertip micromanometer (Millar Instruments, Houston, TX) was inserted through the carotid artery and advanced through the mitral valve to record left ventricular (LV) pressure and its first derivative (dp/dt). Arterial blood pH, pO$_2$ and pCO$_2$ were monitored at various times

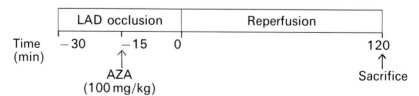

Figure 2 AZA in anaesthetized swine: diagrammatic sketch describing the coronary artery (LAD) occlusion (30 min) – reperfusion (120 min) protocol used in the study. AZA (100 mg/kg i.v.) was given 15 min post LAD occlusion. At the end of the study, animals were sacrificed, hearts excised at 120 min post-reperfusion for biochemical measurements of tissue myeloperoxidase activity.

during the experiment using an acid-base analyzer (ABL 30; Radiometer, Copenhagen). Throughout the experiment, the animals were kept on a heated operating table in order to maintain body temperature around 37°C.

Treatment groups

Group I: Control (n = 17): Saline 1 ml/kg i.v. 15 min post-LAD occlusion.
Group II: AZA alone (n = 19): AZA 100 mg/kg i.v. 15 min post-LAD occlusion.

Experimental protocol (see Figure 2). AZA was administered (100 mg/kg i.v.) 15 min after the LAD occlusion. The LAD was released after 30 min and the artery was reperfused for 120 min. Ventricular fibrillation (VF) occurred in swine either at later periods post-LAD occlusion or early post-reperfusion. Epicardial direct current shock (10 watt) was applied usually within 5 sec of the onset of VF and repeated if necessary (using ISD defibrilator, Electronics For Medicine Inc., Pleasantville, NY). Hearts defibrillated within the first minute resumed normal beating rates and maintained prefibrillation haemodynamics. Haemodynamic parameters were monitored and recorded (using a Gould recorder, Model 2800S: Gould Inc., Cleveland, OH) throughout the study. At the end of the study, the area at risk was delineated by infusing monastral blue dye into the left ventricle. This was followed by an i.v. dose of potassium chloride until asystole was observed. The heart was then excised, divided into mapped epi- and endocardium pieces for the biochemical determination of tissue myeloperoxidase (MPO) activity. The protocol of the study is diagrammatically sketched in Figure 2.

An index of neutrophil migration

Myeloperoxidase (MPO) assay Myeloperoxidase is a neutrophil-specific enzyme[16]. MPO was assayed in the blister fluid in the autologous serum and in cardiac tissues (normal area, area at risk including central and border zones from epi- and endocardium pieces) for the determination of the extent of migrated or activated neutrophil upon topical inflammation or myocardial ischaemia/reperfusion injury. The assay technique was as previously described by Mullane *et al.*[17]. The tissues were homogenized in 50 mM phosphate buffer containing 0.5% hexadecyltrimethyl ammonium bromide to solubilize MPO. The homogenates were then centrifuged at $40000\,g$ for 15 minutes. The supernatant, containing the MPO enzyme, was separated by decantation. To a 100 μl samples of tissue supernatant or blister fluid or autologous serum, 2.98 ml of 50 mM phosphate buffer (pH 6.0) containing 0.167 mg/ml of 0-dianisidine HCl + 0.003% H_2O_2 was added. The changes in absorbance at 460 nm at 25°C was monitored for 2–3 min. Data were expressed as a percent of normal (non-ischaemic) tissue or as a percent of basal MPO activity.

2. Neutrophil function studies

Neutrophil preparation Peripheral blood was drawn from healthy adult donors or anaesthetized animals and mixed with 5% dextran in phosphate buffered saline (pH 7.2) in a 5:1 ratio (blood:dextran). The mixture was incubated at 37°C for one hour. The leukocyte enriched plasma fraction was layered onto ficollpaque (Pharmacia, Piscataway, NJ) and centrifuged at 1500 rpm for 20 min. The pellet was resuspended in an erythrocyte lysing solution (NH_4Cl–0.15M, $KHCO_3$–0.01M and EDTA–0.001M, pH 7.3). PMNs obtained in this manner were >95% pure as determined by Wright stain and microscopic inspection.

Superoxide generation To a series of duplicates of siliconized glass tubes, the following were added: 0.5 ml PMNs (initial concentration 4×10^6/ml), 0.25 ml phorbol myristate acetate (PMA) (final concentration 20 μg/ml), 0.25 ml P-iodonitroterazolium chloride (INT) (initial concentration 5 mM). The samples were incubated at 37°C for 10 min or at room temperature for 40 min and then spun down for 3 min in an eppendorf centrifuge (to stop the reaction). The supernatant was decanted and the reaction rate (superoxide generation) was read spectrophotometrically at 505 nm[25–27].

Calcium mobilization The effects of AZA on hPMN internal calcium stores were determined using Fura2 fluorescence techniques. Briefly, 10^8 hPMN/ml in HBSS with $CaCl_2$ (1.87 mM) were incubated with Fura-2AM (2 μM) at 37°C for 10 min. The cell suspension was then diluted ten fold with warm HBSS and the incubation continued for 20 min. The cells were subsequently washed twice with HBSS and resuspended to a final concentration of 10^7 hPMN/ml. Cells were then incubated with or without AZA (1–100 μM) for 10 min at 37°C. One-ml aliquots were transferred to cuvettes in the sample compartment of a Perkin Elmer fluorescence spectrophotometer (model 650–40). The time drive mode of operation was used with the excitation and emission wavelengths previously determined at 340 and 499 nm respectively. Slit widths were set at 5 nm for excitation and emission. The scan was started at an arbitrary timepoint after recording baseline activity. FMLP (10^{-8}M) was then added and the increase in fluorescence intensity was monitored for 45 sec. The majority of the reaction was over in 10–15 sec.

Graphic recordings were quantified by image analysis of the area under the curve using a 30 sec cut-off point.

3. Analysis of azapropazone plasma levels

Pharmacokinetics of azapropazone Venous blood samples were withdrawn from swine and normal volunteers at different intervals post administration of AZA. AZA blood levels were determined using a previously described high performance liquid chromatographic (HPLC-UV) method[18]. HPLC method for the quantitation of AZA blood levels was as follows:

Column: C18 μ Bondapak reverse phase column

Mobile phase: Methanol 45%/0.1% v/v acetic acid 55%

Flow rate: 1 ml/min

Detection: UV at 254 nm

HPLC system used: Waters HPLC and Column

Internal standard: p-methyl phenytoin

Calculations: the peak heights of AZA were measured and ratioed to the internal standard. The separation of AZA from its 8-hydroxy derivative was not determined under the above listed conditions.

III. STATISTICAL ANALYSIS

The experimental results are given as the mean $\pm$ SE. The statistical significance of the difference between control and azapropazone-treated groups was determined by Student's t-test. Differences were considered statistically significant if $p < 0.05$.

Analysis of the pharmacokinetics of AZA in swine blood was carried out using a NONLIN program (Lexington Consultants, Lexington, KY).

IV. RESULTS

1. Neutrophil migration studies *in vivo*

A. Effect of AZA on PMN migration into topically inflamed sites in swine

AZA given at a dose of 100 mg/kg i.v. 30 min prior to the induction of the blisters inhibited neutrophil migration into the blister fluid as evidenced by a $48 \pm 6\%$ decrease in MPO activity. The blood levels of AZA at the time of the removal of the blister fluid were 115 ± 22 μg/ml.

After the removal of the blister, the neutrophil migration (MPO activity) into the autologous serum chamber was examined. An increase of neutrophil migration (2–3 times above the basal value) with a peak value at 2 hours post-treatment was observed. Addition of FMLP produced a much greater increase in the neutrophil migration (4–5 times above the basal value) into the serum chamber (Figure 3). The neutrophil migration into the skin chambers was significantly inhibited in the AZA-treated animals with MPO activity reduced by $35 \pm 6\%$ in the serum without FMLP and by $69 \pm 5\%$ in the serum with the FMLP (Figure 3). The blood levels of azapropazone ranged from 70–100 μg/ml throughout the study (Figure 3).

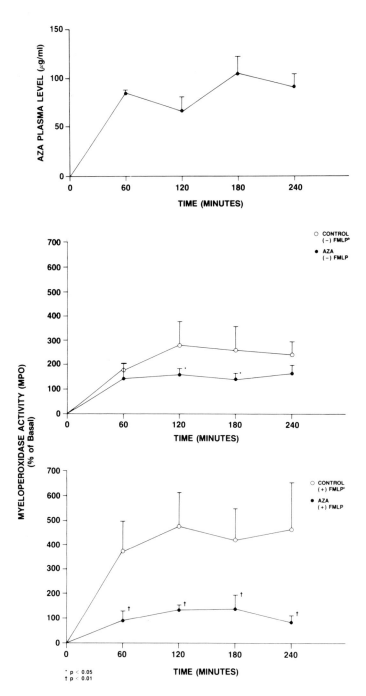

Figure 3 Effect of AZA on neutrophil migration (MPO) into autologous serum (± FMLP) in anaesthetized swine in correlation to AZA blood levels shown.

B. Regional myocardial ischaemia/reperfusion injury model in swine

Effect of azapropazone on neutrophil infiltration. AZA, 100 mg/kg i.v. administered during the LAD occlusion, resulted in a significant inhibition of neutrophil infiltration into the reperfused/ischaemic swine myocardium as compared to the saline-treated group (Table 1). The inhibitory effect of AZA on neutrophil migration was significant in the epicardium central and border zones as well as in the endocardium central and border zones.

Occlusion of the LAD resulted in an anatomical risk area comprising 20–25% of the left ventrical in the control and AZA-treated groups. The area at risk was not statistically different among the two different groups (Table 2).

Effect of azapropazone on the incidence of myocardial fibrillation. AZA reduced the incidence of myocardial fibrillation in 2/14 (14%) as compared to 5/17 (30%) in the saline-treated group. None of the animals from the AZA group fibrillated during the ischaemic phase.

Effects on haemodynamics. AZA had no significant effect on any of the recorded parameters as compared to the control group (Table 3). The lack of effect on the heart rate, blood pressure or on the heart rate-pressure product suggested that AZA has no effect on the oxygen consumption.

Table 1   Effect of azapropazone on neutrophil infiltration in swine myocardium subjected to regional ischaemic/reperfusion

Group	MPO[a] activity (% of normal myocardium)			
	Epicardium AAR		Endocardium AAR	
	Central zone	Border zone	Central zone	Border zone
Control	600 ± 49	426 ± 76	1057 ± 430	789 ± 280
AZA	337 ± 59^b	278 ± 60^c	380 ± 74^b	325 ± 68^b

[a] All values represent the mean $\pm$ SEM.
[b] $p < 0.01$.
[c] $p < 0.05$.

Table 2   Area at risk (AAR) following LAD occlusion/reperfusion in swine

Treatment group	AAR (% of left ventricle)[a]	
	Epicardium	Endocardium
Control (saline)	22.6 ± 1.3	22.5 ± 1.8
Azapropazone	23.9 ± 1.8	25.8 ± 1.7

[a] All values represent the mean $\pm$ SEM.

Table 3 Summarized haemodynamics in anaesthetized swine subjected to a 30 min coronary occlusion (LAD) and 120 min reperfusion: effects of azapropazone

Haemodynamic[a] parameters	Treatment group	Control	Occlusion (15 min)	Post reperfusion (min)				
				5	15	30	60	120
Heart rate (beats/min)	Saline[b]	154 ± 7	160 ± 10	169 ± 8	167 ± 9	169 ± 10	170 ± 9	165 ± 8
	AZA[c]	137 ± 7	146 ± 9	146 ± 7	146 ± 7	150 ± 8	153 ± 8	148 ± 9
Mean arterial blood pressure (mmHg)	Saline	82 ± 3	82 ± 3	82 ± 3	83 ± 3	82 ± 4	86 ± 3	85 ± 4
	AZA	74 ± 2	73 ± 2	77 ± 3	77 ± 4	80 ± 3	84 ± 4	89 ± 4
Left ventricular pressure (mmHg)	Saline	87 ± 4	87 ± 4	87 ± 4	86 ± 4	85 ± 5	90 ± 5	90 ± 6
	AZA	80 ± 3	81 ± 2	83 ± 4	82 ± 3	85 ± 3	88 ± 4	91 ± 5
+dp/dt (mmHg/sec)	Saline	1910 ± 97	1920 ± 154	1995 ± 182	1913 ± 143	1938 ± 185	2050 ± 197	1806 ± 176
	AZA	1682 ± 91	1954 ± 113	1890 ± 91	1926 ± 128	1989 ± 139	2053 ± 136	1980 ± 128

[a] All values represent the mean ± SEM.
[b] Number of animals in the control (saline) group, (n = 17).
[c] Number of animals in the azapropazone treated (AZA) group, (n = 14).

2. Neutrophil function studies

A. Azapropazone and neutrophil function (superoxide generation) in different species

The effect of AZA on PMN function (superoxide generation) was examined *in vitro* and *ex vivo* in blood from different species including rat, swine, canine and human. The IC_{50}s for the inhibition of superoxide by AZA ranged from $0.5–5 \times 10^{-4}$M depending upon the species (Table 4).

B. Potential mechanism

Using the fluorescent probe Fura2, the increase in hPMN cytosolic calcium in response to the addition of FMLP was monitored. Where untreated stimulated controls are equal to 100% of the response, hPMN pretreated with 100 μM AZA were inhibited in their ability to release calcium from intracellular stores (as indicated by reduced fluorescence upon stimulation with FMLP) by 69%. Pretreatment of hPMN with 10 μM AZA also caused a 29% inhibition of Fura2 fluorescence relative to controls. The IC_{50} was estimated to be 50 μM.

3. Pharmacokinetics of azapropazone

Pharmacokinetics of AZA in swine. Pharmacokinetic analysis of the AZA blood levels (μg/ml) over time revealed a biphasic blood clearance pattern ($\alpha t_{1/2} = 2.9$ min and $\beta t_{1/2} = 161$ min, see Table 5). The blood levels of AZA exceeded the determined (40–400 μg/ml) *in vitro* IC_{50}[9,10] required for the inhibition of xanthine oxidase and various neutrophil functions.

Myocardial tissue levels of AZA. An equilibrium in the distribution of AZA between the non-ischaemic and the reperfused/ischaemic myocardium was demonstrated 120 min post reperfusion (Table 6). The tissue levels of AZA approached those required IC_{50}s (40–400 μg/ml as determined in different

Table 4 Effect of azapropazone on neutrophil function (superoxide generation) in different species

Species	IC_{50}[a](M)		Method[b]
	In vitro	*Ex vivo*	
Rat	10^{-4}	—	Cytochrome C
Canine	3.5×10^{-4}	—	NBT
Swine	2×10^{-4}	5×10^{-4}	NBT, INT
Human	0.34×10^{-4}	—	Cytochrome C
	0.75×10^{-4}	—	NBT, INT

[a]IC_{50} was calculated under PMA stimulated condition (*in vitro*).
[b]Ferricytochrome C method[25].
Nitroblue tetrazolium (NBT) method[26].
Iodnitrotetrazolium (INT) method[27].

Table 5   Pharmacokinetic parameters
of azapropazone after i.v. bolus administration of 100 mg/kg of azapropazone
to swine

AUC (μg ml^{-1} min^{-1})	66090
k_α (min^{-1})	0.239
$t_{1/2, \alpha}$ (min)	2.9
k_β (min^{-1})	0.0043
$t_{1/2, \beta}$ (min)	161.4
V_d (ml/kg)	352.2
Cl (ml min^{-1}kg^{-1})	1.51
C_{max} (μg/ml)	647.5

Table 6   Distribution of azapropazone in swine myocardium
subjected to a 30 min LAD occlusion followed by 120 min
reperfusion

Myocardium AZA tissue level[a] (μg/g wet tissue weight)			
Non-ischaemic area		Area at risk	
Epicardium	Endocardium	Epicardium	Endocardium
128 $\pm$ 11	103 $\pm$ 4	114 $\pm$ 3	101 $\pm$ 4

[a] All values are mean $\pm$ SEM.

in vitro studies[9,10]) concentrations for the inhibition of various neutrophil functions.

Pharmacokinetics of AZA in humans. Clinical pharmacokinetic and dose tolerance studies in normal volunteers showed that AZA blood levels of 10^{-3} to 10^{-4}M were achieved at well tolerated doses ranging from 10–30 mg/kg i.v. (Table 7).

V. DISCUSSION

Several reports have suggested the involvement of different free radical species in myocardial ischaemia/reperfusion injury[11,12,19,20]. Oxygen-derived

Table 7   Pharmacokinetics of azapropazone in normal healthy volunteers

Doses[a] (mg/kg i.v.)	AZA blood levels[b] (μg/ml)			$t_{1/2\beta}$ (h)	AUC μg h/ml
	15 min	60 min	240 min		
10	157 $\pm$ 6	89 $\pm$ 6	39 $\pm$ 3	9.3 $\pm$ 1	670 $\pm$ 65
15	220 $\pm$ 21	125 $\pm$ 18	63 $\pm$ 12	10.1 $\pm$ 1.1	1140 $\pm$ 200
20	287 $\pm$ 10	178 $\pm$ 9	118 $\pm$ 13	10.5 $\pm$ 1.3	1960 $\pm$ 340
25	340 $\pm$ 15	214 $\pm$ 8	125 $\pm$ 5	12.5	2140
30	358 $\pm$ 19	242 $\pm$ 17	142 $\pm$ 12	12.1	2485

[a] All doses (bolus i.v. infusion over 10 min period) were given to normal healthy volunteers (n = 5 for each dose) weighing between 70–90 kg.
[b] All values are the mean $\pm$ SE for 5 different determinations at each time point.

118

free radicals have been identified as an important mediator of reperfusion injury[11,12]. Increased production of oxygen free radicals can cause direct tissue injury via lipid peroxidation of cellular and subcellular membranes leading to irreversible injury. Additionally, free radicals can play an important role in releasing chemotactic factors for neutrophil migration into damaged tissue with the subsequent liberation of cytotoxic free radical species (O_2^-, $\dot{O}H$, HOCl). Activation of neutrophils could result in the release of lysosoma enzymes and the obstruction of capillaries and small arterioles[12, 21]. Activated xanthine oxidase and neutrophils upon ischaemia/reperfuson have been shown to be involved in myocardial injury as evident from the different pharmacological intervention studies at either the xanthine oxidase or neutrophil migration and function levels[11,12,21]. It has been demonstrated that infarct size could be reduced in regional myocardial ischaemia/reperfused animal models when animals were made leucopenic before ischaemia[12]. A decreased infarct size was accompanied by a less dense leucocyte infiltration in the risk region and the adjacent myocardium. These studies clearly defined that the inflammatory response can be accepted as one determinant for ischaemic cell death. Because leucocyte depletion before ischaemia is not a reasonable treatment for patients with acute myocardial infarction, compounds that inhibit neutrophil infiltration may be particularly effective against myocardial ischaemia/reperfusion injury.

AZA has been shown to have a dual inhibitory effect on both xanthine oxidase as well as different neutrophil functions *in vitro*[9,10]. In that regard, the role of the oxy-free radical generated via the xanthine oxidase and neutrophils pathways in myocardial ischaemia/reperfusion injuries has been implicated[12,21]. Since it has been reported that the distribution of xanthine oxidase is species dependent and the human heart is devoid of xanthine oxidase[22-24], it was of interest to define the *in vivo* efficacy of AZA on neutrophil migration in a species which is devoid of xanthine oxidase. The present results demonstrated an inhibition of neutrophil migration by AZA into reperfused ischaemic swine myocardium. The presented inhibitory efficacy of AZA on the infiltration of neutrophils into reperfused/ischaemic swine myocardium might explain its cytoprotective efficacy (reduction of the incidence of VF) in the swine heart model which is devoid of the enzyme xanthine oxidase[23,24].

The lack of any apparent haemodynamic effect of AZA indicates that the myocardial protective effects of this drug are not due to haemodynamic changes which improve the myocardial supply-demand ratio. AZA reduced the incidence of VF. The exact mechanism underlying this action is not known.

The pharmacokinetic data (AZA blood and tissue levels) suggested that the inhibitory effect of AZA is not only limited to the neutrophil migration, but might also involve the inhibition of already migrated neutrophils into injured tissues, since AZA tissue levels in the AAR approached the determined IC_{50} for the inhibition of neutrophil functions[9,10].

These data demonstrate that AZA has an inhibitory effect of similar magnitude on both PMN migration and functin at concentrations which are achievable by clinically tolerated doses. In conclusion, these data suggest a clinical potential for AZA in different disease states involving neutrophils.

The inhibitory efficacy of AZA on neutrophils appears to account for the protective efficacy of AZA in regional myocardial ischaemia/reperfusion injury.

References

1. Templeton, JS (1983).In: Huskisson, EC, (ed) *Antirheumatic Drugs*, Vol. 3. (New York: Praeger) p. 97
2. Jones, CJ (1976). The pharmacology and pharmacokinetics of azapropazone (review). *Current Medical Research and Opinion*, **4**, (1), 3
3. McCarty, DJ (1985). In: Gupta, S and Tala, N (eds), *Immunology of Rheumatic Diseases*. (New York: Plenum), p. 425
4. Templeton, JS (1983). In: Huskisson, EC (ed), *Antirheumatic Drugs*. Vol. 3. (New York: Praeger), (1983). p. 110
5. Dutta, SN (1986). In: Pradham, SN, Maikel, RP and Dutta, SN (eds) *Pharmacology in Medicine: Principals and Practice*. (Bethesda, MD: S.P. Press International Inc.), pp. 234–5
6. Dale, MM (1984). In: Dale, MM and Foreman, JC (eds), *Textbook of Immunopharmacology*. (Boston, Mass: Blackwell), pp. 36–52, 167
7. Malech, HL and Gallin, JI (1987). Neutrophils in human diseases. *N Engl J Med*, **317**, 687–94
8. Henson, PM and Johnston, RB Jr (1987). Tissue injury in inflammation: oxidants, proteinases, and cationic proteins. *J Clin Invest*, **79**, 669–74
9. Rakich, SM and Marshall, CL (1986). Inhibition of rat neutrophil functional responses by azapropazone, an anti-gout drug. *Biochem Pharmacol*, **35**, 917–22
10. Jahn, U and Thiele, K (1988). *In vitro* inhibition of xanthine oxidase by azapropazone and 8-hydroxy-azapropazone. *Arzneim-Forsch/Drug Res*, **38**, 507–8
11. McCord, JM (1985). Oxygen-derived free radicals in postischemic tissue injury. *New Engl J Med*, **312**, 159–63
12. Lucchesi, BR and Mullane, KM (1986). Leukocytes and ischaemia-induced myocardial injury. *Ann Rev Pharmacol Toxicol*, **26**, 201–24
13. Montor, SG, Thoolen, MJMC, Mackin, WM and Timmermans, PBMWM (1987). Effect of azapropazone and allopurinol on myocardial infarct size in rats. *Eur J Pharmacol*, **140**, 203–7
14. Knabb, RM, Leamy, AW, Thoolen, MJ and Timmermans, PB (1988). Reduced infarction in dogs given azapropazone prior to coronary thrombolysis. *J Am Coll Cardiol*, **11**, 208
15. Mousa, SA, Cooney, JM, Thoolen, MJMC and Timmermans, PBMWM (1989). Myocardial cytoprotective efficacy of azapropazone in a canine model of regional ischemia/reperfusion. *J Cardiovasc Pharmacol*, **14**, 542–8
16. Bradley, PP, Priebat, DA, Christensen, RD and Rothstein, G (1982). Measurement of cutaneous inflammation: estimation of neutrophil content with an enzyme marker. *J Invest Derm*, **78**, 206–9
17. Mullane, KM, Kraemer, R and Smith, B (1985). Myeloperoxidase activity as a quantitative assessment of neutrophil infiltration into ischemic myocardium. *J Pharmacol Methods*, **14**, 157–67

18. Kline, BJ, Wood, JH, Beightol, LA (1983). The determination of azapropazone and its 6-hydrometabolite in plasma and urine by HPLC. *Arzneim-Forsch/Drug Res*, **33**, 504–6

19. Freeman, BA and Crapo, JD (1982). Biology of disease, free radicals and tissue injury. *Lab Invest*, **47**, 412–5

20. Hess, ML and Manson, NH (1984). Molecular oxygen: friend and foe. The role of the oxygen radical system in the calcium paradox, the oxygen paradox and ischemia/reperfusion injury. *J Mol Cell Cardiol*, **16**, 969–85

21. Rowe, GT, Eaton, LR and Hess, ML (1984). Neutrophil-derived, oxygen free radical-mediated cardiovascular dysfunction. *J Mol Cell Cardiol*, **16**, 1075–9

22. Al-Khaldidi, VA and Chaglassian, TH (1965). The species distribution of xanthine oxidase. *Biochem J*, **97**, 318–20

23. Downey, JM, Miura, T, Eddy, LJ et al. (1987). Xanthine oxidase is not a source of free radicals in the ischemic rabbit heart. *J Mol Cell Cardiol*, **19**, 1053–60

24. Eddy, LJ, Stewart, JR, Jones, HP, Engerson, TI, McCord, JM and Downey, JM (1987). The free radical producing enzyme, xanthine oxidase, is undectable in human hearts. *Am J Physiol*, **253**, H709–11

25. AuClair, C, Voisin, E and Banouth, H (1982). Superoxide dismutase inhibitable NBT and cytochrome C reduction as probe of superoxide anion production. In: Cohen, G and Greenwald, RA (eds), *A Reapraisal in Oxy Radicals and their Scavenger Systems*, Vol. 1. (New York: Elsevier)

26. Bachner, RL and Nathan, DG (1986). Quantitative NBT test chronic granulomatons disease. *N Engl J Med*, **278**, 971–6

27. Podczasy, JJ and Wei, R (1988). Reduction of iodonitrotrazolium violet by superoxide radicals. *Biochem Biophys Res Commun*, **150**, 1294–301

Summary

The purpose of this investigation was to determine the potential inhibitory effects of azapropazone (AZA) on both neutrophil (PMN) migration and function. The effect of AZA on PMN migration was examined in a swine model ($n = 12$) of topical inflammation using the multiblister suction technique (*in vivo*) and in a swine model ($n = 36$) of regional myocardial ischemia/reperfusion injury (*in vivo*).

AZA inhibited PMN migration into swine's topically inflamed sites in the absence and presence of chemoattractant (CAT) by 35 ± 5 and $69 \pm 6\%$, respectively. Similarly, AZA inhibited PMN migration into reperfused/ischemic swine myocardium. This inhibitory effect of AZA on PMN migration was achieved at $2-3 \times 10^{-4}$M AZA blood levels.

The effect of AZA on PMN Function (superoxide generation) was examined *in vitro* and *ex vivo* in blood from different species including rat, swine, canine and human. The IC_{50s} for the inhibition of superoxide by AZA ranged from 0.5 to 5×10^{-4}M depending upon the species.

Clinical pharmacokinetic and dose tolerance studies in normal volunteers showed that AZA blood levels of 10^{-3} to 10^{-4}M were achieved at well tolerated doses ranging from 10 to 30 mg/kg, i.v.

These data demonstrated that AZA has an inhibitory effect of similar magnitude on both PMN migration and function at concentrations which are achievable by clinically tolerated doses. In conclusion, these data suggest a clinical potential for AZA in different disease states involving neutrophil activation.

Zusammenfassung

In der vorliegenden Arbeit wurden mögliche hemmende Wirkungen von Azapropazon (AZA) auf Migration und Funktion der neutrophilen Leukozyten (PMN) untersucht. Die Auswirkungen von AZA auf die PMN-Migration wurden am Schwein ($n = 12$) in einem topischen Entzündungsmodell (nach der Methode der sog-induzierten multiplen Hautbläschen) (*in vivo*) sowie an einem anderen Schweinemodell ($n = 36$) bei durch Ischämie und durch Reperfusion bedingten lokalen

Myokardläsion (*in vivo*) geprüft. AZA hemmte beim Schwein die PMN-Migration in topisch entzündete Bereiche, und zwar um $35 \pm 5\%$ in Abwesenheit chemotaktischer Substanzen (CAT) sowie um $69 \pm 6\%$ in deren Anwesenheit. Die PMN-Migration in reperfundiertes/ischämisches Schweinemyokard wurde in ähnlicher Weise gehemmt. Diese Hemmwirkung von AZA auf die PMN-Migration wurde bei Blutkonzentrationen von $2-3 \times 10^{-4}$ mol/l AZA erzielt.

Die Auswirkungen von AZA auf die Funktion der PMN (Erzeugung von Superoxid) wurde sowohl *in vitro* als auch *ex vivo* im Blut verschiedener Spezies (Ratte, Schwein, Hund, Mensch) untersucht. Die mittleren Hemmkonzentrationen IC50 für die Hemmung von Superoxid durch AZA schwankten je nach Spezies zwischen 0.5 und 5×10^{-4} mol/l.

Klinische Studien über Pharmakokinetik und Dosistoleranz an gesunden Freiwilligen ergaben, dass AZA-Blutkonzentrationen von 10^{-3} bis 10^{-4} mol/l mit gut tolerierten Dosen von 10–30 mg/kg i.v. erreicht werden.

Mit diesen Daten konnte gezeigt werden, dass AZA sowohl die Migration als auch die Funktion der PMN in ähnlichem Ausmass hemmt. Diese Hemmwirkung stellt sich bei Blutkonzentrationen ein, die mit klinisch tolerierten Dosen erreicht werden können. Als Schlussfolgerung weist das Datenmaterial auf ein klinisches Potential von AZA bei verschiedenen Krankheitszuständen hin, an denen neutrophile Leukozyten beteiligt sind.

Resumé

Le but de cette recherche consistait à déterminer les effets potentiellement inhibiteurs de l'azapropazone (AZA) à la fois sur la migration et sur la fonction des neutrophiles (PMN). L'effet de l'AZA sur la migration des PMN a été examiné sur un modèle d'inflammation topique chez le porc ($n = 12$), selon la technique de succion multivésiculaire (*in vivo*) et sur un modèle de lésion localisée du myocarde, ischémie/reperméabilisation chez le porc ($n = 36$) (*in vivo*). L'AZA a inhibé la migration des PMN au niveau des zones d'inflammation topique chez porc, en l'absence et en présence d'agent chimiotactique (ACT), à raison de 35 ± 5 et $69 \pm 6\%$ respectivement. De même, l'AZA a inhibé la migration des PMN dans le myocarde de porc reperméabilisé/ischémique. L'effet inhibiteur de l'AZA sur la migration des PMN s'est manifesté à des concentrations sanguines d'AZA de $2-3 \times 10^{-4}$M.

L'effect de l'AZA sur la fonction des PMN (libération de radicaux superoxydes) a été examiné *in vitro* et *ex vivo* dans le sang de différentes espèces, dont le rat, le porc, le chien et l'homme. La CI_{50} d'inhibition des superoxydes a varié de 0.5 à 5×10^{-4}M selon l'espèce.

Les études des propriétés pharmacocinétiques cliniques et de la tolérance, effectuées chez des volontaires sains, ont montré qu'il était possible d'atteindre des taux sanguins d'AZA de 10^{-3} à 10^{-4}M pour des doses bien tolérées de l'ordre de 10–30 mg/kg i.v.

Ces résultats démontrent que l'AZA a un effet inhibiteur tout aussi important à la fois sur la migration et sur la fonction des PMN, à des concentrations pouvant être atteintes par des doses tolérées en clinique. En conclusion, ces résultats évoquent pour l'AZA des possibilités d'utilisation clinique dans différents états pathologiques faisant intervenir les neutrophiles.

10
Aspects of clinical pharmacology and bioavailability of azapropazone

KK Maggon and GM Lam

I. INTRODUCTION

Clinical testing with azapropazone was begun in 1966 in Europe by Siegfried AG. Currently, azapropazone is available in numerous countries throughout the world for the treatment of arthritic conditions. Clinical development of azapropazone in the United States was initiated by AH Robins. Prior to their decision to terminate clinical development of azapropazone in USA, AH Robins accumulated experience in over 1600 patients on the effectiveness of the drug in rheumatoid arthritis and osteoarthritis. They also completed a preliminary study in patients with acute gout.

du Pont assumed responsibility for the clinical development of azapropazone in the United States from AH Robins. Because of the drug's unique pharmacological properties[1-3] the clinical development of azapropazone under du Pont was solely for the indications of acute and chronic gout.

du Pont filed an US IND for clinical testing with azapropazone in 1984, and studies began shortly thereafter. In September 1986, du Pont suspended clinical investigations with azapropazone for this indication in the USA. The withdrawal of benoxaprofen, followed by several other NSAIDs during that period, indicated a highly unfavourable regulatory climate in the USA. It was considered at that critical moment that FDA approval for azapropazone would take a very long time. The benefit-to-risk ratio based on interim US clinical trials data at that time was judged not sufficiently favourable to justify continued development of the product.

Since the project was discontinued, statistical analysis of the data generated from the four clinical pharmacology studies has been performed. The present chapter will cover the main findings of these four studies.

II. OVERVIEW OF DUPONT'S CLINICAL DEVELOPMENT PROGRAMME IN USA

du Pont's clinical development programme for azapropazone comprised four studies in healthy volunteers and three studies in patients with acute or

Azapropazone – 20 years of clinical use. Rainsford, KD (ed)
© Kluwer Academic Publishers. Printed in Great Britain

chronic gout. The design of these studies, the study medication doses used, and the number of patients or subjects evaluated are listed in Table 1.

In total, 184 patients with gout and 54 healthy volunteers received azapropazone under Du Pont's IND. Three of these four studies (AZ-4, AZ-9, AZ-11) were conducted by Dr JC Kisicki, of Harris laboratories in Lincoln, Nebraska. The cimetidine interaction study (AZ-5) was performed by Dr AJ Dietz in North University, Fargo, N. Dakota.

1. Analytical methods

Azapropazone and cimetidine in the plasma were assayed by the HPLC methods of Kline *et al.*[4] and Greenblatt *et al.*[5] respectively with slight modifications. Standards were linear from 1–100 μg/ml for azapropazone and 0.16 to 10 μg/ml for cimetidine. Inter and intra day coefficients of variations were less than 10% for azapropazone, and less than 8% for cimetidine.

2. Statistical methods

Standard statistical tests like paired Student t test, Wilcoxon test, McNemar test, Kolmogorov–Smirnov test and ANOVA were used for analysis of the

Table 1 **Summary of duPont's clinical development programme in USA for azapropazone**

Study number	Type of gout	Study design	Study duration*	AZA dose (mg)	No. of subj/pts AZA	No. of subj/pts Reference	Reference drug
Patients							
AZ-1	Acute	DB,//	7 days	1200–2400	57	23	Indomethacin
AZ-2	Chronic	DB,//	6 months	300–2400	126	125	Allopurinol
		Open	6 months	300–2400	51**	—	—
AZ-15	Acute	DB	7 days	—	1	-	-
Total patients					184	148	
Subjects							
AZ-4	Nil	Open,//	10 days	900–1800	8	4	Allopurinol
AZ-5	Nil	Open, XO	10 days	600	24	-	-
AZ-9	Nil	DB,XO	12 days	600	14	-	-
AZ-11	Nil	Open, XO	56 days	300–1200	8	-	-
Total subjects					54	4	

AZA = azapropazone; DB = double blind; // = parallel group; XO = cross-over.
*Duration refers to a maximum time on azapropazone therapy; in cross-over designs, duration refers to a maximum time on each period of cross-over.
**Patients who successfully completed double-blind phase could enter open extension.

data. The p limit value for statistical significant differences, allowing to reject the null hypothesis HO, was as usual 0.05 (5%). Any p value $0.05 < p < 0.10$ was considered as a trend, whereas $p > 0.10$ was considered as not significant (NS). The probability values p computed were two-tailed unless otherwise stated.

The pharmacokinetic parameters c_{max} (maximum plasma concentration) and t_{max} (time to maximum plasma concentration) for azapropazone and cimetidine were determined by standard techniques. AUCs (Area under the curve, 0–72 hours) were calculated by the trapezoidal rule. Plasma elimination $t_{1/2}$ (half-lives) were obtained by regressing $\log_{10}$ (concentration) or ln (concentration) on time for detectable concentrations 24 hours or later (3 hours and later for cimetidine) and by using the formulae

$$\log_{10} t_{1/2} = -0.301/\text{slope}; \text{ or } \ln t_{1/2} = -0.693/\text{slope}.$$

All of these parameters were calculated with the help of the software MK-MODEL version 3.36 (Elsevier). Power calculations were performed with PC-SIZE. Tests analysis were performed mainly with the statistical packages SPSSPC+ and BMDPPC r.88. Graphics were generated with STAT-GRAPHICS 2.6 and Harvard Graphics.

III. HYPOURICAEMIC EFFECT PRODUCED BY DAILY AZAPROPAZONE OR ALLOPURINOL TREATMENT

The objective of this study was to compare the extent and time course of the hypouricaemic effects of azapropazone and allopurinol in healthy volunteers, and to explore possible increases in hypoxanthine and xanthine excretion with azapropazone. Only safety data were evaluated in this study. Statistical analysis was not performed because only four subjects were included in each group.

1. Study procedures

The study was designed as an open, parallel group trial in 12 volunteers with a pre-study serum uric acid value of 7.0 mg/dl or greater. Subjects were hospitalized on the evening prior to study day 1 and were to remain hospitalized for the duration of the study.

On study days 1–4, each subject received two placebo capsules immediately before breakfast. On day 5, subjects were randomly assigned to one of three treatment groups; four subjects each received 1800 mg/day azapropazone, 900 mg/day azapropazone, or 300 mg/day allopurinol. On Day 5, medication was administered t.i.d.; the azapropazone being supplied as 300 mg capsules and allopurinol as commercially-available 100 mg capsules.

2. Results and discussions

Prior to study admission, subjects received a physical examination that included measurement of vital signs and weight, as well as various laboratory tests measuring haematological, serum chemistry, and urinalysis parameters. The complete physical examination was repeated at the conclusion of the study. Adverse reactions were monitored throughout the study.

Twelve healthy male volunteers, whose mean age was 33 years, entered the study. There were no clinically meaningful differences in demographic characteristics, pre-study vital signs, or pre-study clinical laboratory parameters among the subjects assigned to the three treatment groups. All subjects completed study days 1–5 and all received the initial dose of the appropriate study medication. No subject completed study days 6–14 because all investigations with azapropazone were halted by the sponsor.

Body temperature was statistically significantly reduced in subjects assigned to 1800 and 900 mg/day azapropazone treatment groups on study day 5 relative to pre-study values. This change was small and averaged 1.1°C across all subjects. The only other statistically significant effect was the reduction in diastolic blood pressure which occurred in subjects assigned to the allopurinol treatment group. There were no statistically or clinically significant changes in any of the urinalysis parameters measured during the study. The only other statistically significant change, apart from uric acid in clinical laboratory tests, was a slight decrease in serum chloride levels in all treatment groups. These changes appear to have no clinical significance.

On study day 5, mean serum uric acid levels were decreased relative to pre-study values in subjects who received 1800 mg/day azapropazone and the reduction in serum uric acid values in the other two treatment groups approached statistical significance ($p < 0.10$). However, there was no change in serum uric acid levels between predose and postdose levels.

The serum uric acid levels are presented in Figure 1. There was a dose-dependent change in serum uric acid levels. Azapropazone, 900 mg, was comparable to 300 mg allopurinol dose in hypouricaemic effect.

The increased urinary clearance of uric acid is shown in Figure 2. These results are in accord with previous published reports[6,7].

No adverse reactions were reported during this study.

IV. MINIMUM HYPOURICAEMIC DOSE OF AZAPROPAZONE

The objective of this study was to establish the minimum hypouricaemic dose of azapropazone in healthy male volunteers.

1. Study procedures

The study was designed as a two-site, open, four-period crossover study using 16 volunteers with a pre-study serum uric acid value of 7.0 mg/dl or

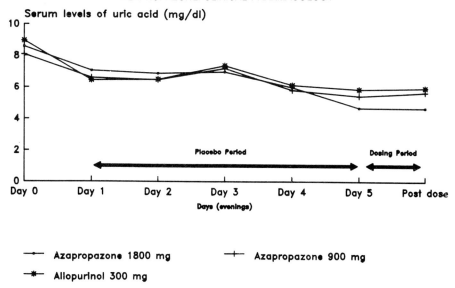

Figure 1 Uricosuric effect of azapropazone and allopurinol. Serum levels of uric acid (mean values).

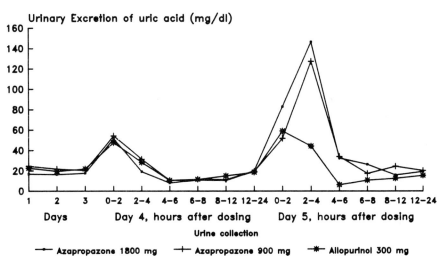

Figure 2 Uricosuric effect of azapropazone and allopurinol. Urinary excretion of uric acid (mean values).

greater. Data from only eight subjects were available for analysis.

Subjects were randomly assigned to one of four treatment groups and medication was administered according to a Latin square design. Each subject received 4 days of treatment at each of four different dosage levels of azapropazone: 300, 600, 900 or 1200 mg/day. Each of the four treatment periods was of 14 days duration, and consisted of two medication-free days during which baseline values were obtained (days 1–2, four days of azapropazone administration (days 3–6), and eight medication-free days (days 7–14). Azapropazone was administered q.i.d. and was supplied as 300 mg capsules.

Prior to study admission, patients received a physical examination which included measurement of vital signs and weight, as well as various laboratory tests measuring haematological, serum chemistry and urinalysis parameters. Laboratory tests were repeated at the conclusion of each treatment period (day 7), and the physical examination was repeated at the conclusion of the study. Adverse reactions were monitored throughout the study.

2. Results and discussions

Eight healthy male volunteers, whose mean age was 43 years, entered the study. None of the subjects showed meaningful differences in demographic characteristics or in pre-study vital signs or clinical laboratory parameters. Two individuals were assigned to each treatment group and all subjects completed each of the four treatment periods.

Clinical laboratory test values were pooled across all eight subjects at each dosage level. Serum uric acid levels decreased significantly at all dose levels on day 7. There were several minor changes in laboratory values but they all returned to normal range (except for uric acid levels, which are depicted in Figure 3. The statistically significant changes in laboratory values at different doses of azapropazone are shown in Table 2. Most of these changes remained within the normal range. These changes have no clinical

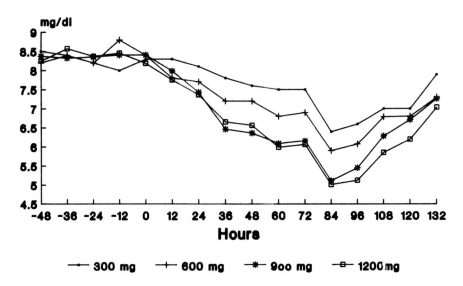

Figure 3 Mean serum uric acid levels. Effect of azapropazone

Table 2   Azapropazone: minimum hypouricaemic dose study. Statistically significant changes in mean laboratory values at each dose level

	Pre-drug screening	300 mg	600 mg	900 mg	1200 mg	n
Uric acid (mg%)	8.14	6.20*	5.41**	4.89**	4.64***	8
Haemoglobin (mg%)	16.68	13.79***	13.66***	13.70***	13.75***	8
Haematocrit (%)	50.88	42.38***	41.88***	42.13***	41.75***	8
RBCs (millions)	5.18	4.63*	4.58**	4.60	4.52*	8
Eosinophils (%)	3.25	3.00	5.13*	3.13	3.38	8
Platelet count (thousands)	224.71	261.50*	238.50	244.50	278.5**	7
BUN (mg%)	14.38	18.63*	17.63*	17.88	17.63*	8
Total bilirubin (mg%)	0.36	0.54*	0.44	0.49	0.55	8
SGOT (U/L)	20.75	16.63*	15.25**	15.25	14.50*	8
Alk. phosphatase (U/L)	54.75	49.50	50.63	48.88	47.63*	8
Creatinine (mg%)	1.19	1.14	1.19	1.19	1.26*	8

* : $0.05 > p > 0.01$.
** : $0.01 > p > 0.001$.
*** : $p < 0.001$.

significance because no dose-response relationship was observed.

Serum uric acid levels are shown in Figures 3–5 and Table 3 on different days of treatment. It is evident that clinically and statistically significant reductions in serum uric acid levels were obtained on the evening of day 6 even at the 300 mg dose. This objective was achieved with higher doses earlier in a dose dependent manner (Table 3, Figure 4). Thus it should be

Table 3   Azapropazone: minimum hypouricaemic dose study. Mean differences between medications days and baseline in serum uric acid levels (mg%; n = 7; mornings and evenings)

		Day 3	Day 4	Day 5	Day 6
300 mg	Mornings	-0.0071	-0.2357	-0.7071	-0.7214*
	Evenings	0.0714	-0.4143	-0.6000	-1.7429***
600 mg	Mornings	0.1464	-0.4964	-1.0250**	-1.3821**
	Evenings	-0.8357*	-1.4357***	-1.9643***	-2.8214***
900 mg	Mornings	0.1143	-1.0286*	-2.0143***	-2.1857***
	Evenings	-0.4286	-1.9429***	-2.3286***	-3.2429***
1200 mg	Mornings	-0.0714	-0.9143*	-1.6143***	-2.1714***
	Evenings	-0.7214**	-1.7500***	-2.4643***	-3.5071***

Percent reduction from baseline in serum uric acid; n = 8

	% Reduction at 84 hour	% Reduction in area under curve	
Dose		0–84 hour	0–144 hour
300	22.03	6.39	9.22
600	29.99	13.97	16.71
900	38.03	18.78	20.83
1200	39.85	19.75	23.44

* : $0.05 > p > 0.01$.
** : $0.01 > p > 0.001$.
*** : $p < 0.001$.

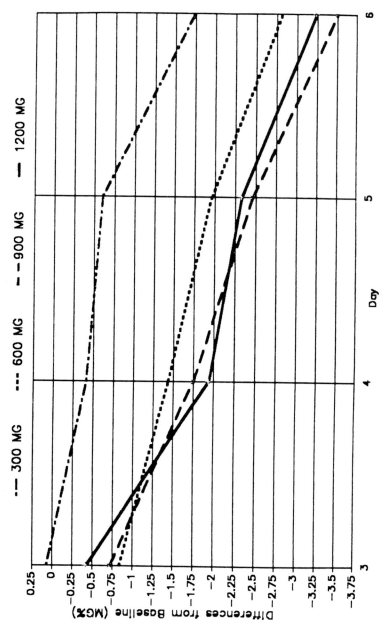

Figure 4 Serum uric acid levels (evening). Mean differences from baseline.

possible to use the 300 mg dose for minimum effectiveness in chronic gout and related indications.

These results substantiate previous results of effectiveness of drug dosages higher than 300 mg[2,3,6-8]. Dieppe and coworkers[7], showed that in a placebo-controlled trial in normal subjects, azapropazone doses from 600–1200 mg daily caused significant hypouricaemia. Similar effects have been reported by Frank[6], Templeton[2], Gibson et al.[9], Higgens and Scott[8]. This topic is reviewed in another chapter in this volume.

The pharmacokinetics of azapropazone were also studied and the parameters obtained are shown in Table 4. These values are in accordance with previously published reports[10-12].

3. Adverse reactions

One subject experienced a single brief episode of mild vasodilation (mild flush) on day 6 of the first treatment period. This subject had been receiving 300 mg/day azapropazone. The subject recovered spontaneously. A relationship to the test drug could be possible.

V. EFFECT OF FOOD ON BIOAVAILABILITY OF AZAPROPAZONE

The aim of this study was to compare the apparent bioavailability of orally administered azapropazone when administered with or without food.

1. Study procedures

In a randomized cross-over pharmacokinetic study, 24 healthy, male subjects were given 2 capsules of 300 mg azapropazone with and without food at a time interval of one week (washout period). Blood samples were taken before dosing and 1, 2, 3, 4, 5, 6, 7, 8, 9, 12, 15, 24, 36, 48, and 72 hours thereafter. Before the study began and at the end, a physical examination with measurement of vital signs, weight and height and a variety of laboratory tests for haematology, blood chemistry and urinalysis; these tests being part of the safety controls.

The treatment frequency was as follows:

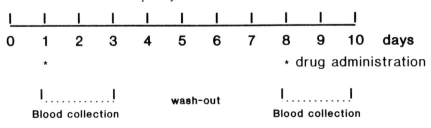

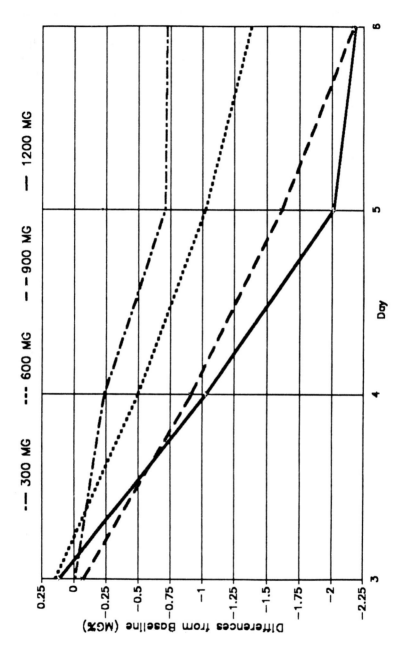

Figure 5 Serum uric acid levels (morning). Mean differences from baseline.

Table 4   Azapropazone: minimum hypouricaemic dose study. Pharmacokinetic parameters of azapropazone after oral administration

Parameters	300 mg Mean ± SD	600 mg Mean ± SD	900 mg Mean ± SD	1200 mg Mean ± SD
c_{max}, g/ml	38.7 ± 4.9	64.3 ± 12.6	91.2 ± 22.1	109.7 ± 27.1
t_{max}, h	3.63 ± 2.33	4.50 ± 0.53	4.62 ± 0.74	4.75 ± 0.46
AUC	450.0 ± 106.5	847.5 ± 232.7	1289.3 ± 439.5	1571.6 ± 539.1
$t_{1/2}$, h	16.93 ± 3.21	14.71 ± 2.58	16.16 ± 2.6	17.57 ± 3.22

AUC from 0 to 24 h (g × h/ml).
Harmonic mean ± pseudo SD.

2. Results and discussions

Several highly significant pharmacokinetic differences were detected due to treatment: c_{max} [$p < 0.001$], t_{max} [$p = 0.002$], AUC [p = 0.004] and $t_{1/2}$ [$p = 0.020$] for the main pharmacokinetics parameters and 11/15 individual time points. Food intake resulted in increases in: c_{max} 34.9 to 50.3 (+ 44%); t_{max} 4.38 to 5.63 (+ 28.5%); AUC 706 to > 854 (+ 20.8%) and a decrease in $t_{1/2}$ 18.6 to 15.8 (–15.4%). The effects of food on plasma levels of azapropazone are shown in Table 5 and in Figure 6.

The ANOVAs performed for the pharmacokinetic parameters and for the individual time points showed significant patient effect for the following items: AUC [$p = 0.009$], $t_{1/2}$ [$p = 0.003$] and 5/15 individual time ponts.

Practically no period effect was found in this cross-over study (Figure 7). The comparisons of the two periods never reached significance for any of the pharmacokinetic parameters taken into account (c_{max}, t_{max}, AUC and $t_{1/2}$). Direct comparison of the individual blood sampling time points were not significant.

The number of subjects enrolled gave an adequate power to detect significant differences in c_{max} and AUC, since the 20% threshold was widely exceeded by the actual values obtained.

Several significant decreases, with however the final values still in the

Table 5   Effects of food on pharmacokinetic parameters of azapropazone

Parameters	With food n = 24	Fasting n = 24	Subject variation p values
c_{max} (μg/ml)	50.3 (7.9)	34.9 (13.5)***	> 0.05, NS
t_{max} (h)	5.63 (0.77)	4.38 (1.53)**	> 0.05, NS
AUC (0–72 h)	854.1 (214.6)	706.9 (227.1)**	0.009**
$t_{1/2}$ (h)	15.77 (3.80)	18.63 (7.25)*	0.003**

* : $0.05 > p > 0.01$.
** : $0.01 > p > 0.001$.
*** : $p < 0.001$.
NS: Not significant.
Mean (SD).
Dose: 600 mg.

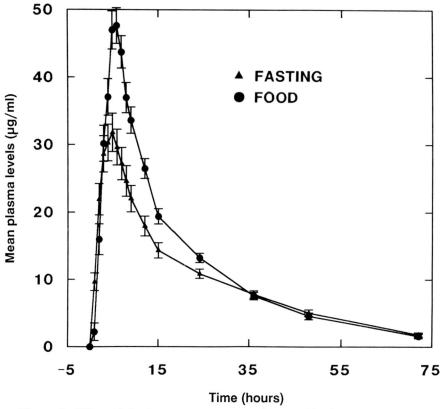

Figure 6 Effect of food on azapropazone pharmacokinetics: mean ($\pm$ SEM) azapropazone levels by treatment (food or fasting) (n = 24).

normal range, were detected by the before with after comparisons (Tables 6 and 7). Body temperature, respiratory frequency, systolic and diastolic BP, pulse rate, and 10/18 laboratory examinations decreased significantly in the majority of subjects. Two laboratory parameters (monocytes and BUN) nevertheless increased significantly during the study period.

On average, there was a 20% increase in AUC but there was a considerable difference, which ranged from 10% to 150%, between individuals. Of 24 subjects, 7 showed no significant change.

In the present study, food slowed the absorption of azapropazone by 28.5% as measured by t_{max}. Food slows gastric emptying and so delays the rate of drug absorption[13]. However, c_{max} and AUC were higher with food. Plasma elimination half-life decreased with food as compared to fasting (Table 5). Brown[14] has compiled the effect of food on NSAIDs. For most of the drugs, food decreased or delayed rate of absorption (ibuprofen, aspirin, difunisal, sulindac, tolmetin, ketoprofen, naproxen, diclofenac). It had little or no effect on the absorption or pharmacokinetics of indomethacin, phenylbutazone, and piroxicam.

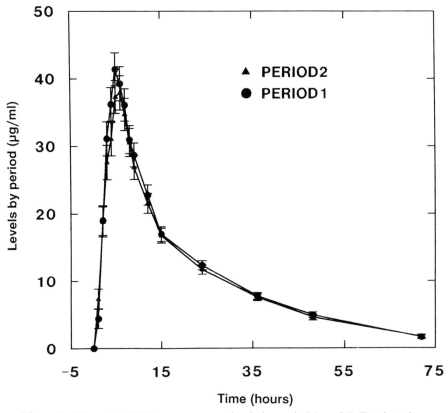

Figure 7 Mean (± SEM) azapropazone levels by period (n = 24). Food study.

Table 6 Effect of food study. Statistically significant changes in physical examination

Parameters	Mean (SD)		
	Before n = 24	After n = 24	Significance # #
Body weight (kg)	74.2 (7.8)	74.4 (7.9)	NS
Temperature (°F)	98.5 (0.6)	97.4 (0.5)	***
Respiratory freq.	17.9 (2.3)	15.1 (3.1)	***
Systolic BP	122.4 (8.6)	109.7 (10.9)	***
Diastolic BP	83.1 (6.0)	71.3 (7.6)	***
Pulse rate	71.4 (12.0)	63.6 (10.4)	**

\# # Paired t-test.
** : $0.01 > p > 0.001$.
*** : $p < 0.001$.
NS : Not significant.

Table 7   Effect of food on azapropazone kinetics: statistically significant changes in laboratory values

Parameters	Mean (SD)		
	Before n = 24	After n = 24	Significance (paired t-tests)
Haemoglobin (g%)	15.77 (0.9)	14.8 (0.8)	***
Haematocrit (%)	46.5 (2.7)	44.7 (2.4)	**
RBCs (10⁶)	5.32 (0.4)	5.0 (0.3)	***
WBCs (10³)	7.22 (1.7)	5.9 (0.9)	***
Neutrophils (%)	57.7 (8.6)	53.0 (6.9)	(*)
Monocytes (%)	1.5 (1.4)	2.5 (1.4)	*
Platelet (10³)	235.5 (44.9)	193.1 (40.2)	**
BUN (mg%)	14.7 (3.0)	20.2 (3.0)	***
Bilirubin (mg%)	0.72 (0.2)	0.5 (0.2)	***
SGOT (U/L)	16.0 (4.1)	14.3 (3.5)	**
SGPT (U/L)	20.8 (6.8)	15.6 (4.5)	***
Alk.phosph. (U/L)	53.8 (11.4)	49.8 (9.1)	***
Specific gravity	1.02 (0.01)	1.02 (0)	**

$p > 0.05$.
(*) : $0.1 > p > 0.05$.
* : $0.05 > p > 0.01$.
** : $0.01 > p > 001$.
*** : $p < 0.001$.

Conflicting evidence has been reported as to whether food effects either the rate or extent of azapropazone absorption. A pilot study by Leach[15] suggested there were no differences in azapropazone levels at 2, 5 and 24 hours after a single 600 mg dose. These preliminary results, however, are in question, as a more detailed study demonstrated a 47% increase in the plasma concentratiron of azapropazone over time when azapropazone was administered with food. The results of the present study could support the findings from the two previous studies depending on the selected population.

There is little public awareness about the effect of food on the bioavailability of azapropazone. To ensure maximum plasma concentrations with a minimum oral dosage, azapropazone must be taken together with food, especially in high risk populations. In view of the large inter-subject variations, the likelihood of an interaction cannot be ruled out.

3. Adverse reactions

During the study period, 6 subjects complained about side-effects of various natures in a total of 14 notifications. In one case the side-effect was found to be directly related to the test drug, for one subject (6 notifications), no positive relationship was found and for all the other notifications, the relationship with the test drug was judged as possible (Table 8).

VI. INTERACTION BETWEEN AZAPROPAZONE AND CIMETIDINE

The objective of the study was to compare the extent of absorption and rate of elimination of azapropazone and cimetidine when administered alone or concurrently.

Table 8 Adverse reactions recorded in the food study

Subject no.	Onset Day	h	Min	Duration h	Min	Maximum intensity	Description	Relationship with test drug	Patient outcome
4	1	11	10	4	5	Mild	Dizziness	Possibly	A
4	1	11	10	4	20	Mild	Tightness in leg muscles	Possibly	A
4	1	11	10	3	20	Mild	Nausea	Possibly	A
11	3	4	00	35	-	Mild	Headache	Possibly	A
12	8	7	10	2	5	Mild	Drowsiness	Possibly	A
16	2	15	00	1	30	Mild	Cramps	Definitely	A
16	8	14	40		40	Mild	Headache on top of skull only	Possibly	A
20	1	7	30	2	34	Mild	Skin crawling	Possibly	A
21	1	8	20		55	Mild	Indigestion	Def. not	A
21	1	9	30	97	30	Moderate	Headache	Def. not	A
21	2	7	00	13	-	Mild	Muscle spasms right arm, tongue/hands	Def. not	A
21	2	7	00	8	-	Mild	Went to sleep	Def. not	A
21	1	19	00	88	-	Mild	Joints ache	Def. not	A
21	1	6	45	100	15	Mild	Temperature	Def. not	A

A: Recovery without therapy.

1. Study procedures

In a randomized cross-over pharmacokinetic study, 12 healthy, male subjects were given 2 capsules of 300 mg azapropazone on day 5 and 12 after a 6-day course of cimetidine 300 mg every 6 hours and after a 6-day course of a placebo with a time interval of one week (washout period). Blood samples were taken before dosing and 0.33, 0.67, 1, 1.5, 2, 2.5, 3, 4, 5, 6, 7, 8, 9, 12, 24, 36, 48 and 72 hours thereafter. Before the study began and at the end of it, a physical examination was performed with measurement of vital signs, weight and height and various laboratory tests for haematology, blood chemistry and urinalysis; these tests being part of the safety controls.

The examination frequency was twice: starting at study day 4 and at study day 11.

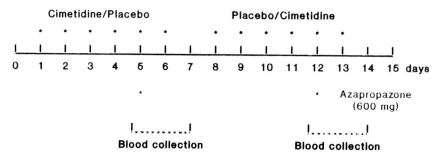

2. Results and discussions

Fourteen healthy male volunteers, whose mean age was 23 years, entered the study. There were no clinically meaningful differences in demographic characteristics, pre-study vital signs, or pre-study clinical laboratory parameters among the subjects assigned to the two treatment groups.

Two subjects were discontinued from the study on day 3 before receiving azapropazone treatment; these two had been entered into the study to ensure an adequate number of subjects (n = 6) in the two treatment groups. The remaining 12 subjects completed both cross-over phases of the study.

Several significant decreases, with values which nevertheless remain in the normal range, were detected in the 'before' with 'after' comparisons. Respiratory frequency, diastolic BP, and 4/18 laboratory examinations decreased significantly during the study period. Five labaratory parameters increased significantly (WBC, % lymphocytes, % monocytes, BUN, SGOT) (Tables 9 and 10).

No significant differences in the before with after comparisons were detected for the following parameters: general appearance; head ENT; eyes; neck; heart; lungs; abdomen; skin; musculoskeletal; neurological. The comparison of the temperature values was not possible since only one measurement was available for the after assessment.

Table 9   Cimetidine interaction study: statistically significant changes in physical examination

| Parameter | Mean (SD) | | Significance comparison |
	Before n = 12	After n = 12	
Body weight (kg)	74.0 (7.5)	73.1 (6.9)	(*)
Respiratory freq.	16.7 (1.8)	13.8 (3.5)	*
Systolic BP	128.8 (9.2)	127.2 (8.8)	NS
Diastolic BP	82.7 (5.9)	77.2 (5.6)	*
Pulse rate	67.3 (9.6)	67.8 (5.4)	NS

All paired t-test.
NS: Not significant.
(*): $0.1 > p > 0.05$.
* : $0.05 > p > 0.01$.

Table 10   Cimetidine interaction study: statistically significant changes in laboratory values

| Parameters | Mean (SD) | | | | Significance comparison |
	Before n = 12		After n = 12		
Haemglobin (g%)	15.3	(1.10)	14.2	(0.72)	***
Haematocrit (%)	45.2	(3.6)	41.4	(2.2)	**
RBCs (10^6)	5.1	(0.38)	4.7	(0.23)	***
WCBs (10^3)	5.8	(1.02)	6.7	(1.42)	**
Neutrophils (%)	55.0	(8.1)	45.6	(8.9)	*
Lymphocytes (%)	34.8	(6.6)	42.8	(9.3)	**
Monocytes (%)	5.5	(2.3)	8.0	(2.4)	*
BUN (mg%)	13.9	(2.5)	18.0	(3.2)	***
SGOT (U/L)	17.8	(5.4)	31.4	(17.4)	*
SGPT (U/L)	21.6	(6.8)	33.8	(26.6)	(*)
Alk.phosph. (U/L)	73.9	(16.1)	79.9	(16.8)	(*)
Specific gravity	1.2	(0.004)	1.0	(0.004)	(*)

(*) : $0.1 > p > 0.5$.
* : $0.05 > p > 0.01$.
** : $0.01 > p > 0.001$.
*** : $p < 0.001$.

No significant differences before–after were detected for the following blood parameters: eosinophils; basophils; total bilirubin; creatinine, as well as for the following urinary parameters: pH, albumin; glucose; microscopic WBC; RBC and casts. For the platelet count, no comparison was carried out, since no numerical data for the after assessment were available. All after figures were nevertheless normal (Table 10). These laboratory changes have no clinical significance.

3. Adverse reactions

A total of four adverse reactions were reported during this study. Three subjects reported headache while receiving only cimetidine; two of these subjects reported headache on study day 4, and one on study day 8. One patient reported pain in his pharynx (sore throat) on study day 6 after receiving azapropazone and cimetidine. All adverse reactions resolved without treatment, except for the patient who took one tablet for his sore throat. For all cases, the relationship with the test drugs was judged as possible (Table 11).

4. Plasma pharmacokinetics

A. Azapropazone

(i) Period effect The comparison of the two periods never reached significance for 3 out of 4 pharmacokinetic parameters (c_{max}, AUC and $t_{1/2}$). A significant difference [$p = 0.036$] was found for t_{max} with a 16.7% increase in the 2nd period. Since no other significant differences were detected for t_{max}, no further investigations were carried out to determine the real impact of this finding over the other pharmacokinetic parameters. Direct comparison of the individual blood sampling time points were not significant with the exception of one (t = 12 hours, $p = 0.0541$, trend). In conclusion, practically no period effect was found in this cross-over study (Figure 8).

(ii) Treatment effect Highly significant differences were detected for AUC [$p = 0.002$] for the main pharmacokinetic parameters and for 9/18 individual time points. The results with cimetidine vs. placebo were as follows:

$$c_{max} = +2.5\%, \text{ NS}$$
$$t_{max} = -5.2\%, \text{ NS}$$
$$AUC = +24.6\% \ p = 0.002$$
$$t_{1/2} = +11.0\%, \text{ NS}$$

The change in AUC ranged from 4–62% in the study population.

The number of subjects enrolled gave an entirely adequate power (> 0.80) to detect differences of 20% for both c_{max} and AUC (Figure 9, Table 12).

B. Cimetidine

(i) Treatment effect Significant differences were detected only for AUC [$p = 0.019$] for the main pharmacokinetic parameters and for 5/11 individual time points. The concomitant administration of azapropazone resulted in a decrease of all the pharmacokinetic parameters of cimetidine:

$$c_{max} = -11.0\%, \text{ NS}$$
$$t_{max} = -12.1\%, \text{ NS}$$
$$AUC = -15.8\%, \ p = 0.019$$
$$t_{1/2} = -2.5\%, \text{ NS}$$

The change in AUC ranged from 4–56% in the study population.

Table 11 Adverse reactions reported in the cimetidine interaction study

Subject no.	Onset			Duration		Maximum intensity	Description	Relationship with test drug	Patient outcome
	Day	h	Min	h	Min				
6	4	16	00	3	30	Mild	Headache	Possibly	A
10	8	13	00	11	00	Mild	Headache	Possibly	A
12	4	12	00	10	00	Mild	Headache	Possibly	A
12	6	24	00		30	Mild	Sore throat	Possibly	A

A: Recovery without therapy.
Headache was reported by three subjects during cimetidine treatment.

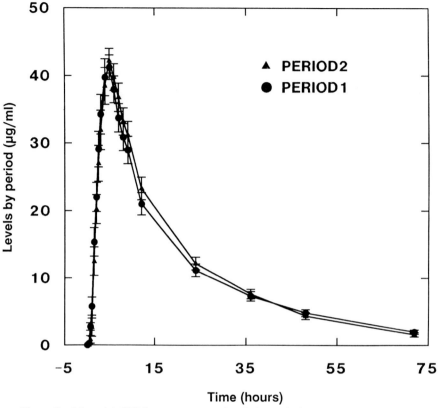

Figure 8 Mean (± SEM) azapropazone levels by period (n = 12). Cimetidine study.

The number of subjects enrolled gave an almost adequate power to detect 20% differences for AUC (0.72) but not for c_{max} (0.40) (Table 13, Figure 10).

(ii) Patient effect The ANOVAs performed for the pharmacokinetic parameters and for the individual time points showed significant patient effect for the following items: AUC [$p = 0.043$] and 5/11 individual time points.

The observed effects were probably due to metabolism and elimination. Rises in plasma levels of azapropazone given concurrently with cimetidine could be attributed to reduced renal elimination due to competition for tubular scretion[16,17]. This is further confirmed by mutual effect exerted by the two drugs upon each other. Thus, 15% of the 25% AUC effect observed in the AUC of azapropazone could be attributed to decreased tubular secretion. The other 10% effect could be due to the inhibition of hepatic microsomal oxidases and hydrolases[18].

Ochs et al.[19] observed a 14% increase in peak concentration of ibuprofen due to concurrent administration of cimetidine. This effect was

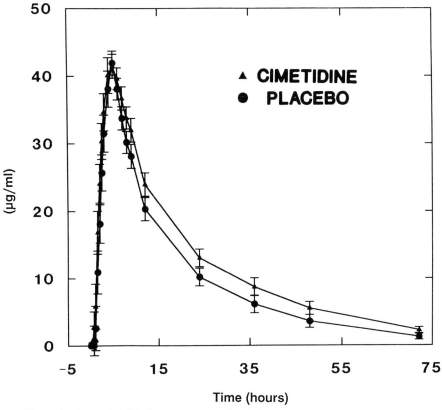

Figure 9   Mean (± SEM) azapropazone levels by treatment. Cimetidine and placebo.

Table 12   Effect of cimetidine on pharmacokinetics parameters of azapropazone

| Parameters | Mean (SD) | | Significance comparison | Subject variations p values |
	Cimetidine n = 24	Placebo n = 24		
c_{max} (g/ml)	44.1 (6.7)	43.0 (7.1)	NS	0.007**
t_{max} (h)	4.6 (1.0)	4.9 (0.6)	NS	> 0.05 NS
AUC (g × h/ml)	887.0 (243.6)	712.4 (165.4)	**	0.002**
$t_{1/2}$ (h)	18.7 (4.4)	16.8 (5.2)	NS	> 0.05 NS

** : $0.01 > p > 0.001$.
NS: Not significant.

attributed to inhibition of liver microsomal oxidases by cimetidine. Delhotal–Landes and coworkers[20] reported increased AUC and decreased clearance of oral cimetidine and ranitidine when co-administered with indomethacin or sulindac. Cimetidine modified the oxidative metabolism of sulindac. The administration of ranitidine significantly reduced the sulindac volume of distribution without modifying its clearance, which caused an increase in the c_{max} and a decrease in $t_{1/2}$.

Table 13 Effect of azapropazone on pharmacokinetics of cimetidine

Parameter	Mean (SD)		Subject variation p values
	Before AZA n = 24	After AZA n = 24	
c_{max} (μg/ml)	2.13 (0.69)	2.39 (0.58)NS	> 0.05, NS
t_{max} (h)	1.21 (0.48)	1.38 (0.70)NS	> 0.05, NS
AUC	5.76 (1.14)	6.84 (1.54)*	0.043*
$t_{1/2}$	2.43 (0.75)	2.49 (0.46)NS	> 0.05, NS

* : $0.05 > p > 0.01$.
AZA = azapropazone.

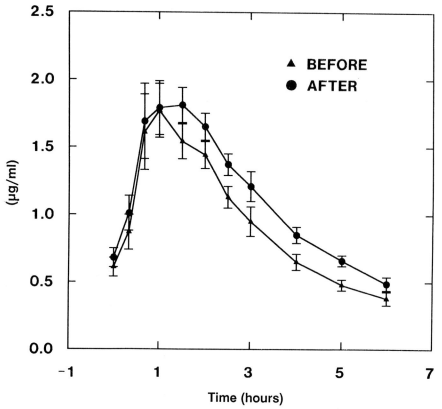

Figure 10 Mean (± SEM) cimetidine levels by treatment, before and after azapropazone.

Cimetidine is also known to interact with phenytoin and theophylline[21]. Over 40% of the oral dose of azapropazone is metabolized to the 8-hydroxy metabolite by hydroxylation in the liver, the remaining 60% is excreted unchanged in the urine[1-3]. Azapropazone inhibits microsomal hydroxylation and therefore reduces the metabolic clearance of phenytoin and theophylline by competitive inhibition[18].

In conclusion, this study shows that there is an interaction between azapropazone and cimetidine. The AUC of azapropazone increased by 25% while that of cimetidine decreased by 15%. The implication of this finding in clinical practice is to use smaller doses of azapropazone, when administered with cimetidine. High risk patient populations such as the elderly, or those with renal hepatic insufficiency receiving azapropazone and cimetidine must be carefully monitored. Dosages for these groups should be titrated for the minimum effective dose of azapropazone, because the interaction could be due to a renal or hepatic mechanism.

VII. OVERVIEW OF ADVERSE DRUG REACTIONS IN USA CLINICAL PHARMACOLOGICAL STUDIES

Seven out of 54 enrolled subjects (13%) reported adverse reactions while receiving azapropazone in duPont's clinical pharmacological studies (Table 14). The most frequently observed adverse reactions that were possibly or probably drug-related in these studies were headache, dyspepsia, abdominal

Table 14 Summary of adverse reactions reported in duPont's clinical pharmacology studies with azapropazone in USA: frequency of adverse reactions

Body system adverse reaction	Subjects (AZ-4, AZ-5, AZ-9, AZ-11) n = 54
Body as a whole	
Fever	1
Headache	2
Cardiovascular	
Vasodilatation	1
Central nervous system	
Dizziness	1
Paraesthesia	2
Somnolence	1
Gastrointestinal	
Abdominal pain, cramp	1
Dyspepsia	1
Nausea, vomiting	1
Musculoskeletal	
Hypertonia	1
Pain	2
Total subjects with adverse reactions	7
Percentage of adverse reactions	13%

pain or cramps, nausea and/or vomiting, diarrhoea, elevated serum BUN and/or creatinine levels, and rash.

In general, all adverse reactions resolved quickly upon discontinuation of azapropazone treatment. The adverse reactions observed during Du Pont's clinical trials with azapropazone are similar to those reported during both European and the earlier US studies with the drug.

1. Clinical laboratory changes

No subject in the above four studies showed a clinically relevant change in clinical chemistry. As predicted from its pharmacological properties, a reduction in serum uric acid levels was apparent following treatment with azapropazone in virtually all subjects.

2. Haematological changes

Statistically significant reductions in haemoglobin, hematocrit and red blood cell counts were evident in studies AZ-5, AZ-9 and AZ-11. These reductions averaged 5–10% relative to baseline values across all subjects or patients in these studies. Haemoglobin, haematocrit, and red blood cell count values returned towards baseline values following cessation of azapropazone treatment.

3. Urinalysis changes

There were no consistent, statistically or clinically significant changes following azapropazone treatment in any urinalysis parameter measured in these studies.

4. Ophthalmic, audiometric and ECG evaluations

There were no clinically significant changes in ECGs or in ophthalmic or audiometric evaluations that were judged as related to azapropazone treatment.

5. Vital signs and body weight

There were no consistent, statistically or clinically significant changes following azapropazone treatment in any vital sign measured or in body weight in these studies.

VIII. CONCLUSIONS

In patients at risk (the elderly, those with renal or liver insufficiency), lowest effective dose should be administered with food to minimize adverse reactions.

This is also true for patients treated with azapropazone and cimetidine. The studies on the hypouricaemic effect of azapropazone support the lower dose recommendations of the past few years.

Acknowledgements

The author wishes to sincerely thank the following colleagues within Du Pont de Nemours, USA:

Paul J Widner for monitoring the studies and to Tom B Lisi for providing preliminary study reports.

Dr B Bigelow, for carrying out preliminary statistical analysis.

In the Frankfurt/Geneva office:

Dr KP Klein, for his critical comments on the manuscript.

Dr KV Martensson, for his constant encouragement.

At Siegfried AG, Zofingen (Switzerland):

Dr A Von Korponay and Dr JL Heidecker, for all their kind help.

References

1. Eberl, R and Fellman, N (eds) (1985). Standortbestimmung des Azapropazons. *Rheuma Forum* Sondernummer **2**, 1–63
2. Templeton, JS (1983). Azapropazone. In: Huskisson, EC (ed), *Anti-Rheumatic Drugs*. (New York: Praeger Publishers), pp. 97–113
3. Jones, CJ (1976). The pharmacology and pharmacokinetics of azapropazone — a review. *Curr Med Res Opin*, **4**, 3–16
4. Kline, BJ, Wood, JH and Beightol, LA (1983). The determination of azapropazone and its 6-hydroxy metabolite. *Arzneim-Forsch (Drug Res)*, **33**, 504–6
5. Greenblatt, DJ, Abernethy, DR, Morse, DS, Shader, RI and Harmhatz, JS (1984). Clinical importance of the interaction of diazepam and cimetidine. *N Engl J Med*, **310**, 1639–43
6. Frank, O (1977). The treatment of acute gouty arthritis. *Adv Exp Med Biol*, **76B**, 288–90
7. Dieppe, PA, Doherty, M, Whicher, JT and Walters, G (1981). The treatment of gout with azapropazone: clinical and experimental studies. *Eur J Rheum Inflamm*, **4**, 392–400
8. Higgens, CS and Scott, JT (1984). The uricosuric action of azapropazone: dose-response and comparison with probenecid. *Br J Clin Pharmacol*, **18**, 439–43
9. Gibson, T, Simmonds, HA, Armstrong, RD, Fairbanks, LD and Rodgers, AV (1984). Azapropazone — a treatment for hyperuricaemia and gout? *Br J Rheumatol*, **23**, 44–51
10. Ritch, AES, Perera, WNR and Jones, CJ (1982). Pharmacokinetics of azapropazone in the elderly. *Br J Clin Pharmacol*, **14**, 116–9
11. Breuing, KH, Gilfrich, HJ, Meinertz, T and Jähnchen, E (1979). Pharmacokinetics of azapropazone following single oral and intravenous doses. *Arzneimittel-Forschung/Drug Research*, **29**, 6, 971–2
12. Breuing, K–H, Gilfrich, H–J, Meinertz, T, Wiegand, U–W and Jähnchen, E (1981). Disposition of azapropazone in chronic renal and hepatic failure. *Eur J Clin Pharmacol*, **20**, 147–55

13.   Markus, FWHM (1980). Drugs to be taken with meals. *Pharm-Int*, **ii**, 1–8
14.   Brown, CH and Pharm, MS (1988). Key pharmacokinetics of arthritis drugs. Effective counselling and clinical monitoring of patient response to these drugs will help avoid adverse reactions and ensure effective therapy. *US Pharmacist*, **13**, 49–67
15.   Leach, H (1976). The determination of azapropazone in blood plasma. *Curr Med Res Opin*, **4**, 35–43
16.   Powell, RJ and Donn, KH (1984). Histamine H_2-antagonist in perspective: mechanistic concepts and clinical implications. *Am J Med*, **77** (Suppl. 58), 57–84
17.   Greene, W (1984). Drug interactions involving cimetidine — mechanisms, documentation, implications. *Rev Drug Metab Drug Interact*, **5**, 25–51
18.   Geaney, DPl, Carver, JG, Davies, CL and Aronson, JK (1983). Pharmacokinetic investigation of the interaction of azapropazone with pnenytoin. *Br J Clin Pharmacol*, **15**, 727–34
19.   Ochs, Hr, Greenblatt, DJ, Matlis, R and Weinbrenner, J (1985). Interaction of ibuprofen with the H-2 receptor antagonists ranitidine and cimetidine. *Clin Pharmacol Ther*, **38**, 648–51
20.   Delhotal–Landes, B, Flouvat, B, Liote, F *et al.* (1988). Pharmacokinetic interactions between NSAIDs (indomethacin or sulindac) and H_2 receptor antagonists (cimetidine or ranitidine) in human volunteers. *Clin Pharmacol Ther*, **44**, 442–52
21.   Somogyi, A and Muirhead, M (1987). Pharmacokinetic interactions of cimetidine 1987. *Clin Pharmacok*, **12**, 321–66

Summary

Results of the four clinical pharmacology studies in 54 healthy, male subjects are discussed. These comprised single and multiple dose hypouricemic effect, effect of food and cimetidine interaction study.

Twelve healthy male volunteers with elevated serum uric acid levels of > 7 mg/dl received 300 mg allopurinol of 900 or 1800 mg azapropazone/day (4 subjects per dose). Prior to treatment, all subjects were on placebo for four days. There was a dose-dependent reduction in serum uric acid levels and increased urinary excretion of uric acid.

The minimum hypouricemic dose of azapropazone was determined in 8 healthy male subjects in an open four-period crossover study. Each subject received four days of treatment at each of four different dosage levels of azapropazone 300, 600, 900 and 1200 mg/day. Each treatment period was of 14 days duration and consistent of two therapy-free days to establish baseline values. After four days of drug administration, there were another 8 drug-free days. Clinical and statistical reduction in serum uric acid was achieved with 300 mg/day on day 6 and earlier at higher doses.

The apparent bioavailability of oral azapropazone was compared with or without food. In a randomized crossover study, 24 healthy, male subjects received 600 mg of azapropazone p.o. with and without food one week apart.

Food intake resulted in increased C_{max} by 44%, T_{max} by 28.5% and AUC by 20.8%. The plasma elimination half-life decreased by 15.4% with food. The changes varied with subjects, no change was observed in 7 out of 24 subjects. In the other 17 subjects, the increase in AUC varied from 10 to 15%.

Interaction with cimetidine was studied in 12 healthy, male subjects in a randomized crossover study. Subjects were given 600 mg of azapropazone p.o. after a 6 day treatment with cimetidine (300 mg ever 6 hours) and after placebo after one week washout period. Cimetidine increased the AUC of azapropazone by 24.6% (range 4–62%). Azapropazone decreased the AUC of cimetidine by 15.8% (range 4–56%). Changes in other pharmacokinetic parameters were less significant between treatment groups. The above results show that 300 mg/day is the minimum effective hypouricemic dose.

In high risk patient populations like the elderly, renal and hepatic insufficiency, lowest effective dose of azapropazone should be administered with food to minimise adverse reactions. Due to interaction of azapropazone and cimetidine, patients on cimetidine should be titrated for minimum effective dose.

Lowest effective dose should be used for chronic administration.

Zusammenfassung

Im folgenden werden die Ergebnisse der vier pharmakologischen Studien an insgesamt 54 gesunden männlichen Freiwilligen besprochen. Diese Studien befassten sich mit der hypourikämischen Wirkung von Einzel- und Mehrfachdosen, dem Einfluss der Nahrungsaufnahme und der Interaktion mit Cimetidin.

Zwölf gesunde männliche Freiwillige, deren Harnsäurekonzentration im Serum auf über 7 mg/dl erhöht war, erhielten entweder 300 mg Allopurinol oder 900 bzw. 1800 mg Azapropazon täglich (je vier Versuchspersonen pro Therapieschema). Vorgängig wurden alle Teilnehmer vier Tage lang mit Placebo behandelt. Es ergab sich eine dosisabhängige Senkung der Serum-Harnsäure-Konzentration sowie eine Erhöhung der Harnsäureausscheidung im Urin.

Die minimale hypourikämische Dosis von Azapropazon wurde in einer offenen, gekreuzten, vierphasigen Studie an acht gesunden männlichen Versuchspersonen ermittelt. Alle Teilnehmer durchliefen die vier Dosisstufen mit Tagesdosen von 300, 600, 900 und 1200 mg Azapropazon während vier Tagen. Die Behandlungsphasen dauerten je 14 Tage; während zwei therapiefreien Tagen zu Beginn wurden die Ausgangswerte bestimmt, dann folgten die vier Tage Therapie und schliesslich weitere acht therapiefreie Tage. Eine klinische und statistische Senkung der Harnsäure-Konzentration im Serum wurde bei 300 mg/Tag am Tag 6, bei höherer Dosierung bereits früher erreicht.

Die effektive orale Bioverfügbarkeit von Azapropazon wurde mit und ohne Nahrungsaufnahme verglichen. In einer randomisierten, gekreuzten Studie wurden 24 gesunde männliche Versuchspersonen mit 600 mg Azapropazon behandelt; eine Dosis wurde mit dem Essen, die andere Dosis eine Woche später ohne Essen verabreicht.

Die Nahrungsaufnahme hatte eine Erhöhung der C_{max} um 44%, der T_{max} um 28.5% sowie der Fläche unter der Kurve (area under the curve, AUC) um 20.8% zur Folge. Bei der Einnahme mit dem Essen verminderte sich die Plasma-Eliminationshalbwertszeit um 15.4%. Diese Veränderungen waren je nach Versuchsperson unterschiedlich stark ausgeprägt, wobei 7 von 24 Versuchspersonen gar keine Veränderungen zeigten. Bei weiteren 17 Versuchspersonen schwankte die Zunahme der AUC zwischen 10% und 150%.

Die Interaktion mit Cimetidin wurde in einer randomisierten, gekreuzten Studie an zwölf gesunden männlichen Versuchspersonen untersucht. Die Teilnehmer erhielten 600 mg Azapropazon p.o., nachdem sie sechs Tage lang mit Cimetidin (300 mg alle sechs Stunden) bzw. mit Placebo behandelt worden waren; zwischen den Behandlungsphasen wurde eine Auswaschphase von einer Woche Dauer eingeschaltet. Cimetidin vergrösserte die AUC von Azapropazon um durchschnittlich 24.6% (Streubereich 4–62%), während Azapropazon die AUC von Cimetidin um 15.8% senkte (Streubereich 4–56%). Bezüglich der übrigen pharmakokinetischen Parameter ergaben sich zwischen den Behandlungsgruppen weniger ausgeprägte Unterschiede.

Die obigen Resultate zeigen, dass die minimale wirksame hypourikämische Dosis bei 300 mg/Tag liegt. Bei Patientenkollektiven mit erhöhtem Risiko, wie älteren Patienten und solchen mit Niereninsuffizienz oder Lebererkrankung, soll Azapropazon in der niedrigsten wirksamen Dosis zusammen mit dem Essen verabreicht werden, um die Nebenwirkungen auf ein Minimum zu senken. Angesichts der Interaktion von Azapropazon mit Cimetidin soll die minimale wirksame Azapropazon-Dosis bei unter Cimetidin stehenden Patienten eintitriert werden.

Zur Langzeitbehandlung ist grundsätzlich die niedrigste wirksame Dosis zu wählen.

Resumé

Les résultats de quatre travaux de pharmacologie clinique sont discutés, qui ont porté sur 54 sujets sains de sexe masculin. Ils comportent l'effet hypo-uricémiant de doses uniques et multiples, l'effet de la nourriture et une étude d'interaction avec la cimétidine.

Douze volontaires mâles sains ayant des taux sériques d'acide urique augmentés à > 7 mg/dl ont reçu soit 300 mg d'allopurinol, soit 900 ou 1800 mg d'azapropazone/jour (4 sujets par posologie). Avant le traitement, tous les sujets ont été mis sous placebo pour quatre jours. Il y a eu une diminution dose-dépendante des taux d'acide urique et une augmentation de l'élimination urinaire d'acide urique.

La dose hypo-uricémiante minimale d'azapropazone a été déterminée chez 8 hommes en bonne santé dans une étude ouverte en cross-over et sur quatre périodes. Chaque sujet a reçu quatre jours de traitement à raison de différentes doses d'azapropazone, 300, 600, 900 et 1200 mg/jour. Chaque période de traitement s'est étendue sur 14 jours, à commencer par deux jours sans traitement dans le but d'établir les valeurs de base. Après quatre jours d'administration du médicament, à nouveau 8 jours sans traitement. Une diminution clinique et statistique de l'uricémie a été obtenue au jour 6 avec 300 mg/jour, plus précocement à des doses supérieures.

La biodisponibilité apparente de l'azapropazone par voie orale a été comparée avec nourriture et à jeûn. Dans une étude randomisée en cross-over, 24 sujets de sexe masculin en bonne santé ont reçu 600 mg d'azapropazone per os, avec de la nourriture et à jeûn, avec une semaine d'intervalle.

La prise de nourriture a fait augmenter la C_{max} de 44%, la T_{max} de 28.5% et l'AUC de 20.8%. Le temps de demi-élimination plasmatique a diminué de 15.4% avec la prise de nourriture. Les modifications ont varié d'un sujet à l'autre, aucun ne fut constatée chez 7 de ces 24 patients. Chez les 17 autres, l'augmentation de l'AUC varia de 10 à 150%.

L'interaction avec la cimétidine a été examinée chez 12 sujets de sexe masculin en bonne santé, dans une étude randomisée en cross-over. Les sujets ont reçu 600 mg d'azapropazone per os après 6 jours de traitement par la cimétidine (300 mg toutes les 6 heures), et après placebo suivant une phase d'une semaine de 'wash-out'. La cimétidine fit augmenter l'AUC de l'azapropazone de 24.6% (extrêmes 4–62%). L'azapropazone a fait diminuer l'AUC de la cimétidine de 15.8% (extrêmes 4–56%). Les modifications des autres paramètres pharmacocinétiques furent moins significatives entre les différents groupes.

Ces résultats démontrent que 300 mg/jour est la dose hypo-uricémiante minimale. Pour les populations de patients à risque comme les vieillards, les insuffisants hépatiques et rénaux, la dose efficace minimale d'azapropazone doit être administrée avec un repas, si l'on souhaite limiter à un minimum les effets secondaires. Du fait des interactions entre l'azapropazone et la cimétidine, les patients sous cimétidine ne recevront que la dose efficace minimale.

La dose efficace minimale sera utilisée pour l'administration à long terme.

11
Immunochemical studies on azapropazone

CH Schneider

I. INTRODUCTION: HAPTENIC GROUPS AND EPITOPES ON PROTEINS

Previously, analysis of epitopes on proteins has been beyond the capacity of classical immunochemistry. Instead, ingenious ways have been developed to couple a vast number of low molecular weight chemicals to protein carriers and to assess the antibody response against the artificial structures thus created. The covalent attachment of the haptenic compounds mainly involved azo linkages, but other possibilities such as carboxamide bonds have also been used[1,2]. The studies gained importance when it was realized that immediate-type allergies against low molecular weight drugs and chemicals involved covalent attachment of these entities to proteinaceous carrier structures as an obligatory step. Only above a certain molecular size, around 500 Daltons, is the requirement for covalent attachment not so strict. With peptides, for instance, a number of uncoupled peptides of about 1000 Daltons have been described in the sixties as immunogens or allergens capable of evoking antibody responses[3].

With regard to immunochemical specificity, it has become clear that most small haptenic groups conjugated to proteins induced antibody with only a low order of cross-reactivity. Even slight changes, such as replacing a substituent on a benzene ring by another one, cause reduction in the antibody binding by two or more orders of magnitude. There have been exceptions to this however, particularly when changes near the attachment point of the haptenic structure are considered, but general rules were difficult to formulate[2].

A rarely discussed phenomenon pioneered by Eisen[4,5] relates antibody affinity and cross-reactivity to the time-course of immunization. It was found that antibodies formed initially after injection of hapten-protein conjugates were of low affinity for the haptenic group, whereas considerably higher affinities were obtained in antibodies generated at later times . The increase in affinity was particularly pronounced with IgG antibodies and with immunization schedules using low antigen doses. Cross-reactivity was also increased and was markedly better in the high affinity antibodies. Thus, in

Azapropazone – 20 years of clinical use. Rainsford, KD (ed)
© Kluwer Academic Publishers. Printed in Great Britain

comparing immunochemical specificity of antisera, it is necessary to make certain that immunization intervals and antigen dosages are indeed comparable.

Based on progress in peptide chemistry, assessment of linear, continuous epitopes and to some extent also of discontinuous determinants on proteins could be undertaken since the middle 1970s. The picture that emerges from studies with myoglobin, lysozyme, cytochrome C and serum albumin is that the surface of a protein is to be regarded as a continuum of potential antigenic sites[6]. However, this potential is not fully employed in any individual immune response and only a restricted number of so-called immunodominant antigenic sites normally come into play. The size of an antigenic site seems larger than was previously concluded. Thus, two discontinuous epitopes in lysozyme involve 16 and 13 amino acids respectively[7,8] and a similar number apparently forms an epitope of neuraminidase[9]. It now seems that the shorter sequential epitopes previously defined may frequently represent only portions of larger discontinuous epitopes. Epitope mapping techniques are presently giving new insights into problems of immunochemical specificity[10]. Within sequential epitope portions, some of the amino acid positions may be occupied by a large number (10–19) of alternative amino acids without loss of antibody binding capacity. The majority of positions seem to allow limited replacement (1–9 amino acids) and some positions are not replaceable at all. It thus becomes apparent that within antibody paratopes, some locations are very sensitive to structural changes of the interacting epitope, whereas others are not.

Of special interest is the question of whether epitopes have intrinsic 'immunogenic' properties which are independent of the host in which the antibody response is generated. Such a view was indeed held by pioneers of epitope analysis[11] but seems untenable in the light of more recent evidence, which shows that sequential epitopes are picked up at different positions on a given protein by different species. Furthermore, individual variation can be clearly shown within a group of out-bred animals, e.g. rabbits[12].

The situation with regard to variation of the immune response against small haptens conjugated to proteins is less clear. The notion has been that generally an immune response can be evoked against almost any chemical structure attached to a protein in virtually all mammalian species[13]. However, if two haptens are conjugated to a protein, the response against one of them may be weakened or even abolished. A well-described example is the hapten pair 2,4-dinitrophenyl/p-azophenyl arsonate[14]. Dinitrophenyl on bovine serum albumin, keyhole limpet haemocyanine, or sheep red cell stroma were able to suppress in part or in full the antibody response in rabbits against the arsonate hapten present on the same carrier.

II. IMMUNOCHEMICAL SPECIFICITY OF SELECTED HAPTENIC GROUPS

The molecular weights of haptens related to penicillins and those of the 1,2-diphenyl-pyrazolidine-3,5-dione and 1-phenyl-2,3-dimethyl-3-pyrazolidin-5-

one series are well above minimal size and penicillin haptens reach the size of a tripeptide, which is about half the size of the sequential epitope portion, found in many cases to be a hexapeptide. With the benzylpenicilloyl haptenic structure, good cross-reactivities have been found with a variety of modified haptens. On the other hand, rather strict specificities are noted among the pyrazolidinedione and pyrazolinone compounds.

1. The benzylpenicilloyl (BPO) haptenic structure

Penicilloyl haptens containing a variety of side chains cross-react well with polyclonal anti-benzylpenicilloyl antibody from rabbits[15,16]. Also, the 5-membered thiazolidine can be replaced by a 6-membered dihydrothiazine ring present in cephalosporins without considerable loss of binding power[15].

These cross-reactivities can be explained if the polyclonal anti-BPO response contains specificities against end-group structures, i.e. against the benzyl side chain and in considerable proportion also against the thiazolidine moiety. Such end-group specificity has indeed been found in rabbit antisera[17]. Furthermore, mouse monoclonal antibodies could be raised which react with different portions of the penicilloyl structure, one recognizing the side chain and another one the thiazolidine ring[18]. On the other hand, an early experiment involving a pool of six rabbit antisera against BPO showed antibodies, not against end-groups, but rather against the entire BPO structure, including the lysine and adjacent protein sequences of the carrier to which BPO was attached[19].

This result, although apparently, but not necessarily, at odds with the other findings, may turn out to be very important in the light of data from the protein epitope field where rather large epitopes are postulated, as mentioned already[7,8,9].

2. Haptens of the 1,2-diphenyl-pyrazolidine-3,5-dione and 1-phenyl-2,3-dimethyl-3-pyrazolin-5-one series

Cross-reactivity relationships of these haptens have recently been studied by considering antibody responses in rabbits and guinea pigs[20-22]. Where the data are comparable, no differences between the two species were noted. In actively immunized guinea pigs and in guinea pigs passively sensitized with guinea pig or rabbit antisera, only the homologous pyrazolidinedione or pyrazolinone haptenic reagents elicited reactions. Similarly, in ELISA tests, the interaction of anti-hapten antisera from rabbits with the homologous hapten coat on the plates could be inhibited only with derivatives of the homologous series. But also within each series the antibodies showed rather strict specificities upon interaction with related haptens or drugs.

Haptenic inhibition of ELISA is therefore suitable as an analytical tool for the elucidation of structural relationships between such haptenic structures.

III. AZAPROPAZONE AS A HAPTEN: CROSS-REACTIVITY STUDIES

Azapropazone was included in groups of haptenic inhibitors related to the 1-phenyl-2,3-dimethyl-3-pyrazolin-5-one structure (Figure 1) on one hand, and to the 1,2-diphenyl-pyrazolidine-3,5-dione structure (Figure 2) on the other. The inhibitors were employed in ELISA tests involving rabbit antibodies against the two structures. The question was to what extent azapropazone would participate in the inhibitions.

1. Methodology

A. Human serum albumin (HSA) conjugates for immunization

The hapten 'Phena' (Figure 1) is actually 4-animoantipyrine. It was directly coupled to HSA by means of N-(3-dimethylaminopropyl)-N'-ethylcarbodiim-ide hydrochloride (DECD) to give Phena-HSA. The procedure is described in detail elsewhere[23]. The hapten 'Buta' described as an intermediate previously[20] (Figure 2, structure with $R_2 = H$; $R_3 = -CH_2-COOH$) was reacted with HSA by means of DECD to give Buta-HSA with a haptenic density of about 20 groups per conjugate molecule.

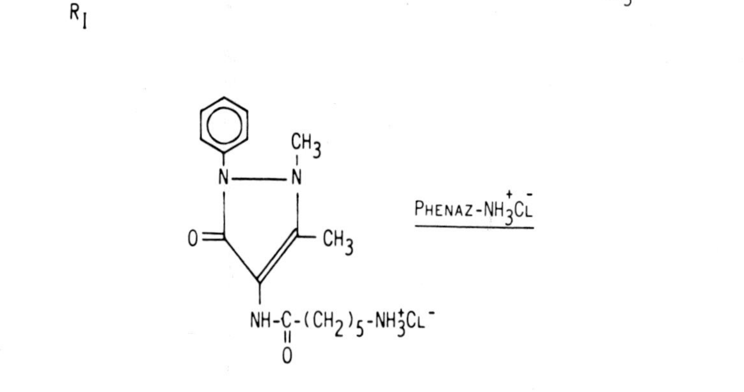

Figure 1 Chemical structures of haptens related to the 1-phenyl-2,3-dimethyl-3-pyrazolin-5-one series.

154

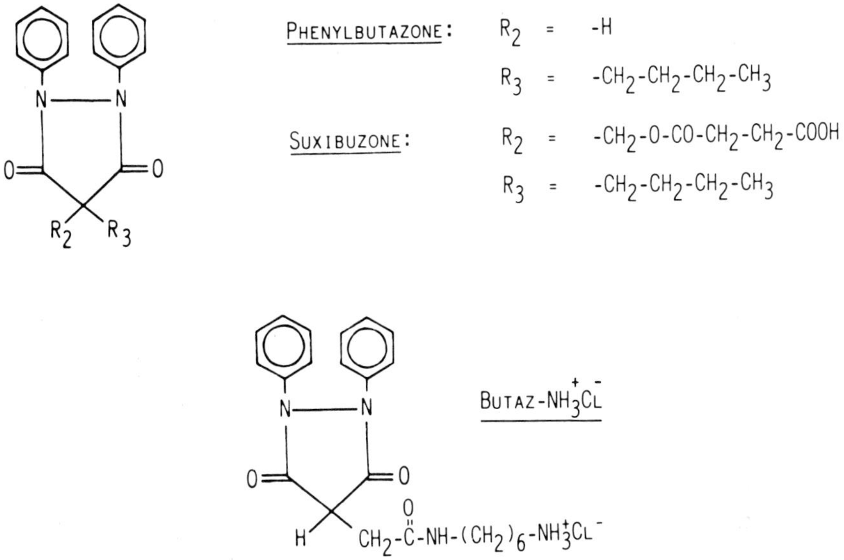

PHENYLBUTAZONE: R_2 = -H

R_3 = $-CH_2-CH_2-CH_2-CH_3$

SUXIBUZONE: R_2 = $-CH_2-O-CO-CH_2-CH_2-COOH$

R_3 = $-CH_2-CH_2-CH_2-CH_3$

BUTAZ-$NH_3^+CL^-$

Figure 2 Chemical structures of haptens related to the 1,2-diphenyl-pyrazolidine-3,5-dione series.

B. Antisera

Phena-HSA and Buta-HSA were incorporated into Freund's complete adjuvant and used for immunizing groups of four rabbits each. The schedule was identical to the one described before[20,21].

C. ELISA

The procedure was as described earlier[20,22]. The microtiter plates were coated with Phenaz-$NH_3^+Cl^-$ (Figure 1) or Butaz-$NH_3^+Cl^-$ (Figure 2). In addition to the antiserum pools, their globulin precipitates obtained by standard ammonium sulphate precipitation were also studied. The optimal conditions for haptenic inhibition were established in pre-experiments.

2. Results and discussion

A total of 11 compounds were evaluated as haptenic inhibitors; antipyrine, 4-aminoantipyrine, propyphenazone and metamizole belong to the 1-phenyl-2,3-dimethyl-3-pyrazolin-5-one series (Figure 1), whereas phenylbutazone, oxyphenbutazone and suxibuzone are drugs of the 1,2-diphenyl-pyrazolidine-3,5-dione series (Figure 2). Also included are Phenaz-$NH_3^+Cl^-$ and Butaz-$NH_3^+Cl^-$, the haptens used for coating the ELISA plates and present on the immunizing conjugates in the form of the Phena and Buta haptens.

Table 1 shows the inhibition of anti-Phena-HSA antibody binding to the Phenaz-$NH_3^+Cl^-$-coated ELISA plates. Generally, the inhibitions of the

Table 1 Haptenic inhibition of anti-Phena-HSA antibody binding to ELISA plates coated with Phenaz-$NH_3^+Cl^-$

Inhibiting hapten	Concentration (M) for 50% of inhibition of*	
	Antiserum	Globulin precipitate
Phenaz-$NH_3^+Cl^-$	2×10^{-5}	6×10^{-4}
Butaz-$NH_3^+Cl^-$	neg	(3×10^{-3})
4-Aminoantipyrine	1×10^{-4}	2×10^{-3}
Antipyrine	5×10^{-4}	3×10^{-3}
Metamizole	2×10^{-4}	5×10^{-3}
Propyphenazone	5×10^{-4}	1×10^{-2}
Phenylbutazone	neg	neg
Oxyphenbutazone	neg	neg
Suxibuzone	neg	neg
Azapropazone	neg	neg
Salicylic acid	neg	neg

*Lacking evidence for significant inhibition at 10^{-2}M is indicated as 'neg'. The values were obtained from graphic displays of the data and refer to pooled antisera from 4 animals and to globulin precipitates from such pools.

globulin precipitate require higher concentrations than those of the antiserum but no pronounced differences between the two data series are apparent. The value for Butaz-$NH_3^+Cl^-$ was put in parenthesis because it is related to a singular inhibition at 10^{-2}M and thus represents possibly an artefact.

It is apparent that the compounds related to the Phenaz-$NH_3^+Cl^-$ structure, namely 4-aminoantipyrine, antipyrine, metamizole and propyphenazone show a distinct inhibitory effect, whereas compounds related to the 1,2-diphenylpyrazolidine-3,5-dione series are negative. This finding is a confirmation of earlier results. Negative results were also obtained with azapropazone and salicylic acid. It is thus possible to state that azapropazone is immunochemically different from the compounds of the 1-phenyl-2,3-dimethyl-pyrazolin-5-one series.

Table 2 shows the inhibition of anti-Buta-HSA antibody binding to Butaz-$NH_3^+Cl^-$-coated ELISA plates. As before, inhibitions of the globulin precipitate require somewhat higher concentrations than inhibitions of antiserum. The difference is not, however, pronounced. Again, no significant discrepancies between the two series of data are apparent.

The anti-Buta–HSA antibody cross-reacts slightly with Phenaz-$NH_3^+Cl^-$ but not with 4-aminoantipyrine, antipyrine, metamizole, propyphenazone and salicylic acid. Azapropazone is also clearly negative, whereas oxyphenbutazone and phenylbutazone are inhibitory. The inhibition by phenylbutazone is rather weak and in the case of the globulin precipitate does not reach the 50% limit.

Generally, it appears that due to lack of immunochemical cross-reactivity, azapropazone is distinct from the series of 1,2-diphenyl-pyrazolidine-3,5-dione derivatives.

A remark with regard to the uniformity of the anti-haptenic responses

Table 2 Haptenic inhibition of anti-Buta-HSA antibody binding to ELISA plates coated with Butaz-NH$_3^+$Cl$^-$

Inhibiting hapten	Concentration (M) for 50% inhibition of*	
	Antiserum	Globulin precipitate
Butaz-NH$_3^+$Cl$^-$	2×10^{-4}	5×10^{-4}
Phenaz-NH$_3^+$Cl$^-$	1×10^{-2}	
4-Aminoantipyrine	neg	neg
Antipyrine	neg	neg
Metamizole	neg	neg
Propyphenazone	neg	neg
Phenylbutazone	1×10^{-3}	$> 10^{-2}$
Oxyphenbutazone	4×10^{-3}	5×10^{-3}
Suxibuzone	1×10^{-3}	
Azapropazone	neg	neg
Salicylic acid	neg	neg

*Cf. footnote to Table 1.

of the present series may be in order. In the experiments described here, the antisera pools from four animals were used similar to pools in experiments already published[20-22]. The cross-reactivity data in all instances were quite similar, indicating that individual specificity variation of antibody responses if present, does not seem very marked with the haptens of the 1-phenyl-2,3-dimethyl-3-pyrazolin-5-one and the 1,2-diphenyl-pyrazolidine-3,5-dione series.

Acknowledgement

The competent technical assistance of Mrs E Gruden is gratefully acknowledged.

References

1. Pressman, D and Grossberg, AL (1968). *The Structural Basis of Antibody Specificity*. (New York: Benjamin)
2. Landsteiner, K (1945). *The Specificity of Serological Reactions*. (Cambridge: Harvard University Press)
3. Schneider, CH (1983). Immunochemical basis of allergic reactions to drugs. In: *Handbook of Experimental Pharmacology*, Vol. 63. (Berlin: Springer), p. 3
4. Eisen, HN and Siskind, GW (1964). Variations in affinities of antibodies during the immune response. *Biochemistry*, **3**, 996–1008
5. Eisen, HN (1973). *Immunology*. (New York: Harper & Row)
6. Benjamin, DC, Berzofsky, JA, East, IA et al. (1984). The antigenic structure of proteins: a reappraisal. *Annu Rev Immunol*, **2**, 67–101
7. Amit, AG, Mariuzza, RA, Phillips, SEV and Poljak, RJ (1986). Three-dimensional structure of an antigen-antibody complex at 2.8 Å resolution. *Science*, **233**, 747—53
8. Sheriff, S, Silverton, EW, Padlan, EA et al. (1987). Three-dimensional structure of an antibody-antigen complex. *Proc Natl Acad Sci US*, **84**, 8075–9

9.   Colman, PM, Laver, WG, Varghese, JN *et al.* (1987). Three dimensional structure of a complex of antibody with influenza virus neuraminidase. *Nature*, **326**, 358–63

10. Geysen, HM, Mason, TJ and Rodda, SJ (1988). Cognitive features of continuous antigenic determinants. *J Mol Recognition*, **1**, 32–41

11. Atassi, MZ (1975). Antigenic structure of myoglobin: the complete immuno-chemical anatomy of a protein and conclusions relating to antigenic structures of proteins. *Immunochemistry*, **12**, 423–38

12. Geysen, HM, Rodda, SJ and Mason, TJ (1986). The delineation of peptides able to mimic assembled epitopes. In: *Ciba Foundation Symposium* 119. (Chichester: Wiley), p. 130

13. Humphrey, JH and White, RG (1964). *Immunology for Students of Medicine*, 2nd edn. (Oxford: Blackwell), p. 162

14. Amkraut, AA, Garvey, JS and Campbell, DH (1966). Competition of haptens. *J Exp Med*, **124**, 293–306

15. Nishida, K, Kinoshita, Y, Atsumi, T, Shibata, K and Horiuchi, Y (1972). The analysis of combining sites of rabbit anti-benzyl-penicilloyl antibodies. *Immunochemistry*, **9**, 1195–202

16. Locher, GW, Schneider, CH and de Weck, AL (1969). Hemmung allergischer Reaktionen auf Penicillin durch Penicilloyl-amide und chemische verwandte Substanzen. *Z. Immun-Forsch*, **138**, 299–323

17. Atsumi, T, Nishida, K, Kinoshita, Y, Shibata, K and Horiuchi, Y (1967). The heterogeneity of combining sites of anti-benzyl-penicilloyl antibodies obtained from individual rabbits: fractionation of antibodies with a specific immuno-adsorbent. *J Immunol*, **99**, 1286–93

18. De Haan, P, de Jonge, AJR, Verbrugge, T and Boorsma, DM (1985). Three epitope-specific monoclonal antibodies against the hapten penicillin. *Int Arch Allergy Appl Immunol*, **76**, 42–6

19. Levine, BB (1963). Studies on the dimensions of the rabbit anti-benzylpenicilloyl antibody-combining sites. *J Exp Med*, **117**, 161–83

20. Kasper, MF, Schneider, CH, Rolli, H, Angst, BD and de Weck, AL (1986). Diagnostic reagents in drug allergy: immunochemical specificity in the 1,2-diphenyl-pyrazolidinedione series. *Immunobiol*, **173**, 98–109

21. Kasper, MF and Schneider, CH (1987). Defined test reagents for the diagnosis of drug-induced allergy: antibody-dependent skin reactions towards pyrazolinone and pyrazolidinedione derivatives in the guinea pig. *J Immunol Methods*, **101**, 235–43

22. Schneider, CH, Kasper, MF, de Weck, AL, Rolli, H and Angst, BD (1987). Diagnosis of antibody-mediated drug allergy: pyrazolinone and pyrazolidine-dione cross-reactivity relationships. *Allergy*, **42**, 597–603

23. Schneider, CH, Rolli, H and Kasper, MF (1990). Note on the immunochemical specificity of pyrazolinone and pyrazolidinedione reactions. Submitted for publication

Summary

Some aspects of B-cell epitope analysis are briefly reviewed including haptenic moieties related to penicillins and to the 1,2-diphenyl-pyrazolidine-3,5-dione and the 1-phenyl-2,3-dimethyl-3-pyrazolin-5-one series. Azapropazone was studied as a hapten in ELISA inhibitory assays. It was found that in these assays azapropazone is immunochemically distinct from the series of 1,2-diphenyl-pyrazolidine-3,5-dione and 1-phenyl-2,3-dimethyl-3-pyrazolidin-5-one derivatives.

Zusammenfassung

Einige Aspekte der B-Zellepitop-Analyse werden kurz dargestellt. Dabei werden Haptengruppen der Penicilline und der 1,2-Diphenyl-pyrazolidin-3,5-dion-Serie sowie der 1-Phenyl-2,3-dimethyl-3-pyrazolidin-5-on-Serie berücksichtigt. Azapropazon wurde als Hapten in ELISA-Inhibitionsversuchen untersucht. Es wurde gefunden, dass sich Azapropazon immunchemisch unterscheidet sowohl von der Serie der 1,2-Diphenyl-pyrazolidin-3,5-dion-Derivate, als auch von jener der 1-Phenyl-2,3-dimethyl-3-pyrazolidin-5-on-Derivate.

Resumé

Certains aspects de l'analyse de l'épitope des cellules B sont brièvement passés en revue y compris les haptènes (semi-antigènes) des pénicillines, des séries 1,2-diphényl-pyrazolidine-3,5-dione et 1-phényl-2,3-diméthyl-3-pyrazoline-5-one. L'azapropazone a été soumise en tant qu'haptène à des tests d'inhibition ELISA. L'auteur a constaté que du point de vue immunochimique, l'azapropazone se distinguait à la fois de la série des dérivés de la 1,2-diphényl-pyrazolidine-3,5-dione et de celle des dérivés 1-phényl-2,3-diméthyl-3-pyrazolidine-5-one.

Section II
THERAPEUTIC ACTIONS

12
Untersuchungen zur Arthrose
[Studies on osteoarthritis]

O. Knüsel, J.L. Heidecker, E.M. Lemmel, M. Waldburger, J.A. Pfister und F.Ch. Geerling

EINLEITUNG

Azapropazon (u.a. Prolixan®, Rheumox®, Tolyprin®) ist ein von der Siegfried AG/Schweiz entwickeltes nichtsteroidales Antirheumatikum aus der Klasse der Benzotriazine. Es weist ausgeprägte anti-inflammatorische, analgetische und antipyretische sowie urikosurische Eigenschaften auf.

Azapropazon hat sich in der Behandlung aller Erkrankungen des entzündlichen und degenerativen rheumatischen Formenkreises, einschliesslich stoffwechselbedingter Arthropathien, bewährt. Ausführliche präklinische Untersuchungen an mehreren Tierarten haben seine geringe Toxizität dokumentiert. Bei Menschen verursacht Azapropazon wenig gastrointestinale Reizungen und besitzt eine geringe ulcerogene Aktivität. Die Inzidenz unerwünschter Nebenwirkungen im allgemeinen und von gastrointestinalen Nebenwirkungen im besonderen war bisher sehr niedrig. Azapropazon wirkt auf die Prostaglandinsynthese nur schwach, was seine relativ gute Verträglichkeit erklärt. Seine Wirksamkeit wird mit der ausgeprägten Hemmung der Freisetzung und Aktivität lysosomaler Enzyme in engen Zusammenhang gebracht. Innerhalb der NSA erscheint die mittlere Eliminations-Halbwertszeit von Azapropazon um 12 Stunden als sehr günstig. Im Blutplasma ist kein Metabolit, sondern nur Azapropazon nachzuweisen. Es wird zu über 90% über die Nieren ausgeschieden. Im Urin findet sich als Hauptbestandteil die unveränderte Substanz und zu etwa 20% 8-Hydroxyazapropazon, ein nicht mehr wirksamer und zugleich untoxischer Metabolit. Die mittlere therapeutische Dosis liegt bei 600 bis 1200 mg täglich[1].

Wirksamkeit von Azapropazon bei der Arthrose

Die degenerativen Krankheiten der grossen und kleinen Gelenke sowie der Wirbelsäule gehören zu den häufigsten Erkrankungen des rheumatischen Formenkreises. Der Verschleiss kann schon in frühen Jahren beginnen,

Azapropazone – 20 years of clinical use. Rainsford, KD (ed)
© Kluwer Academic Publishers. Printed in Great Britain

wenngleich klinische Symptome erst im mittleren und späteren Alter auftreten. Im 40. Lebensjahr sind wenigstens ein bis mehrere Gelenke erkrankt, und ab dem 7. Lebensjahrzehnt ist die Arthrose meistens polyartikulär. NSA sind in dieser Krankheitsgruppe überwiegend im Stadium der akuten entzündlichen Aktivierung (aktivierte Arthrose) indiziert. Somit handelt es sich meist um eine Kurzzeitbehandlung mit Antiphlogistika.

Seit der Veröffentlichung der ersten klinischen Erfahrungen mit Azapropazon im Jahre 1968[2] hat dieses NSA einen festen Platz in der Behandlung entzündlicher und degenerativer rheumatischer Erkrankungen erhalten. Mehrere Übersichten zur klinischen Wirksamkeit und Verträglichkeit sind erschienen[3-6]. In den letzten 20 Jahren sind zahlreiche Studien mit Azapropazon in der Behandlung der Arthrose durchgeführt worden. Einige Studien waren als offene Prüfungen, andere doppelblind mit Vergleich zu Plazebo oder anderen NSA angelegt und haben sowohl Kurzzeit- als auch Langzeittherapien beinhaltet.

In einer offenen Multizenterstudie, an der 149 niedergelassene Aerzte teilnahmen, wurden 1348 Patienten mit Gonarthrose und Coxarthrose sowie Wirbelsäulenbeschwerden behandelt. Die Studie wurde über 14 Tage mit einer Dosierung von 1200 mg Azapropazon täglich durchgeführt. Eine Besserung der klinischen Symptome konnte bereits am 2. Tag bei 85% der Patienten erreicht werden[7]. In anderen Kurzzeituntersuchungen an jeweils kleineren Gruppen von Patienten mit Arthrose wurde über ähnlich gute Ergebnisse berichtet. Hier lag die tägliche Azapropazondosis gewöhnlich bei 600 bis 1200 mg. Von einigen Autoren wurden aber auch versuchsweise Erhaltungsdosen von 200 bis 400 mg oder aber 600 bis 1800 mg täglich verordnet[2,8-16].

In Doppelblindprüfungen wurde die Wirkung von Azapropazon mit anderen symptomatischen Antirheumatika verglichen. So fanden Nagai u. Mitarb.[17] zur Behandlung der aktivierten Kniegelenksarthrose ein etwa gleich gutes Ansprechen auf 1200 mg Azapropazon wie auf 2,25 g Aspirin täglich. Smahet[18] verglich Azapropazon mit Indometacin bei 61 Patienten mit verschiedenen Arthrosen. 32 Patienten erhielten 1200 mg Azapropazon täglich für 5 Tage, gefolgt von 900 mg für 23 Tage. 29 Patienten wurden mit 75 mg Indometacin über einen Zeitraum von 28 Tagen behandelt. Beide Antirheumatika waren wirksam, Indometacin etwas besser, jedoch weniger verträglich. In einer ähnlichen Studie verglichen Frank u. Mitarb.[19] bei 20 Patienten mit Gonarthrose oder Coxarthrose 1200 mg Azapropazon mit 100 mg Indometacin täglich und erzielten vergleichbare Ergebnisse.

Hingorani[20] behandelte in einer Doppelblind-crossover-Prüfung 41 Patienten mit Gonarthrose mit 1200 mg Azapropazon oder 1600 mg Ibuprofen täglich. Nach einer Auswasch-bzw. Vergleichsperiode mit Plazebo wurde jede Substanz 2 Wochen lang gegeben. Beide NSA waren Plazebo in der Wirkung überlegen. Azapropazon wurde von den Patienten signifikant häufiger bevorzugt.

In einer Langzeitstudie von zwei Wochen bis 38 Monate wurden bei

Gonarthrose initial bis zu 1800 mg Azapropazon täglich gegeben. Diese Dosierung wurde dann auf 1200 mg bzw. 900 mg täglich "eingependelt". Der Erfolg der Behandlung bestand zu 54,6% in einem Rückgang der Gelenkschwellung und -steife und in 37,3% noch in einem guten analgetischen Effekt[21]. Die von Wheatley[22] veröffentlichte Studie über 51 Patienten mit Gonarthrose und Coxarthrose wurde ebenfalls offen durchgeführt und dauerte bis zu einem Jahr. An den Untersuchungen nahmen 9 niedergelassene Aerzte teil. Die Initialdosis lag bei 900 mg täglich, sie wurde, der klinischen Symtomatik angepasst, entweder auf 1200 mg erhöht oder auf 600 mg reduziert. Die Studie wurde nach 9 bis 12 Monaten von 70% der Probanden beendet. Es kam zu einer signifikanten Besserung aller klinischen Parameter wie Belastungsschmerz, Nachtschmerz, Bewegungsschmerz und Morgensteife sowohl im Gesamturteil des Arztes als auch des Patienten.

Frank[23] behandelte die klinischen Symptome des akuten und chronischen Zervikal- und Lumbalsyndroms. Azapropazon wurde in einer Dosierung von 600 mg bzw. 1200 bis 1800 mg täglich unter zusätzlicher physikalischer Therapie verabreicht. Der Autor fand bei 55 Patienten in 47% einen sehr guten und in 24% einen guten Erfolg. Die besten Resultate wurden beim akuten Zervikalsyndrom erzielt. Aehnlich waren die Ergebnisse von Beckschäfer[8] und Fiegel[24], die bei ihren Patienten mit Wirbelsäulenbeschwerden in 74 bzw. 87% eine Besserung erzielten.

In einer Doppelblindstudie verglichen Hingorani u. Templeton[25] 1200 mg Azapropazon mit 200 mg Ketoprofen täglich bei 50 Patienten mit akuten Kreuzschmerzen. Azapropazon wurde von den Patienten bevorzugt. In einer Doppelblind-dreifach-crossover-Studie[26] wurden bei Patienten mit Nacken- und Schulterbeschwerden 900 mg Azapropazon, 750 mg Naproxen und Plazebo wechselweise eingesetzt. Jede Therapieform wurde jeweils über eine volle Woche gegeben. Azapropazon und Naproxen zeigten gegenüber Plazebo gleich gute Wirkung.

Bach *u. Mitarb.*[27] setzten 600 mg Azapropazon zur intravenösen Kurzzeitbehandlung bei 80 Patienten mit aktivierter Gonarthrose, Lendenwirbelsäulensyndrom und anderen rheumatischen Erkrankungen ein. Die globale Bewertung des Erfolges gaben die Autoren mit 88% an. Der rasche Wirkungseintritt nach einer Injektion auf den Ruhe- und Bewengungsschmerz wurde speziell hervorgehoben. Hadidi[28] behandelte von 51 Patienten mit Lendenwirbelsäulensyndrom 25 mit 1200 mg Azapropazon i.v. und 26 mit 900 mg Azetylsalizylsäure i.v. Die Injektionen wurden zunächst über drei Tage täglich, dann alle drei Tage bis zu einer Gesamtzahl von 12 über vier Wochen verabreicht. In gleicher Art und Weise sowie Umfang war die Prüfung von El-Badawy[29] bei 50 Patienten mit Gonarthrose angelegt. In beiden Prüfungen zeigten nahezu alle Parameter wie Ruhe- und Bewegungsschmerz, Fingerbodenabstand und Pauschalurteil die Ueberlegenheit der Behandlung mit Azapropazon.

Neuere klinische Prüfungen mit Azapropazon bei Patienten mit verschiedenen Formen der Arthrose haben die früher gezeigten Ergebnisse bestätigt. Im Folgenden soll über eine kontrollierte Vergleichsstudie ausführlich berichtet werden.

I. DIE AKTIVIERTE ARTHROSE UND IHRE THERAPIE

1. Ergebnisse einer multizentrischen Doppelblindstudie zwischen Azapropazon und Diclofenac-Natrium

Die Verabreichung von NSA bei der aktivierten Form der Arthrose hat ihre anerkannte Indikation. In der Folge sollen die Resultate einer multizentrischen Doppelblindstudie zwischen Azapropazon (Prolixan®, Siegfried AG, Zofingen/Schweiz) und Diclofenac-Natrium (Voltaren®, Ciba-Geigy AG, Basel/Schweiz) bei Patienten mit aktivierter Arthrose des Hüft- und Kniegelenkes berichtet werden.

Azapropazon und Diclofenac sind bekannte NSA, die seit langem als Standard-Präparate Eingang in die Therapie rheumatischer Erkrankungen gefunden haben. Es darf von beiden Präparaten die gute Wirkung bei eher leichten und seltenen Nebenwirkungen herausgestrichen werden.

Ziel der vorliegenden Studie war es, die klinische Wirksamkeit sowie die Verträglichkeit dieser beiden NSA zu überprüfen, etwaige Unterschiede zu erfassen und zu interpretieren. Besonders interessant schien die Fragestellung vor allem auch aus dem Aspekt, als mit Diclofenac[30,31] ein ausgesprochen starker Prostaglandinsynthesehemmer zur Verfügung steht, mit Azapropazon[1,32] hingegen eine Substanz, die auf die Prostaglandinsynthese relativ schwach wirkt, die Freisetzung und Aktivität lysosomaler Enzyme hingegen ausgeprägt hemmt.

Um möglichst über ein homogenes Patientengut zu verfügen und um die kontinuierliche Ueberwachung dieser Patienten zu gewährleisten, wurde die Studie in verschiedenen Rheumazentren unter stationären Bedingungen durchgeführt. Jedoch kann unter diesen Umständen die Beobachtung der Patienten nicht beliebig ausgedehnt werden, so dass in der vorliegenden Studie[33] die Beobachtungsdauer auf 2 Wochen beschränkt werden musste.

2. Patienten und Methode

In die Studie einbezogen wurden 123 Patienten (42 Männer, 81 Frauen) im Alter zwischen 28 und 76 Jahren (Durchschnitt 64 Jahre), die an einer mässig stark ausgeprägten aktivierten Arthrose des Hüftgelenkes bzw. Kniegelenkes litten (Tab. 1). Sämtliche Patienten wurden über die Prüfung informiert und gaben vor Studienbeginn ihre Einverständniserklärung ab. Die Studie war doppelblind randomisiert angelegt, wobei die Hälfte der Patienten jeweils 600 mg Azapropazon morgens und abends oder 50 mg Diclofenac morgens und 100 mg dieses Wirkstoffes in retardierter Formulierung am Abend erhielten.

Alle Patienten hatten eine normierte Physiotherapie mit Heilgymnastik und Wassergymnastik, Hochfrequenztherapie sowie Packungen. Der Prüfung vorausgeschaltet war eine Washout-Periode von mindestens 3 Tagen; für den Fall, dass die Patienten eines der beiden Prüfpräparate schon vor der Therapie erhalten hatten, musste eine Washout-Phase von 2 Wochen eingehalten werden. Neben den beiden Prüfpräparaten durfte keine weitere antiphlogistische Medikation verabreicht werden. Bei Schmerzexazerbation, vor allem während der Washout-Periode, konnte zusätzlich Paracetamol, maximal 4 g/die eingenommen werden. Diese Dosis wurde registriert. Die klinischen Befunde wurden unmittelbar vor Therapie sowie nach 7 bzw. 14 Tagen nach Therapiebeginn erhoben. Für die Studie kamen solche Patienten mit aktivierter Coxarthrose bzw. Gonarthrose in Frage, die auf der visuellen Analogskala ihren Ruhe- bzw. Bewegungsschmerz in der rechten Hälfte der Skala angaben. Als weitere Einschlusskriterien dienten die röntgenologische Beurteilung mit den Symptomen subchondrale Sklerosierung, Osteophyten-bildung, Gelenkspaltverschmälerung, Zystenbildung sowie deformierte Gelenkflächen. Mindestens 3 dieser Symptome mussten vorhanden sein. Neben dem Ruhe- und Bewegungsschmerz musste noch mindesten eines der im folgenden aufgeführten klinischen Symptome vorliegen: lokale Empfind-lichkeit, eingeschränkte Beweglichkeit, Steifigkeit, Schwellung, Erguss, Wärme, Rötung, Gelenkvergrösserung infolge von Knochenneubildung sowie Crepitatio.

Als Beurteilungskriterien für den therapeutischen Effekt dienten nach 7 bzw. 14 Tagen Ruhe- und Bewegungsschmerz, Morgensteifigkeit sowie Flexion, Extension und Aussen- und Innenrotation, Abduktion und Adduk-tion im Bereiche des Hüftgelenkes. Die Funktionstests im Kniegelenk beinhalteten die Flexion und Extension. Daneben wurde die Zeit gemessen, die zur Bewältigung einer 15 m Gehstrecke benötigt wurde.

Laboruntersuchungen wurden vor Therapiebeginn und unmittelbar bei Therapieende, also nach 14 Tagen, durchgeführt. Hier wurden Blutbild, Blutsenkungsgeschwindigkeit, Leber- und Nierenfunktion, Blutzucker und Harnsäure bestimmt. Ausserdem erfolgte ein kompletter Urinstatus sowie eine Blutbestimmung im Stuhl. Einfache kardiovaskuläre Parameter wurden bei jedem Untersuchungszeitpunkt ermittelt. Neben klinischem Befund und Laborparametern wurde zusätzlich die Beurteilung der jeweiligen Medikation durch Prüfarzt und Patienten erfragt.

Ausschlusskriterien bildeten die bekannten Kontraindikationen gegen NSA sowie andere rheumatische Erkrankungen als die zur Studie zugelasse-nen.

3. Ergebnisse

Von den 123 Patienten, die ursprünglich in die Studie aufgenommen waren, erfüllten 110 die Einschlusskriterien (Tab. 1). Die Patienten wurden randomisiert in 2 Gruppen eingeteilt, die vergleichbar waren hinsichtlich Geschlecht, Grösse, Körpergewicht, Krankheitsdauer und Alter bei Ausbruch

Tabelle 1   Demographische Daten der beiden Versuchsgruppen

	Mittelwerte (Bereich)	
	Azapropazon	Diclofenac
Anzahl	55	55
Alter (Jahre)	63,5 (40–75)	64,5 (28–76)
Grösse (cm)	163,3 (146–181)	160,9 (146–186)
Gewicht (kg)	73,5 (43–115)	74,1 (52–109)
Krankheitsdauer (Jahre)	7,3 (0.2–35)	8,2 (0.2–40)
Alter bei Krankheitsausbruch (Jahre)	56,5 (16–74)	55,9 (19–75)

der Krankheit. Dies betrifft auch die oben aufgeführten Einschlusskriterien für die Prüfung. Der Verlauf der klinischen Prüfparameter ist in den folgenden Tabellen dargestellt. Die Dauer der Morgensteifigkeit ging ebenso signifikant zurück wie die benötigte Zeit, um eine Gehstrecke von 15 m zurückzulegen. Auch der Ruhe- sowie der Bewegungsschmerz verringerte sich signifikant unter beiden Medikationen. Der Verlauf der klinischen Parameter unter der Medikation (Tab. 2) bei den Patienten mit Coxarthrose zeigte bei allen Bewegungsrichtungen ausser der Extension eine signifikante Verbesserung. Bei den Patienten mit Gonarthrose (Tab. 3) konnte ebenfalls die Flexion signifikant verbessert werden, während die Extension fast unverändert blieb. Der zwischen den Präparaten durchgeführte Vergleich gab bei allen Prüfparametern keine relevanten Unterschiede. Der zusätzliche Verbrauch an Paracetamol war sowohl qualitativ wie quantitativ bei beiden Präparaten gleich häufig. Insgesamt wurde bei Therapieende bei 11 Patienten unter Azapropazon und 9 Patienten unter Diclofenac ein durchschnittlicher Verbrauch von 8,5 bzw. 7,0 Tabletten Paracetamol pro Woche registriert.

Tabelle 2   Klinische Parameter (Mittelwerte in Grad) bei den Coxarthrosepatienten im Verlauf der Therapie

Prüfparameter Hüftgelenk	Azapropazon			Diclofenac		
	−1	7	14	−1	7	14
Flexion	91.9	97.8	101.4*	85.9	91.5	93.4*
Extension	3.9	4.6	4.8	5.0	5.2	6.2
Innenrotation	11.5	14.1	17.0*	7.2	9.6	11.6*
Abduktion	23.0	27.2	27.8*	9.1	21.9	24.4*
Adduktion	15.4	19.1	20.2*	14.4	16.7	20.6*

* $p < 0.01$ (Tag-1 im Vergleich zu Tag 14) gemäss Friedman's Test und 2 Weg-Varianz-Analyse

Tabelle 3   Klinische Parameter (Mittelwerte in Grad) bei den Gonarthrosepatienten im Verlauf der Therapie

Prüfparameter Kniegelenk	Azapropazon			Diclofenac		
	−1	7	14	−1	7	14
Flexion	108.6	113.4	118.4*	98.9	105.2	110.4*
Extension	4.6	5.0	5.4	7.9	8.2	8.0

* $p < 0.01$ (Tag-1 im Vergleich zu Tag 14) gemäss Friedman's Test und 2 Weg-Varianz-Analyse

Insgesamt berichteten 12 Patienten unter Azapropazon und 13 Patienten unter Diclofenac über eine oder mehrere unerwünschte Wirkungen (Tab. 4). In jeder Gruppe musste bei 3 Patienten die medikamentöse Therapie abgebrochen werden, in erster Linie wegen aufgetretener Oedeme, gastrointestinaler Störungen oder Nichtansprechens auf die Therapie.

Unter beiden Präparaten kam es zu einer Abnahme der Blutsenkungsreaktionsgeschwindigkeit, des Serumbilirubins und der Serumharnsäure. Die Senkung der Harnsäure war nur unter Azapropazon statistisch signifikant. Unter dem selben Präparat war ein Anstieg der eosinophilen und basophilen Leukozyten, der alkalischen Phosphatase, des Harnstoffs und des Kreatinins zu beobachten. Unter der Therapie mit Diclofenac wurde ein Anstieg von SGOT und SGPT, des Serumharnstoffes und des Serumkupfers registriert, wobei letzgenannte Untersuchung lediglich vom Autor E.M. Lemmel durchgeführt wurde. Die Urinanalyse aller Patienten zeigte keine klinisch bedeutsamen Veränderungen. Während der Hämoccult-Test bei allen Patienten unter Azapropazon negativ blieb, kam es bei 3 Patienten in der Diclofenac-Gruppe zu Anzeichen eines fäkalen Blutverlustes.

4. Diskussion der Ergebnisse

Die therapeutische Wirksamkeit und Verträglichkeit der beiden Prüfpräparate Azapropazon und Diclofenac sind durch zahlreiche klinische Studien und durch ihren breiten Gebrauch in der täglichen Praxis belegt[1,30-32]. Inwieweit und ob sie sich in Wirksamkeit und Verträglichkeit bei Patienten mit vergleichbaren rheumatischen Erkrankungen, nämlich bei aktivierter Coxarthrose und Gonarthrose unterscheiden, sollte durch die vorliegende doppelblind durchgeführte Prüfung an einer grossen Patientanzahl beantwortet werden.

Die jeweils 55 in die Auswertung der Ergebnisse einbezogenen Patienten pro Gruppe waren bezüglich demographischer Merkmale vergleichbar. Die

Tabelle 4 Anzahl Patienten mit Nebenwirkungen (zum Teil Mehrfachnennungen)

	Azapropazon		Diclofenac	
Art der Nebenwirkungen	7	14	7	14
Schwindel	1	—	—	1
gastrointestinal*	3	2	4	6
Cephalea	—	—	1	—
Schlaflosigkeit	—	—	1	—
Ödembildung	—	—	3	2
Pruritus/Exanthem	1	3	1	1
Thrombozytopenie intermitt.	—	1	—	—
Müdigkeit	1	—	1	1
Andere	1	1	—	—

*Obstipation, Nausea, Diarrhoe, Sodbrennen, epigastrischer Schmerz, Melaena

klinischen Prüfparameter, nämlich Dauer der Morgensteifigkeit und Zeit, die zur Bewältigung einer 15 m langen Gehstrecke benötigt wurde, verliefen unter Azapropazon und Diclofenac in etwa parallel. Die Reduktion der Dauer der Morgensteifigkeit lag bei Azapropazon um 40,8%, bei Diclofenac 33,2% des Ausgangswertes. Hinsichtlich der Zeit der Gehstrecke konnte eine Verbesserung um 72,6 resp. 69,2% des Ausgangswertes erreicht werden.

Die klinischen Prüfparameter der Beweglichkeit besserten sich bei zum Teil leicht differierenden Ausgangswerten in beiden Behandlungsgruppen in etwa parallel, so dass zwischen den Gruppen keine Signifikanz zu ermitteln war. Die Analyse des Verlaufes der visuellen Analogskala der beiden Schmerzparameter ergab in beiden Behandlungsgruppen eine signifikante Linderung der Schmerzen.

Interessant im Zusammenhang mit dem Schmerzverlauf ist auch der Verbrauch an zusätzlichem Paracetamol. Am Ende der Behandlung nahmen 11 der 55 Azapropazon-Patienten und 9 der 55 Diclofenac-Patienten zusätzlich Paracetamol ein, so dass auch hieraus in etwa ein gleicher analgetischer Effekt beider Präparate abgeleitet werden kann. Es scheint, dass Diclofenac eher über die Prostaglandinsynthesehemmung analgetisch wirkt, anderseits Azapropazon über die Hemmung der Feisetzung und Aktivität lysosomaler Enzyme, was wiederum zu einer Verminderung deren destruierender Wirkung führt.

Was die häufigsten Nebenwirkungen, nämlich die seitens des Gastrointestinaltraktes anbelangt, wurden diese häufiger unter Diclofenac (8mal) als unter Azapropazon (5mal) angegeben. Es ist möglich, dass sich die im Tiermodell für Diclofenac beschriebene stärkere Hemmung der Prostaglandin-E_2-Synthese im Bereiche der gastrointestinalen Mucosa negativ auswirken könnte. Auch die Ergebnisse dieser Studie im Hämoccult-Test deuten auf eine bessere gastrointestinale Verträglichkeit des Azapropazons hin. Andererseits traten Unverträglichkeitserscheinungen seitens der Haut unter Azapropazon häufiger auf, unter Diclofenac wurde vermehrte Oedembildung festgestellt. Der stark urikosurische und urikostatische Effekt unter Azapropazon ist bekannt und schon früher beschrieben worden[32].

Insgesamt konnte in dieser vorliegenden Studie gezeigt werden, dass der analgetische und antiphlogistische Effekt von Azapropazon und Diclofenac bei Patienten mit aktivierter Gonarthrose beziehungsweise Coxarthrose vergleichbar gut ist.

Aus den bisher durchgeführten offenen Studien mit Azapropazon kann der Schluss gezogen werden, dass eine tägliche Dosis von 1200 mg bei der Behandlung der aktivierten Arthrose therapeutisch wirksam ist, während für die Erhaltungstherapie oft 900 mg Azapropazon täglich ausreichen und zufriedenstellende Resultate ergeben. Die Ergebnisse der kontrollierten Vergleichsstudien zeigen eine vergleichbare Wirksamkeit von 1200 mg Azapropazon mit der empfohlenen Tagesdosis anderer nichtsteroidaler Antirheumatika wie Ibuprofen, Ketoprofen, Diclofenac, Naproxen oder Aspirin. Nur in besonders schweren Fällen mag eine Initialtherapie mit 1800 mg Azapropazon angezeigt sein.

In zahlreichen Fällen wurde Azapropazon wegen der besseren Verträglichkeit gegenüber anderen Therapieformen bevorzugt. Die Veträglichkeit von Azapropazon in der Langzeitbehandlung ist gleich gut wie unter kurzen Perioden der Therapie.

References

1. Bach, GL, Eberl, R, Mutschler, E, Dunky, A, Fellmann, N, Jahn, U und Thiele, K (1985). Standortbestimmung des Azapropazons. In Eberl, R und Fellmann, N (eds.) *Rheuma-Forum* Sonder-Nr.**2**. (Karlsruhe: G Braun)
2. Kiesewetter, E (1968). Klinische Ergebnisse mit der neuen antiphlogistisch wirkenden Substanz Azapropazon. *Wien Med Wschr*, **118**, 941–3
3. Brooks, PM und Buchanan, WW (1976). Current management of rheumatoid arthritis. In Buchanan, WW und Dick, WC (eds.) *Recent Advances in Rheumatology*, Vol. 1, part II, p. 34. (Churchill Livingstone, Edinburgh–London–New York)
4. Hart, FD (1978). Azapropazone: a review of the literature. *Eur J Rheumatol*, **1**, 142–6
5. Sondervost, M (1979). Azapropazone. *Clin Rheum Dis* **5**, 465–480
6. Fenner-H. und Eberl, R (eds.) (1977). Azapropazon bei Erkrankungen des rheumatischen Formenkreises. *Rheuma-Forum* Sonder-Nr.**1**, 7–10. (Karlsruhe: G Braun)
7. Fassl, H und Neubauer, E (1978). Offene Feldstudie mit Dolo-Prolixan, einem neuen Antirheumatikum. *Therapiewoche*, **28**, 6314–16
8. Beckschäfer, W (1969). Zur klinischen Beurteilung der Wirkung von Azapropazon, einem neuen Antiphlogisticum, bei Erkrankungen des rheumatischen Formenkreises. *Arzneim-Forsch*, **19**, 52–3
9. Nakagawa, T (1969). Clinical trial of Mi-85 for gonitis deformans. *Med Cons New Rem*, **6** (Japan)
10. Hammer, O (1970). Kurbehandlung rheumatischer Erkrankungen in einem klinischen Sanatorium. *Therapiewoche*, **20**, 2891
11. Zicha, K (1972). Zur Bewertung des therapeutischen Effekts bei der Coxarthrose. *Phys Med Rehab*, **13**, 132–5
12. Neumann, M (1973). Clinical and biological study of Azapropazone, a new analgesic-antiphlogistic agent. *Ars Medici* (Belgium) **28**, 231–9
13. Gomez, G, Asensi, E, Obach, J und Barcelo, P (1975). Azapropazone in Rheumatology. *Rev Esp Reum*, **18**, 178–89
14. D'Omezon, Y, Bouvenot, G und Godde, JL (1978). Trial with azapropazone in rheumatology. *Provence Med*, **46**, 30–2
15. Sfikakis, P, Charalabopoulos, D, Siamopoulos, K und Daikos, G (1978). Azapropazone in the treatment of osteoarthritis of the knee. Presented at the *4th Panhellenic Medical Congress*, May 1978, Athens
16. Dieppe, PA, Doherty, M, Whicher, JT und Walters, G (1981). The treatment of gout with azapropazone: clinical and experimental studies. *Eur J Rheum Inflamm*, **4**, 392–400
17. Nagai, S, Taguchi, A, Morooka, H, und Ujuki, K (1969). Therapeutic effect of azapropazone on chronic articular rheumatism. Presented at the *13th Congress of Japanese Rheumatic Society*, May 16–17
18. Smahel, O, Grafnetterova, J, und Truhlar, P (1977). Klinische Pharmakologie und kontrollierte klinische Prüfung von Azapropazon. In: Fenner, H und Eberl, R (eds.) Azapropazon bei Erkrankungen des rheumatischen Formenkreises.

Rheuma-Forum Sonder-Nr. **1**; pp. 37–41, (Karlsruhe: G Braun)

19. Frank, AJM, Moll, JMH und Hort, JF (1982). A comparison of three ways of measuring pain. *Rheumatol Rehab*, **21**, 211–217

20. Hingorani, K (1976). A comparative study of azapropazone and ibuprofen in the treatment of osteoarthritis of the knee. *Curr Med Res Opin*, **4**, 57–64

21. Thune, S (1976). Azapropazon in der Langzeitbehandlung rheumatischer Erkrankungen. *Curr Med Res Opin*, **4**, 80–8

22. Wheatley, D (1984). Azapropazone in arthritis: a long-term treatment. *Curr Med Res Opin*, **9**, 86–92

23. Frank, O (1972). Zur kombinierten physikalischen und medikamentösen Therapie degenerativer Wirbelsäulenerkrankungen. *Praxis*, **61**, 1564–65

24. Fiegel, G (1973). Pharmakologische Eigenschaften und therapeutische Wirkung des Azapropazon beim rheumatischen Formenkreis. *Z Allgemeinmed*, **49**, 592–4

25. Hingorani, K und Templeton, JS (1975). Vergleich von Azapropazon mit Ketoprofen bei der Behandlung von akuten Rückenschmerzen. In: Fenner, H und Erberl, R (eds.) Azapropazon bei Erkrankungen des rheumatischen Formenkreises. *Rheuma-Forum* Sonder-Nr.1, 17–21 (Karlsruhe: G Braun)

26. Berry, H, Bloom, B, Mace, BEW, Hamilton, EBD, Fernandes, L, Molloy, M und Williams, IA (1980). Expectation and patient preference – does it matter? *J Roy Soc Med*, **73**, 34–8

27. Bach, GL, Neubauer, M und Gmeiner, G (1984). Azapropazon intravenös bei Erkrankungen des rheumatischen Formenkreises. 1. Behandlung der aktivierten Arthrose, des LWS-Syndroms und anderer rheumatischer Erkrankungen mit 600 mg Azapropazon i.v. *Arthritis Rheuma*, **6**, 16–21

28. Hadidi, T (1984). Intravenous Azapropazone vs. Acetylsalicylic Acid in the Treatment of Low Back Pain. *Arthritis Rheuma*, **6**, 1–6

29. El-Badawy, SA und Haeberli, E (1984). Intravenous Azapropazone vs. Injectable Acetylsalicylic Acid in the Treatment of Osteoarthritis of the Knee. *Arthritis Rheuma*, **6**, 1–7

30. Voltaren – 10 Jahre klinische Bewährung. (1981). (Basel: Ciba-Geigy)

31. Voltaren – Neue Ergebnisse (1982). In Kass, E (ed). (Bern: Huber)

32. Dunky, A, Bartsch, G und Eberl, R (1984). The intravenous applications of azapropazone in the treatment of acute gout. *Arthritis Rheum*, **6**, 1–6

33. Knüsel, O, Lemmel, EM, Waldburger, M, Pfister, JA und Geerling, FCh (1988). Die Aktivierte Arthrose und ihre Therapie. *Therapiewoche Schweiz* **5**, 402–13

Summary

Degenerative diseases of the large and small peripheral joints and the spinal column are among the most frequent problems in therapy owing, among other things, to the rising proportion of the elderly in the total population. In the last 20 years azapropazone, a non-steroidal anti-inflammatory drug (NSAID) which is one of the benzotriazines, has secured a firm place in the treatment of osteoarthritis. Numerous clinical trials have investigated the efficacy and tolerability of azapropazone in this indication. A daily dose of 1200 mg has been shown to be therapeutically effective in the treatment of active osteoarthritis, while 900 mg has often proven sufficient in maintenance therapy. Efficacy of 1200 mg azapropazone has been demonstrated to be comparable with the recommended daily dose of other non-steroidal anti-inflammatory drugs such as ibuprofen, ketoprofen, diclofenac, naproxen or aspirin.

The results of a multicentre, randomized, double-blind trial of azapropazone and diclofenac sodium in 110 patients with active osteoarthritis of the hip and osteoarthritis of the knee are presented and discussed. Azapropazone and diclofenac showed a comparable analgesic and anti-inflammatory effects, with relatively few adverse reactions which were invariably mild.

Zusammenfassung

Die degenerativen Erkrankungen der grossen und kleinen peripheren Gelenke wie auch der Wirbelsäule gehören unter anderem wegen der progredienten Überalterung der Bevölkerung zu den häufigsten Behandlungsproblemen. In den letzten 20 Jahren hat Azapropazon, ein nichtsteroidales Antirheumatikum (NSA) aus der Gruppe der Benzotriazine, einen festen Platz in der Behandlung der Arthrose erhalten. Die Wirksamkeit und Verträglichkeit von Azapropazon in diesem Indikationsgebiet wurde in zahlreichen klinischen Prüfungen untersucht. Für die Behandlung der aktivierten Arthrose hat sich eine tägliche Dosis von 1200 mg als therapeutisch wirksam gezeigt, während sich für die Erhaltungstherapie oft 900 mg als ausreichend erwiesen haben. Eine vergleichbare Wirksamkeit von 1200 mg Azapropazon mit der empfohlenen Tagesdosis anderer nichtsteroidaler Antirheumatika wie Ibuprofen, Ketoprofen, Diclofenac, Naproxen oder Aspirin konnte aufgezeigt werden. Es werden schliesslich die Resultate einer multizentrischen randomisierten Doppelblindstudie von Azapropazon mit Diclofenac-Natrium an 110 Patienten mit aktivierter Coxarthrose and Gonarthrose vorgelegt und besprochen. Es zeigte sich ein vergleichbarer analgetischer und antiphlogistischer Effekt zwischen Azapropazon und Diclofenac bei relativ wenigen und fast durchwegs schwachen Nebenwirkungen.

Resumé

Les maladies dégénératives qui affectent les grosses et petites articulations périphériques et la colonne vertébrale comptent parmi les problèmes thérapeutiques les plus fréquents, notamment en raison du vieillissement progressif de la population. L'azapropazone, un anti-inflammatoire non stéroïdien (AINS) du groupe des benzotriazines, a pris une place importante dans le traitement de l'arthrose au cours des 20 dernières années. De nombreuses études cliniques ont porté sur l'efficacité et la tolérance de l'azapropazone dans cette indication. Elles ont permis d'établir qu'une dose quotidienne de 1200 mg était efficace dans le traitement de l'arthrose active alors qu'une dose de 900 mg se révélait souvent suffisante pour le traitement d'entretien. Il a été démontré que l'efficacité de 1200 mg d'azapropazone était comparable à celle des doses quotidiennes recommandées pour d'autres AINS tels que l'ibuprofène, le kétoprofène, le diclofénac, le naproxène ou l'aspirine. L'auteur présente et commente également les résultats d'une étude multicentrique randomisée en double insu portant sur 110 patients souffrant de coxarthrose et de gonarthrose actives et traités avec l'azapropazone et le diclofénac sodique. L'azapropazone et le diclofénac ont exercé un effet analgésique et antiphlogistique comparable en entraînant un nombre relativement restreint d'effets secondaires, qui ont été presque toujours bénins.

13
Azapropazone in gout and hyperuricaemia

G Nuki, F Grinlinton, J Palit and R Wallace

I. INTRODUCTION

After 20 years of clinical use as a non-steroidal anti-inflammatory drug (NSAID) azapropazone is now well established as both a useful agent for treating attacks of acute gouty arthritis and as single agent interval therapy for the management of patients with hyperuricaemia and recurrent gouty arthritis where uric acid lowering drug therapy is indicated.

II. HYPOURICAEMIC EFFECT

As long ago as 1971 Frank[1] demonstrated that azapropazone had uricosuric properties after observing a fall in serum urate (SUA) levels in a clinical trial of azapropazone in patients with rheumatoid arthritis. Single doses of azapropazone 600 mg produced no significant fall in SUA or change in uric acid excretion 6 hours after administration but serum urate was reduced by 43–77% and urate clearance increased by 133–436% in 8 patients with gout and hyperuricaemia after 5 days of treatment with 900 or 1800 mg of azapropazone daily. The fall in SUA with azapropazone 900 mg daily was less than that with oxyphenbutazone 300 mg/day in a double blind comparison in 25 RA patients over one month[1]. Our own early studies[2] in asymptomatic patients with gout and hyperuricaemia showed that azapropazone 1200 mg daily lowered serum urate and increased uric acid clearance to a greater extent than phenylbutazone 300 mg daily in a 7-day cross-over comparison. Significant changes in serum urate and urine uric acid clearance were observed within 24 hours of starting drug therapy (Table 1)[2]. Azapropazone 1200 mg daily was similarly effective in lowering SUA and augmenting uric acid excretion in a short-term open study in France[3] in patients with asymptomatic hyperuricaemia and Dieppe et al.[4] were able to show sustained lowering of SUA over six months in patients with chronic 'interval' gouty arthritis treated with this dose. This group demonstrated a uricosuric effect within four hours of administration of a single dose of 600 mg of azapropazone[4] and Higgens and Scott[5] subsequently showed that the hypouricaemic effect of azapropazone increased with dosage between

Azapropazone – 20 years of clinical use. Rainsford, KD (ed)
© Kluwer Academic Publishers. Printed in Great Britain

Table 1 SUA and urine uric acid clearance data from crossover study in 7 hyperuricaemic patients treated with azapropazone (300 mg q.d.s.) and phenylbutazone (100 mg t.d.s.) (from ref. 2)

Day	Azapropazone (A)*	Phenylbutazone (P)*	Statistical analysis (p values)		
			A vs Initial value	P vs Initial value	A vs P
Serum uric acid (mmol/L)					
0	0.59 ± 0.07	0.59 ± 0.10			NS
1	0.45 ± 0.13	0.55 ± 0.06	< 0.001	NS	< 0.01
3	0.40 ± 0.14	0.49 ± 0.07	< 0.001	< 0.01	< 0.05
7	0.45 ± 0.12	0.48 ± 0.11	< 0.01	< 0.01	NS
Uric acid clearance (ml/min)					
0	4.31 ± 2.06	4.19 ± 1.72			NS
1	9.37 ± 5.77	5.70 ± 1.97	< 0.05	NS	NS
3	8.26 ± 4.20	6.07 ± 1.93	< 0.02	< 0.01	< 0.05
7	6.90 ± 3.39	6.08 ± 5.39	< 0.02	NS	NS

* means ± 1 SD

900 mg and 2400 mg daily. Azapropazone 1800 mg and 2400 mg daily had a uricosuric effect comparable to probenecid 1 g daily but a dose of 1200 mg/day was less effective[5].

III. PHYSIOLOGICAL AND BIOCHEMICAL BASIS FOR REDUCTION OF SERUM URATE

Since the uricosuric effect of azapropazone and the fall in SUA could be blocked by prior administration of pyrazinamide Frank attributed the drug induced uricosuria to enhanced tubular secretion of urate[1]. This interpretation of the effects of pyrazinamide suppression assumes that secreted urate is not further reabsorbed. With the clear demonstration of substantial post-secretory reabsorption of urate in man[6] it now seems more likely that azapropazone increases urate excretion by inhibiting urate reabsorption at a post-secretory site[6].

An increase in filtered urate following drug induced displacement of urate from protein binding is a further theoretical possibility. Whitehouse and colleagues demonstrated that a number of drugs with uricosuric properties will reduce the binding of urate to albumin in vitro[7] and the increases in uric acid removal during haemodialysis following administration of salicylates have been taken as evidence for in vivo urate protein binding[8]. Albumin binding of urate at physiological temperature is however vanishingly small so that significant changes in urate filtration following drug administration are unlikely to be significant.

Azapropazone is a weak inhibitor of xanthine oxidase in vitro[9]. Xanthine and hypoxanthine excretion are not however increased during drug therapy ruling out the possibility of significant inhibition of this enzyme in vivo[10]. Nevertheless the uricosuric response to treatment with azapropazone was not consistent in this[10] and some previous studies[3,3] suggesting the possibility of an additional mechanism for lowering of serum urate[10].

We have confirmed these findings. Ten men with gout discontinued all drug therapy for two weeks before taking azapropazone 600 mg b.d. for 2 further weeks. Plasma urate, urinary uric acid and urinary oxypurine excretion were measured by HPLC[11]. The results are shown in Table 2 and Figures 1–3. There was a significant fall in plasma urate ($p < 0.001$) but urine uric acid excretion only rose in half the patients and there was no evidence of an increase in xanthine or hypoxanthine excretion. The small decrease in total oxypurine excretion (uric acid + xanthine + hypoxanthine) following treatment with azapropazone could indicate some suppression of *de novo* purine biosynthesis but inhibition of purine absorption from the gut or enhancement of extrarenal urate disposal would be alternative possibilities. Sorensen[12] has demonstrated that about one third of total urate excretion in normal individuals is via extrarenal routes and this increased to 70% in patients with chronic renal insufficiency. In our study creatinine clearance fell markedly from 1.2 ml/s to 0.69 ml/s in one patient with marginally depressed creatinine clearance following administration of azapropazone although creatinine clearance was not affected in the rest of the group whose renal function was intact. This emphasises the need for caution before giving NSAIDs to patients with renal insufficiency. Preliminary attempts to examine the effect of azapropazone therapy on salivary and biliary urate excretion have been technically unsuccessful to-date because of the extreme variability of salivary and biliary flow rates.

IV. ACUTE GOUTY ARTHRITIS

In common with the majority of NSAIDs azapropazone is consistently effective in resolving the inflammation associated with an acute attack of gouty arthritis. This was first demonstrated by Frank in 1976[13]. Our own early studies in hospital in-patients with acute gouty arthritis suggested that azapropazone, in the relatively high dose of 600 mg q.d.s., was as effective as previous agents used for the management of individual patient's acute gout with resolution of pain in 2–21 days depending on the severity and chronicity of the acute attack[2]. Dieppe *et al.*[4] achieved symptomatic remission within 72 hours in 8 patients with acute gouty arthritis using azapropazone 600 mg

Table 2 Plasma urate, urinary uric acid and oxypurine excretion following azapropazone 600 mg b.d. in 10 patients with gout

	Plasma urate (mmol/L)[†]	Urine uric acid (mmol/24 h)[†]	Urine oxypurines* (mmol/24 h)[†]
Pre-study	0.43 ± 0.06	4.74 ± 2.56	0.35 ± 0.46
Week 1	0.27 ± 0.03	4.62 ± 1.59	0.15 ± 0.07
Week 1	0.27 ± 0.04	3.97 ± 1.74	0.16 ± 0.09

* Oxypurine = xanthine + hypoxanthine
[†] mean ± SD

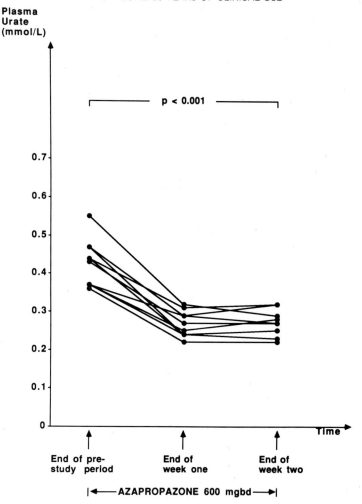

Figure 1 The effect of azapropazone 600 mg b.d. on plasma urate

8-hourly for 24 hours followed by 600 mg b.d. Treatment was commence
within 72 hours of onset in all cases. With intravenous azapropazone 600 n
b.d. Dunky and colleagues[14] obtained significant pain relief after 75 minut
and resolution of acute gouty arthritis in 4 days in 15 patients. Azapropazo
and indomethacin were equally effective in a randomised double-blir
comparison of azapropazone 600 mg t.d.s. for three days followed by 300 n
q.d.s. with indomethacin 50 mg t.d.s. for three days followed by 25 mg q.d
in 30 patients[15].

V. MECHANISM OF ANTI-INFLAMMATORY EFFECT

Although most NSAIDs are consistently effective in resolving the inflar
mation associated with acute gouty arthritis the biochemical basis for the

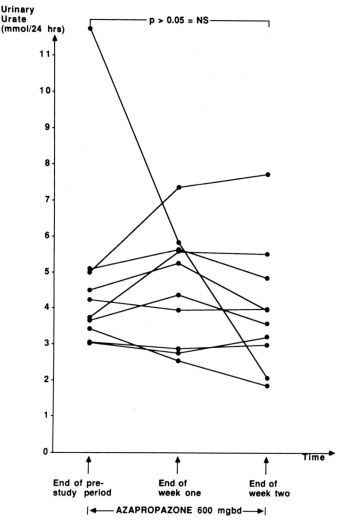

Figure 2   The effect of azapropazone 600 mg b.d. on urinary uric acid excretion

anti-inflammatory action in crystal-induced arthritis may not be identical for each drug.

Azapropazone reduces rat foot pad oedema induced experimentally by monosodium urate crystals in the rather high dose of 100 mg/kg[4]. Despite relatively weak activity as an inhibitor of prostaglandin synthesis[16] azapropazone is effective in inhibiting inflammation in many animal pharmacological models. Increasingly it is becoming apparent that NSAIDs can inhibit the cellular activation of phagocytic cells in the absence of effects on prostaglandin synthesis by inserting into the lipid bilayer of plasma membranes and

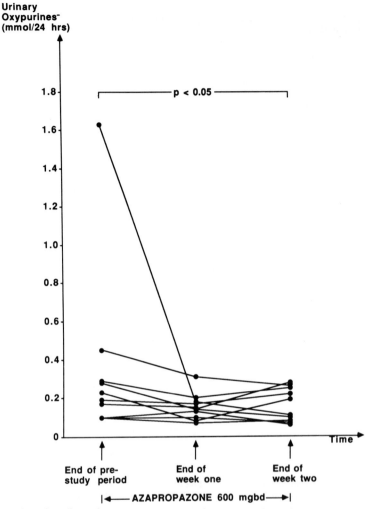

Figure 3   The effect of azapropazone on urinary excretion of oxypurines (xanthine + hypoxanthine)

so interfering with normal signal transduction. As long ago as 1971[17] azapropazone was shown to stabilise lysosomal membranes. More recently Mackin and his colleagues[18] have shown that azapropazone will inhibit neutrophil migration, aggregation and degranulation in response to chemotactic peptides at physiologically relevant concentrations without interfering with peptide binding. It also inhibits superoxide anion generation in response to phorbol esters in rat polymorphs[18]. We have found that azapropazone will inhibit superoxide anion generation by human peripheral blood monocytes in response to urate crystals *in vitro* in a dose-responsive manner in concentrations of $10^{-5}-10^{-3}$mol/L[19]. Of five NSAIDs tested diclofenac and piroxicam inhibited superoxide anion generation in response to serum treated zymosan *in vitro* while benoxaprofen, indomethacin and phenylbutazone did not[20].

VI. SINGLE AGENT THERAPY FOR THE PREVENTION OF RECURRENT GOUTY ARTHRITIS

Although highly effective drugs for the management of patients with hyperuricaemia and recurrent gouty arthritis exist, uricosuric agents such as probenecid, sulphinpyrazone and benzbromarone, and xanthine oxidase inhibitors such as allopurinol, all require co-administration of small doses of colchicine or NSAIDs during the early phases of treatment if troublesome 'breakthrough' attacks of acute gouty arthritis are to be avoided. Phenylbutazone combines uricosuric with anti-inflammatory activity but it cannot be recommended for long-term prophylactic therapy in gout because of the risks of bone marrow toxicity.

Evidence suggesting that azapropazone might be used as a single agent for the management of gout and hyperuricaemia has gradually accumulated since it was mooted 10 years ago[21]. Dieppe *et al.*[4] treated 10 patients with 'interval gout' with azapropazone 1200 mg/day for six months. Each had had at least four attacks of acute gouty arthritis in the preceding year. Not only did the azapropazone produce sustained lowering of the serum urate but only a single episode of gouty arthritis was recorded in one patient in the six-month period. Templeton[22] conducted a 24-centre comparison of azapropazone and allopurinol in 278 gouty patients previously treated with allopurinol. Half the patients continued with their allopurinol in previously prescribed doses and half were switched to azapropazone 1200 mg/day. Control of serum urate was equally good in both groups but acute attacks of gout occurred in 23 patients on allopurinol and only 10 receiving azapropazone.

Further evidence that azapropazone might be unusual among uric acid lowering drugs in not being associated with an increased risk of precipitating acute attacks of gouty arthritis in the early phase of treatment comes from a multi-centre study in hospital and general practice[23]. Ninety-three patients presenting with acute gouty arthritis were randomly allocated to receive either azapropazone (600 mg t.d.s.) alone or indomethacin for 28 days followed by allopurinol (150 mg b.d.) for a further 30 weeks. Azapropazone and indomethacin appeared to be equally effective in controlling the acute gouty arthritis and there was a substantial fall in SUA in azapropazone-treated patients after four days. SUA levels were similar in both azapropazone- and allopurinol-treated groups after day 28 but there were fewer breakthrough attacks of acute gouty arthritis in the azapropazone-treated patients (12 *vs* 21) over the course of the trial. Further studies need to be undertaken to assess whether monotherapy with azapropazone is as effective in preventing further episodes of gouty arthritis as allopurinol combined with small prophylactic doses of colchicine or an NSAID.

Further studies are also required to look at the overall risk/benefit of these alternative management regimes. Azapropazone may be associated with a higher incidence of gastrointestinal and cutaneous rections than allopurinol alone but data are simply not available on the comparative toxicity of azapropazone and allopurinol or standard uricosuric drug therapy combined with colchicine or another NSAID.

All drugs currently used for the management of gout are potentially more toxic in patients with renal insufficiency and data are required to examine their relative effects on renal function, the control of hypertension, hyperlipidaemia and the cardiovascular morbidity frequently associated with gout.

References

1. Frank, K.O. (1971). Investigation of the uricosuric action of azapropazone. Z. Rheumaforsch., 30, 368–373
2. Thomas, A.L., Majoos, F.L. and Nuki, G. (1983). Preliminary studies with azapropazone in gout and hyperuricaemia. Eur. J. Rheumatol. Inflamm., 6, 149–154
3. Herne, N., Hugny, D., Hauteville, D., Desbaumes, J., De Muizon, H. and Andran, M. (1977). L'azapropazone, Etude de son activite hypouricemiante. Nouv. Presse. Med., 6, 1657–1658
4. Dieppe, P.A., Doherty, M., Whicher, J.T. and Walters, G. (1977). The treatment of gout with azapropazone: clinical and experimental studies. Eur. J. Rheumatol. Inflamm., 4, 392–400
5. Higgen, C.S. and Scott, J.T. (1984). The uricosuric action of azapropazone: dose response and comparison with probencid. Br. J. Clin. Pharmacol., 18, 439–443
6. Steele, T.H. (1973). Urate secretion in man: the pyrazinamide suppression test. Ann. Intern. Med., 79, 734–737
7. Kippin, I., Whitehouse, M.W. and Klinenberg, J.R. (1974). Pharmacology of uricosuric drugs. Ann. Rheum. Dis., 33, 391–393
8. Postelethwaite, A.E., Gutman, R.A. and Kelley, W.N. (1974). Salicylate mediated increase in uric acid removal during haemodialysis: evidence for urate binding in vivo. Metabolism, 23, 771–777
9. Jahn, U. and Thiele, K. (1988). In-vitro inhibition of xanthine oxidase by azapropazone and 8-hydroxy azapropazone. Arzneim. Forsch., 38, 507–508
10. Gibson, T., Simmonds, H.A., Armstrong, R.D., Fairbanks, L.D. and Rogers, A.V. (1984). Azapropazone – a treatment of hyperuricaemia and gout? Br. J. Rheumatol., 23, 44–51
11. Rylance, H.J., Wallace, R.C. and Nuki, G. (1983). Analysis of human plasma and urine purines using high performance liquid chromatograghy. Ann. Rheum. Dis., 42, (Suppl)., 85
12. Sorenson, C.B. (1965). Role of the intestinal tract in the elimination of uric acid. Arthritis Rheum., 8, 694–703
13. Frank, O. (1976). The treatment of acute gouty arthritis. J. Clin. Chem. Clin. Biochem., 14, 290
14. Dunky, A., Bartsch, G. and Eberl, R. (1984). The intravenous application of azapropazone in the treatment of acute gout. Arthritis Rheum., 6, 1–6
15. Thompson, M., Sanders, P.A., Walker, D.J. and Templeton, J.S. (1985). Abst. XVIth International Congress Rheumatology, Sydney

16. Brune, K., Rainsford, K.D., Wagner, K. and Peskar, B.A. (1981). Inhibition by anti-inflammatory drugs of prostaglandin production in cultured macrophages. *Naunyn Schmiedeberg's Arch. Pharmacol.*, **315**, 269–281

17. Lewis, D.A., Capstick, R.B. and Ancill, R.J. (1971). The action of azapropazone, oxyphenbutazone and phenylbutazone on lysosomes. *J. Pharm. Pharmacol.*, **23**, 931

18. Mackin, W.M., Rakich, S.M. and Marshall, C.L. (1986). Inhibition of rat neutrophil functional responses by azapropazone, an anti-gout drug. *Biochem. Pharmacol.*, **35**, 917–922

19. Palit, J., Nuki, G. (Unpublished observations)

20. Bell, A.L., Hurst, N.P., French, J.K., Adamson, J. and Nuki, G. (1987). Effects of non-steroidal anti-inflammatory drugs and antimalarial agents on blood monocyte superoxide anion production in vitro and ex vivo in rheumatoid arthritis. In: A.J.G. Swaark and J.K. Forster, (eds.) *Free Radicals and Arthritis Diseases., Topics in Ageing Research in Europe.* **11**, 151–160

21. Thomas, A. and Nuki, G. (1979). The hypouricaemic effects of azapropazone and phenylbutazone. XIXth European Congress Rheumatology, Wiesbaden

22. Templeton, J.S. (1983). Longterm comparison of azapropazone with allopurinol in control of chronic gout and hyperuricaemia. *Ann. Rheum. Dis.*, **42** (Suppl. 1), 92–93

23. Fraser, R.C., Harvard-Davis, R. and Walker, F.S. (1987). Comparative trial of azapropazone and indomethacin plus allopurinol in acute gout and hyperuricaemia. *J. Roy. Coll. Gen. Practit.*, **37**, 409–411

Summary

Azapropazone is now well established as a useful agent for the treatment of acute gouty arthritis and for the management of patients with hyperuricaemia and recurrent gouty arthritis where uric acid lowering drug therapy is indicated.

In common with the majority of non-steroidal anti-inflammatory agents it is consistently effective in resolving the inflammation of an acute attack of gouty arthritis although the biochemical basis for the inhibitory effects may not be the same for all NSAIDs. Experimentally induced crystal inflammation is inhibited by azapropazone in rat and in man but the mechanisms relevant to its anti-inflammatory effects remain uncertain.

Azapropazone is one of a relatively small number of NSAIDs with serum urate lowering potential and currently the only such agent which can be considered as an acceptable alternative to allopurinol or uricosuric agents for the prophylactic management of patients with hyperuricaemia and recurrent gouty arthritis. Azapropazone has a dose dependent uricosuric effect which is probably secondary to inhibition of tubular reabsorption of urate. Inhibition of xanthine oxidase which is seen at high doses *in vitro* does not occur *in vivo* but some clinical studies do point to the possibility of an additional mechanism for the hypouricaemic effect of the drug. Clinical trials suggest that azapropazone has the advantage of not being associated with the induction of the acute attacks of gout which can be troublesome after the initiation of other hypouricaemic drugs but its use may be associated with a higher incidence of rashes and gastrointestinal intolerance than with allopurinol. Further studies are required to establish the relative costs and benefits of azapropazone and other currently available hypouricaemic drugs and also to examine their effects on hypertension, hyperlipidaemia and the cardiovascular morbidity frequently associated with gout.

Zusammenfassung

Azapropazon hat sich mittlerweile bestens etablieren können und wird als wirksames Mittel für die Behandlung der akuten Arthritis urica sowie für die Behandlung von an Hyperurikosämie und rekurrierender Arthritis urica leidenden Patienten eingesetzt, bei denen eine medikamentöse Behandlung zur Senkung der Harnsäurewerte indiziert ist.

Gemeinsam mit der überwiegenden Zahl nichtsteroidaler entzündungshemmender Substanzen zeigt Azapropazon konsistente Wirksamkeit bei der Beseitigung der während des akuten Schubs einer Arthritis urica auftretenden Inflammation, auch wenn die biochemische Grundlage für die inhibitorische Wirkung nicht für alle nichtsteroidalen, anti-inflammatorisch wirkenden Pharmaka die gleiche sein mag. Experimentell induzierte Kristallinflammation wird bei der Ratte und beim Menschen durch Azapropazon inhibiert, auch wenn der für die entzündungshemmende Wirkung relevante Mechanismus weiterhin ungeklärt bleibt.

Azapropazon zählt zu der relativ kleinen Gruppe nichtsteroidaler, anti-inflammatorisch wirksamer Substanzen, die über ein Potential zur Senkung der Serumuratwerte verfügen. Azapropazon stellt gegenwärtig das als einzige Pharmakon dar, das als akzeptable Alternative zu Allopurinol-haltigen Mitteln oder Urikosurika für die Basistherapie von Hyperurikosämie und rekurrierender Arthritis urica angesehen werden kann. Azapropazon weist eine dosisabhängige die Harnsäureausscheidung durch die Niere steigernde Wirkung auf, die möglicherweise der Inhibierung der tubulären Rückresorption des Urats zuzuordnenist. Die bei hohen Dosen in vitro beobachtete Inhibierung der Xanthin-oxidase tritt in vivo nicht auf, obwohl einige klinische Studien auf die Möglichkeit verweisen, daß ein zusätzlicher Mechanismus für die den Harnsäuregehalt des Blutes senkende Wirkung des Pharmakons vorläge. Klinische Prüfungen legen nahe, daß Azapropazon den Vorzug aufweist, nicht mit der Auslösung akuter Gichtanfälle in Zusammenhang zu stehen, die nach Einstellung auf andere, den Serum-Harnsäurewert absenkende Pharmaka auftreten können. Seine Verabreichung kann möglicherweise mit im Vergleich zu Allopurinol vermehrtem Auftreten von Ausschlägen und gastrointestinale Unverträglichkeit einhergehen. Es müssen weitere Untersuchungen durchgeführt werden, um die relativen Kosten und Vorzüge des Azapropazons sowie anderer, gegenwärtig verfügbarer den Serum-Harnsäurewert absenkender Pharmaka abzuwägen und darüber hinaus ihre Auswirkung auf Hypertonie, Hyperlipidämie und die häufig mit der Gicht assoziierte kardiovaskuläre Morbidität abzuklären.

Resumé

L'azapropazone est maintenant bien établie comme agent thérapeutique dans le traitement de l'arthrite goutteuse et chez les malades souffrants d'hyperuricémie et de rechute d'arthrite goutteuse quand une thérapie visant à diminuer l'acide urique est recommandée.

Comme c'est le cas avec la plupart des agents anti-inflammatoires non stéroïdiens, elle est généralement efficace pour combattre l'inflammation lors d'une attaque sévère d'arthrite goutteuse bien que la base biochimique pour les effets inhibiteurs ne soit pas la même avec tous les AINS. L'inflammation cristalline provoquée à titre d'expérience est inhibée par l'azapropazone chez le rat et l'homme mais le mécanisme associé à ses effets anti-inflammatoire reste incertain.

L'azapropazone est l'un des rares AINS ayant un potentiel de réduction du taux de l'acide urique dans le sang et, à présent, le seul agent qui puisse être considéré comme alternative acceptable à l'allopurinol ou aux agents uricosuriques dans le traitement prophylactique de malades souffrant d'hyperuricémie et de rechute d'arthrite goutteuse. L'azapropazone a un effet uricosurique associé au dosage qui résulte probablement de l'inhibition de la réabsorption tubulaire de l'urate. L'inhibition de la xanthine-oxydase que l'on relève à hautes doses in vitro ne se produit pas in vivo mais certaines études cliniques semblent indiquer la possibilité d'un mécanisme additionnel causant l'effet hypo-uricémique du produit. Des essais cliniques avancent que l'azapropazone a l'avantage de ne pas être associée aux sévères attaques de goutte parfois très pénibles provoquées au début d'un traitement avec d'autres produits hypo-uricémique mais son utilisation peut être liée à une plus haute incidence d'éruption et d'intolérance gastrointestinale qu'avec l'allopurinol. Des études plus approfondies sont nécessaires pour établir les avantages et inconvénients relatifs de l'azapropazone et des autres médicaments hypo-uricémiques et aussi pour examiner leur effet sur l'hypertension, l'hyperlipidémie et morbidité cardiovasculaire fréquemment associées à la goutte.

14
Die Analgetische Wirksamkeit von Azapropazon
[Analgesic effects of azapropazone]

H Spring, JL Heidecker, A Wright, I ab I Davies,
FS Walker, JG Riddell, FU Bauer, D Eggli, E Gillemann
and J Steens

I. EINLEITUNG

Azapropazon ist ein nichtsteroidales Antirheumatikum aus der Klasse der Benzotriazine. Der antiphlogistische und analgetische Wirkungsmechanismus von Azapropazon beruht insbesondere auf Inhibition von Freisetzung und Aktivität lysosomaler Enzyme, wogegen die prostaglandinhemmenden Eigenschaften weniger ausgeprägt sind[1,2]. Dies bewirkt, dass die destruierende Wirkung der lysosomalen Enzyme gemindert und gleichzeitig die Schutzfunktion bestimmter Prostaglandine, wie im Bereich der Magen-Darm-Mucosa, erhalten bleibt[3].

Obwohl Azapropazon die Prostaglandin-Synthese, im Vergleich zu anderen nichtsteroidalen Antiphlogistika, nur gering hemmt, hat es sich in der Klinik nicht nur als potentes Antiphlogistikum, sondern auch als ein gutes Analgetikum bewährt, indem es den Reflexbogen Schmerz-Spannung-Schmerz unterbricht.

II. DIE ANALGETISCHE WIRKUNG VON ORALEM UND INTRAVENÖSEM AZAPROPAZON IN DER KLINISCHEN PRÜFUNG

Parameter wie Belastungsschmerz, Nachtschmerz, Ruheschmerz, Druckschmerz oder Bewegungsschmerz wurden in den meisten klinischen Prüfungen zum Nachweis der Wirksamkeit und Verträglichkeit einer Therapie mit Azapropazon in diversen Indikationen mit untersucht. Die Erfassung der Schmerzintensität erfolgte zumeist semiquantitativ mit Verfahren, die sich bei der klinischen Prüfung von Antiphlogistika eingebürgert haben. So kamen Skores in verschiedenen Abstufungen (z.B. Schmerzintensität viel stärker-stärker-gleich-schwächer-viel schwächer) oder Visuelle Analog-Skalen zur Anwendung.

Azapropazone – 20 years of clinical use. Rainsford, KD (ed)
© Kluwer Academic Publishers. Printed in Great Britain

Zahlreiche klinische Untersuchungen bei Patienten mit Schmerzen verschiedener Genese belegen die analgetische Wirksamkeit von Azapropazon. Zwei Studien seien hier stellvertretend für die intravenöse Applikation sowie für die kombinierte intravenöse und orale Anwendung von Azapropazon aufgeführt.

Achtzig ambulante Patienten mit akuten Schmerzen infolge einer Gonarthrose (55 Personen), akuter Lumbalgien (17 Personen) und anderer rheumatischer Beschwerden (8 Personen) wurden in einer offenen Prüfung mit Azapropazon intravenös behandelt[4]. 33 Patienten erhielten eine Injektion von 600 mg Azapropazon pro Tag, 47 Patienten erhielten 1200 mg am Tag.

Ein wesentlicher Rückgang der Score-Werte für den Ruheschmerz trat bei 40% der Patienten nach 30 Minuten, bei 90% nach 45 Minuten auf. Eine anhaltende Besserung wurde bei 85% der Patienten bei weiterer Befragung registriert. Beim Bewegungsschmerz wurde der analgetische Effekt nach 45 Minuten bei 85% der Patienten erzielt. Das Maximum der Schmerzabnahme zeigte sich zwei bis zweieinhalb Studen nach der Injektion. Am darauffolgenden Tag ergab sich eine andauernde Besserung bei mehr als 80% der Patienten. Die Abbildung 1 zeigt den raschen Wirkungseintritt nach einer Injektion auf den Ruheschmerz anhand einer Visuellen Analog-Skala. Vergleichbare Resultate wurden beim Bewegungsschmerz gefunden.

In eine Doppelblindstudie[5] wurden 40 Patienten aufgenommen, die nach unterschiedlichen Traumata die orthopädische Ambulanz aufgesucht hatten und Schwellungen sowie Schmerzen aufwiesen. Je 20 Patienten wurden randomisiert einer Azapropazon- und einer Placebo-Gruppe zugeteilt. In der Azapropazon-Gruppe erhielten die Patienten am ersten Tag zwei Injektionen von 600 mg Azapropazon i.v. An den nächsten 6 Tagen wurde ihnen täglich zweimal je eine Tablette zu 600 mg Azapropazon oral verabreicht. Die Kontrollgruppe wurde im gleichen Zeitraum mit Placebo-Injektionen und Tabletten in gleicher Dosierung und Anwendungsweise behandelt.

Nach der siebentägigen Behandlungsperiode beurteilten Arzt und Patienten die Schmerzlinderung anhand einer Vier-Punkte-Skala (keine, leichte, mässige, völlige Schmerzlinderung). Die Schmerzintensität wurde mit einer Visuellen Analog-Skala zu festgesetzten Zeitpunkten ermittelt.

Die Azapropazon-Gruppe schnitt hinsichtlich der analgetischen Wirksamkeit signifikant besser ab. Die Schmerzintensität nahm innerhalb einer Stunde nach der ersten Azapropazon-Injektion und im weiteren Verlauf der Behandlung deutlich ab, wogegen die Schmerzintensität in der Kontroll-Gruppe nur langsam und in einem geringeren Ausmass zurückging (Abb. 2).

III. QUANTIFIZIERUNG DES ANALGETISCHEN EFFEKTES VON ORALEM AZAPROPAZON BEI PROBANDEN[6]

1. Einleitung

Eine Methode, den Gelenkschmerz auf nicht-invasive Art zu erzeugen, wurde von Wright und Davis[7] entwickelt. Sie benutzten einen strahlenförmig

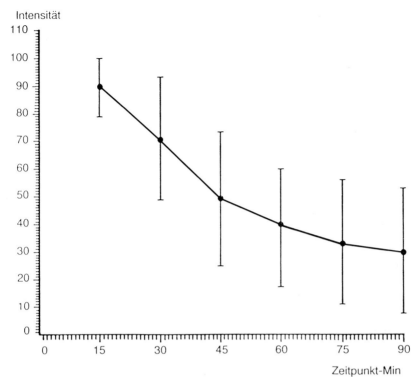

Abb. 1 Visuelle Analog-Skala: Verlauf der Schmerzintensität beim Ruheschmerz nach einer Injektion von 600 mg Azapropazon.

gebündelten Ultraschall zum Setzen eines Reizes. Das dadurch im Gehirn evozierte Potential widerspiegelt objektiv den empfundenen Schmerz und kann durch die Verabreichung eines Analgetikums reduziert werden. Bromm[8] hat schon gezeigt, dass ein oberflächlicher elektrischer Hautreiz ebenso ein Potential im Gehirn hervorzurufen vermag, das wiederum mit dem empfundenen Schmerz korreliert und dessen Amplitude durch Analgetika vermindert werden kann. Die Qualität des empfundenen Schmerzes zeigt jedoch wesentliche Unterschiede. Im ersten Fall werden tiefliegende Schmerz-rezeptoren, insbesondere des Gelenkes, stimuliert, im zweiten Fall ein oberflächlich empfundener Hautschmerz verursacht. Wright und Davis fanden eine statistisch signifikante Korrelation zwischen der Amplitude des evozierten Potentials und der subjektiven Schmerzempfindung, gemessen mittels computergestützter Visuellen Analog-Skala (VAS). Eine wiederholte Anwendung des Tests verursachte zwar Abweichungen zwischen den Ampli-tuden der evozierten Potentiale und den mittleren Messwerten der VAS, diese waren jedoch für die Testperiode von 5 Stunden nicht signifikant. Da die vorliegende Methode mit Induktion eines tiefen Gelenkschmerzes besser die klinische Situation bei aktivierten Phasen von rheumatischen Erkran-kungen widerspiegelt und auch die Analgesie in solchen Fällen rasch nach

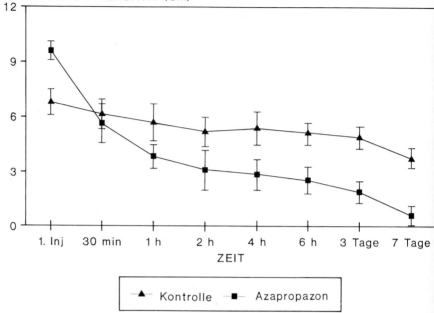

Abb. 2 Visuelle Analog-Skala: Verlauf der Schmerzintensität nach einer Initialtherapie mit 2 × 600 mg Azapropazon i.v. am ersten Behandlungstag und anschliessender Weiterbehandlung mit 2 × 600 mg Azapropazon oral im Vergleich zur Kontrolle mit Placebo.

der Medikation einsetzen sollte, wurde der Einfluss von oral verabreichtem Azapropazon auf den Gelenkschmerz in diesem Modell untersucht.

2. Material und Methode

In einer doppelblinden Versuchsanordnung wurde die analgestische Wirkung einer Einzelgabe von oral verabreichtem Azapropazon (600 mg), Pethidin (100 mg) und Placebo an 8 gesunden Probanden untersucht. Die Probanden wurden erst nach einer umfassenden medizinischen Untersuchung in die Studie aufgenommen. Probanden mit Arthritis oder Rheumatismus in der Familienanamnese wurden ausgeschlossen.

Der Ultraschall-Reiz wurde durch einen 500 kHz Frequenz-Generator erzeugt. Dieser war durch einen Kraftverstärker mit einem speziell entwikkelten fokussierten Ultraschall-Umwandler (Durchmesser 5,5 cm, Fokuslänge 4 cm) verbunden. Die randomisierten Zeit-Intervalle von 10–20 Sekunden zwischen den Impulsen, Impulsdauer und -Intensität sowie die Erfassung und Bildung von Mittelwerten aus den EEG-Signalen und die Umwandlung in Potentiale wurden durch einen Apple 11e Mikrocomputer gesteuert. Eine speziell adaptierte Version des DAN-Software-Pakets (Data Acquisition in Neurophysiology, Dept. Mental Health, Queen's University, Belfast) kam zur Anwendung. Segmente des EEG eine Sekunde vor bis eine Sekunde nach Setzen eines Ultraschall-Reizes wurden aufgenommen und im Computer gespeichert. Ein gleichzeitig aufgenommenes EEG ermöglichte den automatischen Ausschluss von EEG-Signalen, die durch Augenbewegungen überlagert waren. Der Mittelwert eines EEG-Segmentes von 80 Reizen ergab ein Potential, aus dem die Amplitude berechnet wurde. Die Amplitude des Potentials wurde vor der Verabreichung der Medikamente oder des Placebos und anschliessend in regelmässigen Intervallen festgehalten.

Die subjektive Beurteilung des Schmerzes erfolgte anhand des VAS, das ebenfalls per Computer erfasst und in die Auswertung mit einbezogen wurde. Auf dem Monitor wurde der Versuchsperson jeweils 3 Sekunden nach Setzen eines Reizes eine 10 cm lange Linie präsentiert, deren Enden die Gegensätze in der Schmerzempfindung repräsentierten. Der Proband steuerte von Hand den Cursor auf denjenigen Punkt dieser Linie, der für ihn der Schmerzempfindung nach den jeweiligen Reizen entsprach.

Für den Versuchsablauf wurde die nicht-dominante Hand der Versuchsperson in ein Wasserbad von 37°C getaucht und der Zeigefinger leicht an der Grundplatte der stereotaktischen Einrichtung befestigt. Der Strahl des Ultraschalls wurde vertikal auf das proximale Interphalangealgelenk gerichtet. Die Schmerzgrenze jedes Probanden wurde durch graduelle Erhöhung der Reizintensität bei gleichbleibender Frequenz bis zur Schmerzempfindung festgestellt. Für die eigentliche Untersuchung gelangten das 1,5–und 2-fache der so ermittelten, über der Schmerzgrenze liegenden Reizintensitäten in Intervallen zwischen 10 und 20 Sekunden zur Anwendung, wobei sowohl die Reizintensität als auch der Intervall randomisiert variierten. Potential und VAS-Werte wurden vor der Verabreichung der Medikamente oder des Placebos und anschliessend in regelmässigen Abständen während 4 Stunden festgehalten. Blutproben wurden regelmässig entnommen, um den Serumspiegel der Medikamente zu bestimmen.

3. Resultate

Eine statistisch signifikante Veränderung sowohl im Potential als auch in den VAS-Werten wurde 2,5 und 3,5 Stunden nach oraler Verabreichung einer Einzeldosis von 600 mg Azapropazon gefunden. Ein vergleichbarer Effekt wurde nach der Gabe von 100 mg Pethidin festgestellt (Abb. 3 und 4). Placebo zeigte in diesem Modell keine Wirkung.

Die analgetische Wirkung von Azapropazon korreliert nur in der Anfangsphase der Versuches mit der Serumkonzentration des Wirkstoffes. Obwohl der Serumspiegel noch weiter ansteigt, zeigt die Analgesie sowohl im Potential als auch in den VAS-Werten einen 'Sättigungseffekt' d.h. es wird rasch ein Maximum der Analgesie erreicht und anschliessend gehalten (Abb. 5 und 6).

Es wird allgemein angenommen, dass Pethidin seine Wirkung durch das Zentralnervensystem entwickelt. Demgegenüber erscheint es unwahr-

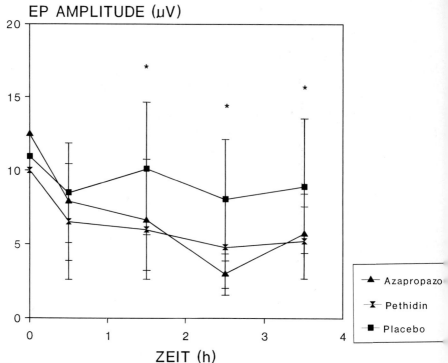

Abb. 3 Evoziertes Potential: Vergleich der analgetischen Wirksamkeit einer oralen Einzelgabe von 600 mg Azapropazon und 100 mg Pethidin sowie Placebo (*$p < 0,025$).

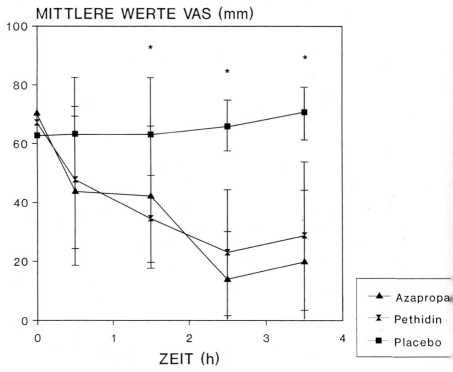

Abb. 4 Visuelle Analog-Skala: Vergleich der analgetischen Wirksamkeit einer oralen Einzelgabe von 600 mg Azapropazon und 100 mg Pethidin sowie Placebo (*$p < 0,025$).

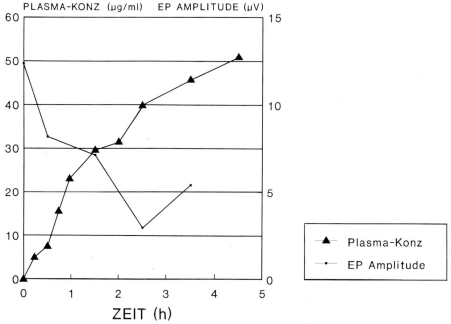

Abb. 5   Verlauf der Plasmakonzentration von Azapropazon sowie der Schmerzintensität gemäss evoziertem Potential.

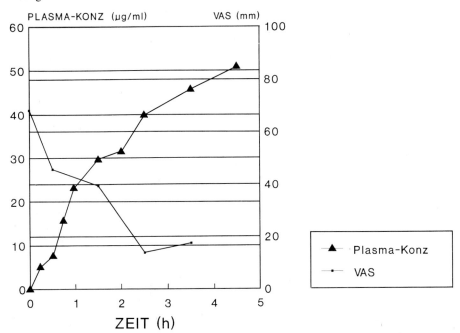

Abb. 6   Verlauf der Plasmakonzentration von Azapropazon sowie der Schmerzintensität gemäss Visueller Analog-Skala.

scheinlich, dass Azapropazon eine ähnliche analgetische Wirkungsweise aufweist. Eine periphere Wirkungsweise von Azapropazon scheint wahrscheinlicher, entweder an den Schmerzrezeptoren selbst oder an den Synapsen, die an der Reizübermittlung ins Zentralnervensystem beteiligt sind.

IV. QUANTIFIZIERUNG DES ANALGETISCHEN EFFEKTES VON INTRAVENOESEM AZAPROPAZON BEI SUBAKUTEN LUMBALGIEN

1. Einleitung

Das Auftreten von akuten und subakuten lumbalen Schmerzen ohne Vorliegen einer radikulären Symptomatik ist häufig[9]. Diese lumbalen Syndrome sind gekennzeichnet durch das subjektive Empfinden von störenden Schmerzen und die objektivierbare Verminderung der funktionellen Leistungsfähigkeit des Rückens. Die Beweglichkeit der Wirbelsäule ist sowohl global wie segmental eingeschränkt und die Kraftleistung der Rumpfmuskulatur herabgesetzt. In kurzer Zeit wird eine muskuläre Dysbalance mit Verkürzung der im Becken- und Lendenwirbelsäulenbereich ansetzenden tonischen und Abschwächung der phasischen Muskulatur auftreten. Eine weitere Einbusse der Leistungsfähigkeit des Rückens ist die Folge.

Die Therapie wird in einer ersten Phase aus analgetischen Massnahmen bestehen. Dabei kommen Analgetika und nichtsteroidale Antirheumatika zum Zug, die des raschen Wirkungseintrittes wegen oft parenteral appliziert werden. Zusätzlich wird die physikalische Therapie mit Mobilisationstechniken unterstützt durch reizmindernde passive Therapieformen eingesetzt.

Ziel dieser Studie war es, bei Patienten mit subakutem Lumbalsyndrom den Soforteffekt des auch intravenös zu applizierenden Antirheumatikums Azapropazon (Prolixan) mit Hilfe einer isokinetischen Kraftmesseinheit (Cybex-Back-System) zu untersuchen. Für dieses System ist eine quantitative Messung der Rückenfunktion gut belegt[10-13].

Für das Azapropazon liegen bis jetzt vor allem aus den Bereichen der Orthopädie und Traumatologie Studien vor, die die rasche analgetische Wirksamkeit der i.v.-Gabe beschreiben[4,5,14-17].

2. Methode

Es wurden fünf Patienten (Alter 35–58 Jahre, Durchschnittsalter 47,6 Jahre, Durchschnittsgewicht 74 kg) mit der Diagnose eines subakuten lumbalen Schmerzsyndromes untersucht. Ausgeschlossen waren Patienten mit einer radikulären Symptomatik, ossären Läsionen der Wirbelkörper und entzündlichen oder neoplastischen Veränderungen der Wirbelsäule.

Die Behandlung erfolgte mit 600 mg Azapropazon i.v., die in 5 ml Wasser gelöst und über 5 Minuten langsam i.v. injiziert wurden.

Unmittelbar vor der Injektion und eine Stunde nach der Injektion wurde auf einer isokinetischen Messeinheit für den Rücken (Trunk Extension/ Flexion Unit, Cybex, Division of Lumex Inc., Ronkonkoma, NY, USA) die Maximalkraft und die Leistung für die Flexion und Extension der Rumpfmuskulatur gemessen.

Der Ausdruck *Maximalkraft* wird in diesem Zusammenhang gebraucht, um das bei einer vorgegebenen Winkelgeschwindigkeit gemessene maximale Drehmoment (Peak Torque) bezogen auf den ganzen Bewegungsumfang anzugeben (Masseinheit foot pound). Die *mittlere Leistung* (Average Power) wird berechnet, indem die geleistete Arbeit (Fläche unter der Kurve) in einem Bewegungszyklus durch die entsprechende Kontraktionszeit dividiert wird (Massenheit: Watt).

Die Patienten wurden bei beiden Tests in der gleichen, genau definierten aufrechten Stellung in der Messeinheit fixiert (Abb. 7). Es wurden bei einer Winkelgeschwindigkeit von 60°/sec drei vollständige Bewegungszyklen (Flexion/Extension über den ganzen Bewegungsumfang) und nach einem Pausenintervall von 30 sec nochmals 3 Wiederholungen bei einer Winkel-

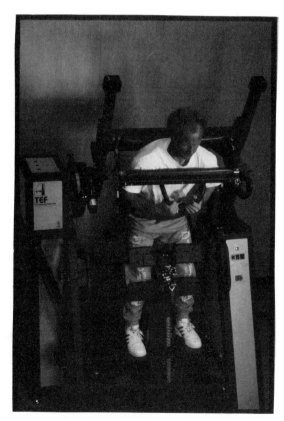

Abb. 7 Trunk Extension/Flexion Unit (TEF).

193

Tab.1 Maximalkraft für Flexion und Extension bei 60°/sec und 120°./sec (Peak Torque in foot-pounds). Test 1 = Ausgangswert, Test 2 = 1 Stunde nach i.v. Azapropazon-Gabe

| | Flexion 60°/sec | | Flexion 120°/sec | | Extension 60°/sec | | Extension 120°/sec | |
	Test 1	Test 2	Test 1	Test 2	Test 1	Test 2	Test 1	Test 2
HF	44	106	13	114	58	126	0	141
BH	130	159	162	169	145	179	151	178
RE	75	79	51	58	75	91	57	83
RC	147	160	152	161	123	165	172	159
GF	193	202	193	199	197	200	197	203
x̄	118	141	114	140	120	152	115	153
▲%	+19.5%		+22.8%		+26.7%		+33.0%	

geschwindigkeit von 120°/sec durchgeführt. Nach dem Test 1 und der erfolgten intravenösen Gabe von Azapropazon ruhten die Patienten für eine Stunde, dann erfolgte Test 2.

3. Resultate

In der Tab. 1 und der Abb. 8 sind die für die Flexion und Extension bei einer Winkelgeschwindigkeit von 60°/sec und 120°/sec vor und eine Stunde nach der intravenösen Azapropazon-Gabe gemessenen Maximalwerte für die Kraft (Peak Torque in foot pound) angegeben. Die entwickelte Kraft bei der Flexion nahm dabei um 19,5% bei 60°/sec, bzw. 22,8% bei 120°/sec zu. Für die Extension betragen die entsprechenden Werte 26,7% und 33,0%.

Die Werte für die mittlere Leistung bei der Flexion und der Extension finden sich in der Tab. 2 und Abb. 9. Bei 60°/sec wurden für die Flexion eine

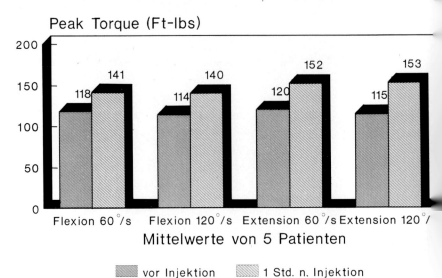

Abb. 8 Maximalkraft für Flexion und Extension bei 60°/sec und 120°/sec.

Tab.2 Mittlere Leistung für Flexion und Extension bei 60°/sec und 120°/sec (average power in watts). Test 1 = Ausgangswert, Test 2 = 1 Stunde nach i.v. Azapropazon-Gabe

	Flexion 60°/sec		Flexion 120°/sec		Extension 60°/sec		Extension 120°/sec	
	Test 1	Test 2	Test 1	Test 2	Test 1	Test 2	Test 1	Test 2
HF	39	109	5	221	44	123	0	277
BM	137	179	299	336	114	176	263	364
RE	75	84	95	103	75	95	89	159
RC	165	196	288	322	123	173	327	310
GF	235	235	422	428	218	221	400	422
$\bar{x}$	130	161	222	282	115	158	216	306
▲%	+23.8%		+27.0%		+37.4%		+41.7%	

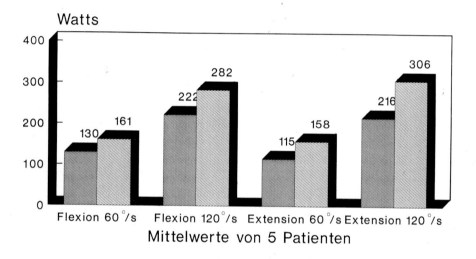

Abb. 9 Mittlere Leistung für Flexion und Extension bei 60°/sec und 120°/sec.

Steigerung um 23,8%, für die Extension um 37,4% gemessen. Bei einer Winkelgeschwindigkeit von 120°/sec erhöhte sich die Leistung bei der Flexion um 27,0%, bei der Extension um 41,7%.

Die grösste Kraft- und Leistungszunahme durch die Medikamentengabe wurde beim Patienten HF gemessen. Die Abb. 10 zeigt die Kraftentwicklung bei 60°/sec vor und nach der Azapropazon-Gabe. Die Maximalwerte wurden dabei mehr als verdoppelt. Bei der höheren Geschwindigkeit von 120°/sec war der Patient vor der Medikamentengabe kaum in der Lage, eine messbare Kraft weder in der Flexions- noch der Extensionsrichtung zu entwickeln. Die Beweglichkeit der Wirbelsäule war deutlich eingeschränkt. Nach der Azapropazon-gabe normalisierte sich der Kurvenverlauf und es bestand eine praktisch normale Kraftentwicklung über das ganze Bewegungsausmass (Abb. 11).

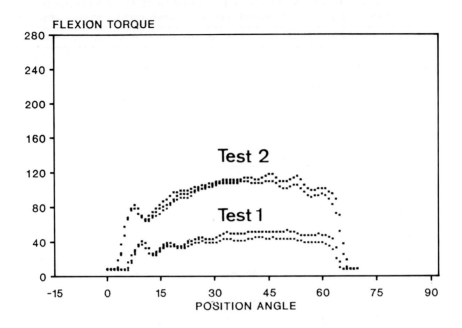

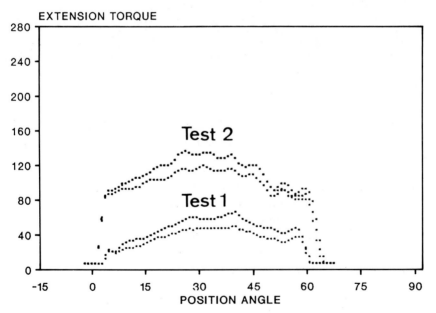

Abb. 10 Maximalkraft für Flexion und Extension bei 60°/sec bei Patient HF. Test 1 = Ausgangswert, Test 2 = 1 Stunde nach i.v. Azapropazon-Gabe.

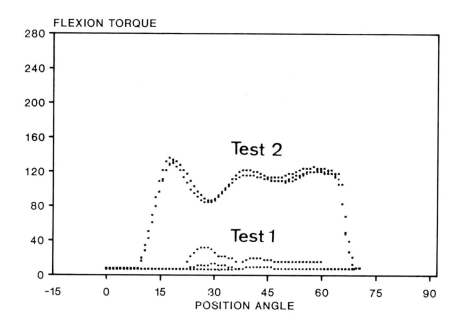

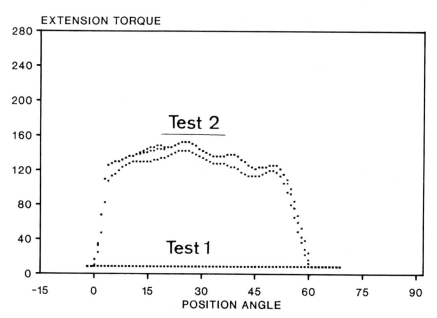

Abb.11 Maximalkraft für Flexion und Extension bei 120°/sec bei Patient HF. Test 1 = Ausgangswert, Test 2 = 1 Stunde nach i.v. Azapropazon-Gabe.

V. DISKUSSION

Die funktionelle muskuläre Kapazität des Rückens lässt sich durch isokinetische Kraftmessgeräte objektiv beurteilen[10-13]. Der Vorteil solcher Messungen liegt darin, dass die Kraftentwicklung, die geleistete Arbeit und erbrachte Leistung über den ganzen Bewegungsablauf und bei verschiedenen Bewegungsgeschwindigkeiten gemessen werden kann. Nicht möglich ist eine Aussage über die Kraftentwicklung in den einzelnen Bewegungssegmenten, die Messwerte beziehen sich auf die Globalfunktion der Rumpfmuskulatur.

In dieser Arbeit wird die Rumpfflexions- und Extensionsbewegung bei Patienten mit subakutem Lumbalsyndrom vor und nach i.v.-Applikation des steroidfreien Antirheumatikums Azapropazon analysiert.

Azapropazon wird heute zu den bewährten nichtsteroidalen Antirheumatika gezählt, dessen Wirkung und Verträglichkeit in adäquater Dosierung gewährleistet ist und das ohne grösseren Probleme breit einzusetzen ist[18].

Therapeutische Wirksamkeit und Verträglichkeit der oralen und der intravenösen Darreichungsformen von Azapropazon sind sowohl durch die Literatur als auch den klinischen Einsatz belegt[19].

Unter den zur Verfügung stehenden nichtsteroidalen Antirheumatika zeichnet sich Azapropazon dadurch aus, dass es auch intravenös verabreicht werden kann, was rasch zu hohen Wirkstoffkonzentrationen in Serum und Gewebe führt. Während nach oraler Gabe von Azapropazon vergleichbare analgetische und antiphlogistische Eigenschaften wie bei anderen nichtsteroidalen Antirheumatika, so z.B. Diclofenac, beschrieben sind[20], ist nach der i.v.-Gabe ein besonders rasch einsetzender, sowohl analgetischer als auch antiphlogistischer Effekt zu erwarten.

Die intravenöse Gabe ist daher vor allem bei akuten Schmerzzuständen rheumatischer Erkrankungen verschiedener Genese als Initialtherapie angezeigt. Für die Weiterbehandlung bietet sich die orale Gabe von Azapropazon an. Dies wird durch zahlreiche Untersuchungen belegt[4,5,14-17,21].

Bei allen in dieser Studie untersuchten Patienten führte die i.v.-Azapropazon-Gabe innerhalb einer Stunde zu einer deutlichen Kraftzunahme in der Rumpfflexion und der Rumpfextension. Die durch das Lumbalsyndrom bedingte Schmerzhemmung schränkte die Kraftentwicklung sowohl bei der langsamen Bewegungsgeschwindigkeit wie auch in grösserem Ausmass bei der schnelleren Geschwindigkeit ein. Der analgetische Effekt des Medikamentes erlaubte, dass neben dem höheren Kraftniveau bei der langsamen Geschwindigkeit nun auch wieder erheblich mehr Kraft bei der koordinativ anspruchsvolleren höheren Bewegungsgeschwindigkeit entwickelt werden konnte. Entsprechend ist die Kraftzunahme bei einer Bewegungsgeschwindigkeit von 120°/sec prozentual höher ausgefallen als bei 60°/sec. In den Abbildungen 10 und 11 ist dieser Medikamenteneffekt eindrücklich dargestellt.

Dic nun vorliegenden Befunde aus der Studie zur analgetischen Wirsamkeit von oralem Azapropazon bei Probanden (ultraschall-evoziertes

Potential) sowie die zuletzt dargestellten Ergebnisse mit dem Cybex-Back-System bei Patienten mit subakutem Lumbovertebralsyndrom untermauern objektivierbar die in den klinischen Prüfungen erzielten Ergebnisse.

Referenzen

1. Mutschler, E, Jahn, U und Thiele, K (1985). Stellung des Azapropazons in Bezug auf die Kategorien nichtsteroidaler Antirheumatika. In: Eberl, R und Fellmann, N (eds), *Rheuma-Forum* Sonder-Nr. **2** (Karlsruhe: G Braun), pp. 13–17

2. Walker, FS (1985). Azapropazone and related benzotriazines. In: Rainsford, KD (ed), *Anti-Inflammatory and Anti-Rheumatic Drugs*, Vol. II: *Newer Anti-Inflammatory Drugs*. (Florida: CRC Press Inc.), pp. 1–32

3. Rainsford, KD (1984). Side-effects of anti-inflammatory analgesic drugs: epidemiology and gastrointestinal tract. *TIPS*, **5**, 156–9

4. Bach, GL, Neubauer, M und Gmeiner, G (1984). Azapropazon intravenös bei Erkrankungen des rheumatischen Formenkreises. 1. Behandlung der aktivierten Arthrose, des LWS-Syndroms und anderer rheumatischer Erkrankungen mit 600 mg Azapropazon i.v. *Arth Rheum*, **6**, 16–21

5. Köchermann, D und Holtfreter, KCh (1987). Posttraumatische orthopädische Behandlung. Untersuchung der antiphlogistischen und analgetischen Wirkung von Azapropazon. *Z Allg Med*, **63**, 156–8

6. Wright, A, Davies I, Walker, FS und Ridell, JG (1989). Azapropazone analgesia in a joint pain model. *Br J Rheumatol* (in press)

7. Wright, A und Davies, I ab I (1989). The recording of brain evoked potentials resulting from intra-articular focused ultrasonic stimulation: a new experimental model for investigating joint pain in humans. *Neuroscience Letters*, **97**, 145–50

8. Bromm, B (1985). Modern techniques to measure pain in healthy man. *Meth Find Expl Clin Pharmacol*, **7**, 161–9

9. Moser, H und Ackermann–Liebrich, U (1986). Die Epidemiologie rheumatischer Erkrankungen in der Schweiz und angrenzenden Ländern. *Editiones 'Roche' Basel*, 47–9

10. Smith, SS, Mayer, TG, Gatchel, RJ und Becker, TJ (1985). Quantification of lumbar function. Part 1: Isometric and multispeed isokinetic trunk strength measures in sagittal and axial planes in normal subjects. *Spine*, **10**, 757–64

11. Mayer, TG, Smith, SS, Keeley, J und Mooney, V (1985). Quantification of lumbar function. Part 2: Sagittal plane trunk strength in chronic low-back pain patients. *Spine*, **10**, 765–72

12. Mayer, TG, Gatchel, RJ, Kishino, N *et al.* (1985). Objective assessment of spine function following industrial injury. A prospective study with comparison group and one-year follow-up. *Spine*, **10**, 482–93

13. Mayer, TG und Gatchel, RJ (1988). Functional restoration for spinal disorders: the sports medicine approach. (Philadelphia: Lea & Febiger)

14. Arquint, A (1987). Analgetisch-antiinflammatorische Therapie bei Operationen im Gelenkbereich. *Therapiewoche Schweiz*, **3**, 266–70

15. Pfeil, J, Niethard, F und Kauth, J (1987). Azapropazon in der Traumatologie und Orthopädie. *Therapiewoche*, **37**, 895–8

16. Esch, PM, Kapphan, J und Gerngross, H (1988). Objektive Schwellungsmessung am oberen Sprunggelenk im prä- und postoperativen Verlauf bei Aussenbandrupturen unter Prüfung der Wirksamkeit von Azapropazon. *Wehrmed Mschr*, **2**, 75–83

17.   Christ, H und Frenkel, G (1985). Tolyprin zur Behandlung von schmerzhaften Schwellungen und Entzündungen nach kieferchirurgischen Eingriffen. *ZWR*, **12**, 986–9

18.   Chlud, K (1986). Die Rheumapyramide. Ein Beitrag zur Klärung von aktuellen Problemen mit nichtsteroidalen Antirheumatika. *EULAR Bulletin*, **3**, 83

19.   Fellmann, N (1985). Standortbestimmung des Azapropazons. Einleitung und Uebersicht. In: Eberl, R und Fellman, N (eds), *Rheuma-Forum* Sonder-Nr.2 (Karlsruhe: G Braun), pp. 5–11

20.   Knüsel, O, Lemmel, EM, Waldburger, M, Pfister, JA und Geerling, FCh (1988). *Therapiewoche Schweiz*, **5**, 402–13

21.   Dunky, A und Eberl, R (1985). Azapropazon bei akuter und chronischer Gicht. In: Eberl, R und Fellmann, N (eds), *Rheuma-Forum* Sonder-Nr. **2**. (Karlsruhe: G Braun), pp. 53–60

Summary

The analgesic efficacy of the non-steroidal anti-inflammatory azapropazone was investigated in clinical trials with semi-quantitative methods of measurement, including pain scales or visual analog scales. Pain regressed substantially within the first hour after intravenous administration of azapropazone; maximum analgesic effect was evident after two to two and one-half hours. Following an intravenous loading dose on the first day, oral administration of azapropazone proved advantageous in further treatment.

The analgesic efficacy of azapropazone was quantified using two different objective methods of investigation. Deep pain receptors in the interphalangeal joint were stimulated by means of ultrasonography in the first study. The potential thus evoked in the brain objectively reflects the pain sensation. The subjects' subjective pain sensation was determined by means of a computer-aided visual analog scale. The analgesic effect of a single oral dose of 600 mg azapropazone was significantly better than that of the placebo and was comparable to the effect of an oral dose of 100 mg pethidine. In the second study, the analgesic effect of azapropazone administered intravenously in patients with subacute low-back pain was investigated with the aid of an isokinetic dynamometer (Cybex Back System). A perceptible improvement in back function occurred owing to reduction in subjective pain. One hour after the i.v. injection of 600 mg azapropazone an increase of 23.8% (flexion) and 37.4% (extension) was measured for average capacity at an angular velocity of 60°/sec. At 120°/sec. flexion capacity increased by 27.0% and extension by 41.7%.

Zusammenfassung

Die analgetische Wirksamkeit des nichtsteroidalen Antirheumatikums Azapropazon wurde in klinischen Prüfungen mit semiquantitativen Messmethoden, u.a. Schmerzskalen oder Visuelle Analog-Skalen, untersucht. Ein wesentlicher Rückgang der Schmerzen wurde innerhalb der ersten Stunde nach intravenöser Verabreichung von Azapropazon erreicht; die maximale analgetische Wirkung wurde nach zwei bis zweieinhalb Stunden festgestellt. Nach der intra-venösen Initialtherapie am ersten Tag hat sich die orale Weiterbehandlung mit Azapropazon als günstig gezeigt.

Die analgetische Wirksamkeit von Azapropazon konnte mit zwei unterschiedlichen objektiven Untersuchungsmethoden quantifiziert werden. Mittels Ultraschall wurden im ersten Modell bei Probanden tiefliegende Schmerzrezeptoren des Interphalangealgelenkes gereizt. Das dadurch evozierte Potential im Gehirn widerspiegelt objektiv den empfundenen Schmerz. Die subjektive Schmerzempfindung der Probanden wurde mittels computergestützter Visuellen Analog-Skala erfasst. Die analgetische Wirkung einer oralen Einzelgabe von 600 mg Azapropazon war signifikant besser als diejenige von Placebo und war mit der Wirkung von 100 mg Pethidin p.o. vergleichbar. In der zweiten Studie wurde bei Patienten mit subakutem Lumbovertebralsyn-drom die analgetische Wirkung von intravenös verabreichtem Azapropazon mit Hilfe einer isokinetischen Kraftmesseinheit (Cybex-Back-System) untersucht. Durch Verminderung der subjektiv empfundenen Schmerzen trat objektivierbar eine Verbesserung der funktionellen

Leistungsfähigkeit des Rückens ein. Eine Stunde nach der Injektion von 600 mg Azapropazon i.v. wurde für die mittlere Leistung bei einer Winkelgeschwindigkeit von 60°/sec eine Steigerung von 23.8% (Flexion) bzw. 37.4% (Extension) gemessen. Bei 120°/sec erhöhte sich die Leistung bei der Flexion um 27.0%, bei der Extension um 4.17%.

Resumé

L'efficacité analgésique de l'azapropazone, anti-inflammatoire non stéroïdien (AINS), a été mesurée à l'aide de méthodes semi-quantitatives (incluant échelles de douleur ou échelles visuelles analogues). Les douleurs ont régressé considérablement au cours de la première heure après l'administration intraveineuse d'azapropazone; l'effet analgésique maximum a été observé après 2–2.5 heures. Après la dose d'attaque administrée par voie i.v. le premier jour, la poursuite du traitement avec l'azapropazone par voie orale a eu un effet favorable.

L'efficacité analgésique de l'azapropazone a pu être quantifiée à l'aide de deux méthodes d'évaluation objective. Dans le premier modèle, les récepteurs profonds de la douleur au niveau de l'articulation phalangienne ont été stimulés par ultra-sons. Le potentiel évoqué au niveau du cerveau reflète objectivement la sensation douloureuse. La douleur subjective éprouvée par les sujets a été déterminée à l'aide d'une échelle visuelle analogue contrôlée par ordinateur. L'effet analgésique d'une dose orale unique de 600 mg d'azapropazone a été significativement supérieur à celui du placebo et comparable à celui d'une dose de 100 mg de péthidine p.o. Dans le deuxième essai, l'effet analgésique de l'azapropazone administrée par voie i.v. a été analysé par dynamométrie isocinétique (Cybex-Back-System) chez des patients souffrant de lombalgie subaiguë. Une amélioration sensible de la capacité fonctionelle dorsale a pu être objectivée grâce à la diminution de la douleur subjective. Une heure après l'injection i.v. de 600 mg d'azapropazone, on a enregistré un accroissement de la capacité moyenne de 23.8% (flexion) et de 37.4% (extension) à une vitesse angulaire de 60°/sec. A 120°/sec, la capacité de flexion a augmenté de 27.0% et celle d'extension de 41.7%.

15
Überblick über die Anwendung von Azapropazon nach operativen Eingriffen und bei traumatisierten Patienten

[Review of application of azapropazone in post-operative and traumatic conditions]

E Schneider and FU Niethard

I. HISTORISCHER ÜBERBLICK

Azapropazon, das zur Gruppe der Benzotriazine gehört, hat sich nunmehr 20 Jahre in der klinischen Anwendung bewährt.

In einer Reihe von experimentellen Studien konnte belegt werden, dass hauptsächlich die Freisetzung lysosomaler Enzyme[1], die Prostaglandinsynthese und Monozytenmigration[2] unter Einfluss dieser Substanz gehemmt werden. Daraus lässt sich eine antiphlogistische Wirkung ableiten. Dieser Effekt, Weichteilschwellungen entweder zu verhindern oder zumindest abzumildern, spielt sowohl in der Traumatologie als auch in allen operativen Fächern eine hervorragende Rolle. Nicht selten hängen einerseits die Erfolge operativer Eingriffe, andererseits aber auch eine rasche Rehabilitation von der Wirksamkeit verabreichter antiphlogistischer Substanzen ab.

Aufgrund seiner Eigenschaften wird Azapropazon vorzugsweise bei Erkrankungen des rheumatischen Formenkreises eingesetzt und hat sich in dieser Indikation bereits als gut wirksam erwiesen.

Seit nunmehr 20 Jahren liegen auch Resultate über die Anwendung dieses Medikaments in der Traumatologie und in verschiedenen operativen Fachrichtungen vor. Unsere Ausführungen sollen einen Überblick darüber geben, welche Erfahrungen hier in zwei Jahrzehnten gesammelt werden konnten. Dabei möchten wir neben einer kritischen Sichtung der früheren Studien die Ergebnisse eigener Forschungsarbeit sowie aktuelle Untersuchungen mitberücksichtigen.

Danach soll versucht werden, die Erkenntnisse aus 20 Jahren klinischer Anwendung darzustellen und daraus ein aktuell gültiges Behandlungskonzept sowohl für die Traumatologie als auch für die postoperative Nachsorge zu erarbeiten.

Azapropazone – 20 years of clinical use. Rainsford, KD (ed)
© Kluwer Academic Publishers. Printed in Great Britain

Vorausgeschickt sei, dass bei der Durchsicht sämtlicher relevanter Arbeiten im wesentlichen folgende Fachgebiete Berücksichtigung fanden:

1. hals-nasen-ohrenärztliche- bzw. mund-, zahn- und kieferchirurgische Eingriffe und deren Folgezustände;

2. die Versorgung nicht operativ behandlungs pflichtiger Verletzungen;

3. die Nachsorge nach operativen Eingriffen aus der Orthopädie, Traumatologie und Allgemeinchirurgie.

Selbstverständlich kann ein Überblick wie der hier vorliegende keinen Anspruch auf vollständige Erfassung der Resultate sämtlicher Arbeitsgruppen erheben.

Aus den Jahren 1969 bis 1971 liegen im wesentlichen vier Berichte vor (s. Tabelle 1), deren wichtigste Aussagen im folgenden zusammengefasst werden sollen: Tominaga[3] berichtete über 22 Patienten nach orthopädischen Eingriffen, die nicht näher bezeichnet wurden. Die Patienten erhielten 5 Tage lang je 3 × 200 mg Azapropazon oral. Ohne die Ergebnisse näher zu spezifizieren, wurde die Wirksamkeit der Substanz bezüglich Spontan-, Druckschmerz, Schwellung, Rötung, Wärmegefühl und Ausmass einer Blutung bzw. Sekretion in knapp 80% der Fälle als positiv eingestuft.

Oyamada[4] verabreichte 24 Patienten 2 Tage prä- und 2 Wochen postoperativ täglich 2–4 Tabletten Azapropazon. Eine positive Wirkung bezüglich postoperativer Schmerzen wurde ebenso festgestellt wie in ca. 70% ein deutlich abschwellender Effekt.

Vokner[5] dehnte die Indikation für eine postoperative Antiphlogese mit Azapropazon auf ein breites allgemeinchirurgisches Spektrum aus. Neben einigen konservativ behandelten Fällen (z.B. Kontusionen, Frakturen und Luxationen) wurde über die Behandlungsergebnisse bei Patienten nach operativ versorgten Knochenbrüchen, Hernien, Wunden etc. berichtet. Nach oraler Gabe von 4 × 200 bis 4 × 400 mg pro Tag über durchschnittlich 7 bis 8 Tage zeigten etwa 86% der Patienten einen Erfolg im Sinne eines Schwellungsrückgangs. Die analgetische Wirksamkeit war gering.

Schmökel[6] (1971) konnte ein Kollektiv von 71 Patienten aus dem traumatologisch-chirurgischen Bereich vorstellen, von denen 44 operativ versorgt werden mussten. Die durchschnittliche Therapiedauer betrug 7 Tage bei einer Dosis zwischen 600 und 1200 mg Azapropazon oral pro Tag. Beurteilt wurden Schwellungsrückgang und Schmerzreduktion, ohne jedoch im einzelnen eine Aufschlüsselung vorzunehmen. Knapp 90% der Patienten wiesen sehr gute bis gute, 9% mässige und 3% schlechte Resultate auf.

Die genannten Arbeiten können weder bezüglich Studiendesign noch statistischer Aufarbeitung heutigen Ansprüchen genügen. Allen Studien gemeinsam war die ausschliesslich perorale Verabreichung des Medikaments. Kontroll- bzw. Vergleichsgruppen wurden nicht berücksichtigt.

Dennoch konnten aus den Erfahrungen, die mit 166 Patienten gewonnen wurden, bezüglich der Charakteristika von Azapropazon wichtige

Table 1 First studies about the application of azapropazone in operative and traumatic conditions

Authors	Dosage Administration Duration of therapy	Indication	Method a. Kind of study b. Number of patients (n) c. Judgement of therapeutic effect	Results	Side-effects
M Tominaga (1963)[3]	3 × 200 mg oral for 5 days (1 dose pre-op)	Postoperative pain	a. Uncontrolled study b. n = 22 c. The patients judged the symptoms: spontaneous pain; local oppressive pain; swelling; reddening & hot sensation	Effective in 77% of the cases relative to all symptoms	Gastric discomfort in 2 patients (= 9%)
Y Oyamada (1969)[4]	2–4 tab/day (dosage was not given) 2 days pre-op and 2 weeks post-op	Swelling before and after orthopaedic surgery; postoperative pain	a. Uncontrolled study b. n = 24 c. Judgement of pain and swelling	Good response; excellent efficacy in 71% of the cases relative to both symptoms	Abdominal pain in 1 patient generalized exanthema in 1 patient (total = 8%)

continued

Table 1 *continued*

Authors	Dosage Administration Duration of therapy	Indication	Method a. Kind of study b. Number of patients (n) c. Judgement of therapeutic effect	Results	Side-effects
J Vokner (1970)[5]	Children: 3 × 200 mg/day oral Adults: 4 × 200 mg/day oral for 4–17 days (average 7.4 days)	Pain and inflammation (surgical indications: 43 patients; rheumatic diseases: 6 patients)	a. Uncontrolled study b. n = 49 (among these 18 patients were treated conservatively and 31 operatively) c. Judgement of pain and swelling	Good response; excellent reduction of swelling in 86% of the cases: little analgesic effect	Extraordinary safety
W Schmökel (1971)[6]	3 × 200 mg/day or 3 × 400 mg/day oral for 3–30 days (average 7 days)	Post-traumatic and postoperative inflammation and swelling	a. Uncontrolled study b. n = 71 c. Judgement of the reduction of swelling and inflammation by the physician; judgment of pain by the patient	In 88% of the cases good response; very good antiphlogistic efficacy	Gastric disturbances in 4 patients, exanthema in 2 patients (total = 9%)

Table 2 Application of azapropazone in ENT therapeutics and maxillo-facial surgery

Authors	Dosage Administration Duration of therapy	Indication	Method a. Kind of study b. Number of patients (n) c. Judgement of therapeutic effect	Results	Side-effects
J Gabka and E Foltin (1971)[7]	4 × 300 mg/day oral for 5 days post-op (control: physical post-op treatment)	Swelling and inflammation following maxillo-facial surgery	a. Controlled study b. Control n = 25, azapropazone n = 25c. Reproducible pre- and post-op measurement of the swelling from certain points of the face	Significant reduction in the duration and the extent of swelling; good analgesic efficacy.	—
F Perrini and G Cocchi (1979)[8]	4 × 300 mg/day oral 3 days post-op (1 dose pre-op)	Swelling and pain after extended dental surgery	a. Uncontrolled study b. n = 58 c. Judgement of the symptoms: pain, swelling and haemorrhage	Good antiphlogistic and analgesic efficacy in 99% of the patients	—
J Gabka (1983)[9]	Azapropazone vs. Lysin-ASS and placebo azapropazone: 300, 600, 900 and 1200 mg i.v.; Lysin-ASS: 900 mg i.v.; Placebo: (0.9% NaCl) i.v.	Pain	a. Controlled randomized, single-blind cross-over study b. n = 12 c. Determination of the individual threshold of pain by electrical stimulation of the dental pulpa	* Dose-dependency of the analgesic effect of azapropazone * Max. of analgesic effect after 50–60 min	Tiredness in 4 test persons; heart beating after 600 and 900 mg azapropazone in 1 test person

continued

Table 2 continued

Authors	Dosage Administration Duration of therapy	Indication	Method a. Kind of study b. Number of patients (n) c. Judgement of therapeutic effect	Results	Side-effects
H Christ and G Frenkel (1985)[10]	600 mg/day i.v. 1 day pre-op 2 × 600 mg/day oral 5 days post-op	Pain and swelling following maxillo-dental surgery	a. Uncontrolled study b. n = 40 c. Judgement of the analgesic effect by the patients and of the swelling by the physician	Complete analgesy in more than 60%; complete reduction of swelling in more than 90% of the patients	—
H Gastpar (1988)[11]	Azapropazone vs. control (physical treament) 2 × 600 mg i.v. 1–2 days post-op; 2 × 600 mg/day oral 4–5 days post-op	Pain and swelling following ENT surgery	a. Controlled, open, double-blind study b. Control n = 40, azapropazone n = 40 c. Judgement of swelling and pain by the physician and the patients	Excellent antiphlogistic efficacy in 85–90% (azapropazone) vs. 60% (control); no difference in the analgesic effect between both groups	—

G

Schlüsse gezogen werden.

1. Nach Verletzungen bzw. Operationen schien die abschwellende Potenz deutlich zu sein.

2. Der analgetische Effekt war geringer.

3. Eine Auswirkung auf relevante Laborparameter wurde nicht festgestellt; lediglich 10 Patienten klagten über Nebenwirkungen, vornehmlich im Magen-Darmtrakt.

Es blieb nun weiteren Arbeitsgruppen vorbehalten, das Wirkprofil der Substanz anhand weiterer Studien zu verifizieren.

Gabka und Foltin[7] wiesen 1971 ebenfalls darauf hin, dass vor allem bei Operationen im Gesichtsbereich eine rasche Abschwellung über den Erfolg entscheiden kann. Erfreulicherweise stellte er die Behandlungsergebnisse mit Azapropazon einer nur mit physikalischen Massnahmen nachbehandelten Kontrollgruppe gegenüber. Er verabreichte 5 Tage postoperativ 1200 mg Azapropazon pro Tag oral. Der Schwellungszustand wurde an definierten Punkten reproduzierbar gemessen. Sowohl das Ausmass der Schwellung als auch die durchschnittliche Schwellungsdauer waren in der Versuchsgruppe geringer. Ein ganz erheblicher analgetischer Effekt wurde beschrieben. Die Ergebnisse konnten dann bei über 200 ambulanten Patienten mit kleineren operativen Eingriffen bestätigt werden. Nebenwirkungen wurden nicht beobachtet.

Aus den Jahren 1979, 1983, 1985 und 1988 (Tab. 2) liegen weitere Erfahrungsberichte aus dem Bereich der Zahnheilkunde vor. Perrini und Cocchi[8] (1979) stellten 58 Patienten, bei denen grössere zahn-chirurgische Eingriffe vorgenommen worden waren, vor. Er führte eine Nachbehandlung über 3 postoperative Tage mit 4 × 300 mg Azapropazon per os durch. Seine Kriterien: Schmerz, Schwellung, und Blutung.

Da auch hier eine Kontrollgruppe fehlt, können die folgenden Angaben nur hinweisgebend sein: von 58 Patienten waren 43 nahezu schmerzfrei; eine wesentliche Ödemneigung war nur in einem Fall zu erkennen; wesentliche Blutungen wurden bei keinem Patienten festgestellt.

Die analgetische Wirkung von Azapropazon wurde durch die Arbeit von Gabka aus dem Jahre 1983[9] mit einer randomisierten Studie experimentell untersucht. Bei 12 gesunden Probanden wurde elektrisch an der Zahnpulpa ein Schmerz induziert; die Analgesie erfolgte durch intravenös verabreichtes Azapropazon gegen Kontrollgruppen mit Lysin-Acetylsalicylsäure ('Aspisol'®) bzw. Placebo. Beginnend 30 Minuten nach intravenöser Applikation von 300 bis 1200 mg Azapropazon wurde mit einem Maximum zwischen 50 und 60 Minuten ein deutlich schmerzlindernder Effekt festgestellt.

Christ und Frenkel[10] beschrieben 1985 erstmals die Resultate einer gemischt intravenösen/oralen Behandlung von 40 Patienten, die sich kiefer-chirurgischen Eingriffen unterzogen hatten. Eine Kontrollgruppe fehlt. Abgesehen davon, dass keine Nebenwirkungen festgestellt wurden, fand sich bei nahezu zwei Dritteln der Patienten ein guter analgetischer Effekt, während bei 90% ein völliger Schwellungsrückgang innerhalb kurzer Zeit zu beobachten war.

Alle Anforderungen an ein zeitgemässes Studiendesign erfüllt die Untersuchung von Gastpar 1988[11], die im Rahmen einer offenen randomisierten Arbeit die antiphlogistische und analgetische Wirkung von Azapropazon bei 40 Patienten nach maxillo-facialen operativen Eingriffen untersuchte und mit einem gleich grossen Kontrollkollektiv verglich. Die Substanz wurde in der Versuchsgruppe am ersten und zweiten postoperativen Tag intravenös, danach über 4 bis 5 Tage peroral verabreicht (Tagesdosis 1200 mg).

Die Patienten wurden bezüglich Analgesie und Schwellung untersucht. Dabei waren bezüglich des analgetischen Effekts zwischen den Gruppen keine statistisch signifikanten Unterschiede festzustellen. Bezüglich der abschwellenden Wirkung sprachen die Ergebnisse signifikant für die Behandlung mit Azapropazon.

Die neueren Studien, vor allem aus dem Bereich der Hals-Nasen-Ohren-Heilkunde und Kieferchirurgie, bestätigen die Hinweise, die uns aus den 60er und 70er Jahren vorliegen. Von grosser Bedeutung ist die in allen Studien dokumentierte antiphlogistische Potenz, die gerade in den genannten Bereichen für den weiteren Verlauf nach einem operativen Eingriff von ausschlaggebender Bedeutung ist. Nicht einheitlich war die Meinung bezüglich des analgetischen Effekts, wobei möglicherweise zu diskutieren wäre, ob eine Schmerzlinderung über die abschwellende Wirkung der Substanz angenommen werden kann.

Aus den Arbeiten kristallisierte sich ein sehr geringer Prozentsatz von unerwünschten Nebenwirkungen heraus. Zudem bewährte sich das gemischt intravenös/orale Behandlungskonzept, das zweifellos in der unmittelbaren peri- und postoperativen Phase erhebliche Vorteile zeigt: zum einen scheint die Wirkung frühzeitiger einzutreten, zum anderen muss nicht auf anaesthesiologische Gesichtspunkte bezüglich oraler Medikation unmittelbar nach einem Eingriff Rücksicht genommen werden.

Auch aus dem Bereich Orthopädie und Traumatologie liegen aus den vergangenen eineinhalb Jahrzehnten, schwerpunktmässig aus den 80er Jahren, eine Reihe hervorragender Studien vor (Tab. 3). Nach den ersten Erfahrungsberichten, die weiter oben dargestellt wurden, wird mit der Arbeit von Täger und Brunner (1973) die Phase der kontrollierten Studien eingeleitet[12]. Es wurde untersucht, ob zwischen Azapropazon und Oxyphenbutazon bezüglich der Kriterien Schwellung, Rötung, Schmerz und Nebenwirkungen signifikante Unterschiede herauszuarbeiten sind. 64 Patienten waren am Haltungs- und Bewegungsapparat operiert worden, bei weiteren 10 wurden konservative Behandlungskonzepte durchgeführt. Das operative Spektrum umfasste ein orthopädisches und traumatologisches Patientengut (Endoprothetik, Osteotomien, Osteosynthesen etc.).

Die statistische Auswertung ergab, dass die beiden verglichenen Substanzen hinsichtlich der genannten Kriterien keine signifikanten Unterschiede zeigten. Gastrointestinale Unverträglichkeit führte bei 4 mit Azapropazon behandelten Patienten zum Abbruch der Medikation. In der Oxyphenbutazongruppe mussten 11 Patienten die Therapie abbrechen; 7 ebenfalls aufgrund gastrointestinaler Unverträglichkeit sowie 4 aufgrund von Hautreaktionen.

Aus 1987 liegen uns drei Arbeiten vor, die die Eigenschaften von Azapropazon in der Akutphase nach Verletzungen bzw. in der peri- und postoperativen Zeitspanne nach orthopädisch traumatologischen Eingriffen dokumentieren. Studiendesign und Behandlungskonzept sind ähnlich:

1. in der Frühphase erfolgt eine intravenöse, später eine orale Applikation der Substanz;

2. Kontrollkollektive sind vorhanden (Arquint: nicht-steroidale Antiphlogistika, Köchermann: Placebo, Pfeil: konservative Behandlung).

Arquint[13] untersuchte 45 Patienten nach Operationen an Schulter-, Hüft- und Kniegelenken hinsichtlich der analgetischen und antiphlogistischen Wirksamkeit sowie der Verträglichkeit von Azapropazon. Die Vergleichsgruppe (40 Patienten) erhielt Oxyphenbutazon. Herausgestellt wird, dass die Schwellungen von beiden Behandlungsmethoden etwa gleich gut beeinflusst wurden, während Häufigkeit und Intensität der Schmerzzustände unter Azapropazon schneller abnahmen.

Köchermann und Holtfreter[14] behandelten 40 Patienten mit posttraumatischen Schwellungen und Schmerzen, die deswegen ihre orthopädische Ambulanz aufgesucht hatten. Die Doppelblind-Studie beinhaltete Folgezustände von Kontusionen, Dislokationen, Luxationen und Distorsionen, die alle konservativ zu behandeln waren.

Die antiphlogistische Wirksamkeit von Azapropazon wurde durch vergleichende Umfangsmessung der verletzten Extremität am ersten und am letzten Tag der Untersuchung überprüft. Unter Azapropazon wurde ein mässiger bis vollständiger Schwellungsrückgang in 89% der Fälle beobachtet, im Gegensatz zum 42%igen Abschwellungserfolg in der Placebogruppe. Auch die Schmerzlinderung, die die Patienten anhand einer visuellen Analogskala angeben konnten, war unter Azapropazon vergleichsweise grösser. Lediglich zwei Patienten klagten über Nebenwirkungen nach der Injektion, die vornehmlich den Gastrointestinaltrakt betrafen.

Über die Erfahrungen an unserer Klinik haben wir (Pfeil *et al.*[15]) im selben Jahr berichtet. Um den Stellenwert von Azapropazon bei der Behandlung von postoperativen und posttraumatischen Schwellungszuständen zu erarbeiten, wurde eine offene vergleichende klinische Studie durchgeführt. Beurteilungskriterien waren die abschwellende Wirkung einerseits sowie die Analgesie und Verträglichkeit andererseits.

62 Patienten mit unterschiedlichen Verletzungen, vor allem im Bereich der Extremitäten (Kontusion, Distorsionen, Luxation, Frakturen etc.) fanden Eingang in die Studie und wurden randomisiert einer Azapropazon- (n = 40) sowie einer Kontrollgruppe (n = 22) zugeteilt. Die Versuchsgruppe erhielt am ersten Tag 1200 mg der Substanz intravenös, danach 6 Tage lang 2 × täglich

Table 3 Application of azapropazone in surgery and traumatology

Authors	Dosage Administration Duration of therapy	Indication	Method a. Kind of study b. Number of patients (n) c. Judgement of therapeutic effect	Results	Side-effects
KH Täger and E Brunner (1973)[12]	Azapropazone vs. oxyphenbutazone (dosage not given)	Pain and swelling following surgery and traumata	a. Controlled, double-blind study b. n=74 (control n=37, aza n=37) c. Reduction of reddening, swelling, spontaneous and oppressive pain	No statistically significant differences between aza and oxy (good efficacy of aza in 80%; of oxy in 62%)	Aza: gastrointestinal complaints in 5 patients (14%) oxy: gastrointestinal complaints and exanthema in 11 patients (30%)
A Arquint (1987)[13]	Azapropazone vs. oxyphenbutazone aza: 2 × 600 mg i.v. day of op; 2 × 600 mg/day oral 3–5 days post-op	Pain and swelling following operations of the joints	a. Controlled, open study b. n=85 (control n=40, aza n=45) c. Judgement of the swelling by the physician and the analgesic effect by the patients	No significant difference between both substances concerning the swelling, but better analgesic efficacy of aza	Gastrointestinal complaints in a total of 6 patients (7%); no difference between both substances

aza = azapropazone; oxy = oxyphenbutazone.

continued

Table 3 *continued*

Authors	Dosage Administration Duration of therapy	Indication	Method a. Kind of study b. Number of patients (n) c. Judgement of therapeutic effect	Results	Side-effects
D. Köchermann and K Ch Holtfreter (1987)[14]	Azapropazone vs. placebo 2 × 600 mg/day i.v. for 1 day; 2 × 600 mg/day oral for 6 days	Pain and swelling following traumata	a. Controlled, randomized, double-blind study b. n=40 (control n=20, aza n=20) c. Measurement of the extent of the injured extremity compared to the uninjured; judgement of the analgesic effect by the patient	Antiphlogistic effect: 89% (aza) vs. 42% (placebo) analgesic effect: 100% (aza) vs. 47% (placebo)	Gastrointestinal complaints in 2 patients (10%) of the aza group
J Pfeil, F Neithard and J Kauth (1987)[15]	Azapropazone vs. control azapropazone: 1–2 × 600 mg/day i.v. for 1 day; 2 × 600 mg/day for 6 days	Pain and swelling following orthopaedic surgery and trauma	a. Controlled, randomized, open study b. n=62 (control n=22, aza n=40) c. Judgement of analgesic effect and swelling by the physician and the patients (swelling: comparison to uninjured extremity)	Decrease in swelling: 89% (aza) vs. 48% (control); good analgesic efficacy: 92% (aza) vs. 81% (control)	Gastrointestinal complaints in 3 patients (8%) of the aza group

continued

aza = azapropazone; oxy = oxyphenbutazone.

213

Table 3 *continued*

Authors	*Dosage* *Administration* *Duration of therapy*	*Indication*	*Method* *a. Kind of study* *b. Number of patients (n)* *c. Judgement of* *therapeutic effect*	*Results*	*Side-effects*
PM Esch, J Kapphan and H Gerngross (1988)[16]	Azapropazone vs. placebo azapropazone: 2 × 600 mg i.v. one day before, during and after the op; 2 × 600 mg/day oral for 5 days	Pain and swelling following surgery of the lateral ligament of ankle	a. Controlled randomized double-blind study b. n = 50 (control n = 25, aza n = 25) c. Quantitative measurement of the swelling in a water-filled vessel; judgement of the analgesic effect by the patients	Reduction of swelling: 3 day post op: 38% (aza) vs. 30% (plac); 7 days post-op: 30% (aza) vs. 1% (plac); better analgesic effect of aza compared to plac	No safety problems

aza = azapropazone; plac = placebo.

214

1 Tablette à 600 mg. Die Kontrollgruppe wurde 7 Tage lang rein konservativ behandelt (Physiotherapie, Gipsruhigstellung, etc.).

Zu Beginn der Untersuchung unterschieden sich die Patienten beider Gruppen nicht wesentlich hinsichtlich ihrer Daten und Diagnosen. 57 Patienten konnten ausgewertet werden. Die Resultate: Es konnte gezeigt werden, dass bei den mit Azapropazon behandelten Patienten eine signifikant stärkere Schwellungsabnahme feststellbar war als bei den Patienten der Kontrollgruppe. Nicht so deutlich war der Unterschied der Kollektive bezüglich des analgetischen Effekts, wobei bei 92% der Patienten der Azapropazon-Gruppe eine deutliche bis vollständige Schmerzlinderung, allerdings auch bei 81% der Patienten in der Kontrollgruppe, notiert wurde. 3 Patienten mussten aufgrund von gastrointestinalen Störungen die Studie vorzeitig abbrechen.

1988 verglich die Gruppe um Esch[16] mit ihrer Doppelblind-Studie (Azapropazon gegen Placebo) die Schwellung im prä- und postoperativen Verlauf bei fibularen Kapselbandrupturen. Die Medikation erfolgte hier am Tag vor, während und nach der Operation intravenös, danach für 2 bis 6 Tage oral. Placebo- und Azapropazongruppe umfassten jeweils 25 Patienten. Kriterien waren Schwellung, Schmerz und Verträglichkeit. Einen deutlichen Rückgang der Schwellung beobachtete Esch am 3. Tag postoperativ bei 60% der Patienten in der Azapropazongruppe, jedoch nur bei 30% der Patienten des Kontrollkollektivs. Bei den Patienten, die erfolgreich antiphlogistisch behandelt werden konnten, war auch das Schmerzniveau deutlich geringer.

Eine signifikante analgetische Wirkung per se konnte nicht belegt werden. Das Präparat wurde von sämtlichen Patienten gut vertragen.

Aus dem Überblick der neueren orthopädischen und traumatologischen Arbeiten lassen sich folgende Anforderungen an die Substanz Azapropazon zusammentragen:

1. Gewünscht wird ein schnellwirksames Pharmakon mit effektiver antiphlogistischer Potenz.

2. Eine analgetische Komponente ist erwünscht.

3. Das Medikament soll rasch wirksam sein und eine praktikable Darreichung ermöglichen.

4. Interaktionen mit anderen häufig postoperativ eingesetzten Arzneimitteln sollen nicht auftreten, Nebenwirkungen selten sein.

Die Resultate der neueren Studien belegen eindrucksvoll und nunmehr auch statistisch signifikant die Vermutungen, die aus den früheren Arbeiten abgeleitet werden konnten:

1. Ausgezeichnete antiphlogistische Eigenschaften liegen vor.

2. Eine gewisse analgetische Potenz wird zumindest in einigen Arbeiten unterstrichen.

3. Nebenwirkungen (vor allem im gastrointestinalen Bereich) sind selten.

215

4. Eine Interaktion mit anderen Medikamenten, die postoperativ relevant sind, wurde ebensowenig beschrieben wie signifikante auf die Wirksubstanz zurückzuführende Verschiebungen der Laborparameter.

Als Darreichungsform hat sich am Tage der Verletzung bzw. des operativen Eingriffs die intravenöse Applikation, danach die orale Medikation über etwa 5 Tage mit einer Tagesdosis von 1200 mg bewährt. Hierbei kann sowohl ein rascher Wirkungseintritt zum Bedarfszeitpunkt als auch eine praktikable Weiterführung der Behandlung erreicht werden.

Es ist somit gerechtfertigt, die Indikation zur Verwendung der Wirksubstanz Azapropazon über den entzündlich rheumatischen Formenkreis hinaus auf akut traumatisierte und frisch operierte Patienten dann auszudehnen, wenn erhebliche Schwellungszustände bzw. deren Folgen zu befürchten sind.

Referenzen

1. Arrigoni-Martelli, E and Restelli, A (1972). Release of lysosomal enzymes in experimental inflammations; effects of anti-inflammatory drugs. *Europ J Pharmacol*, **19**, 191–8
2. Mackin, WM, Rakich, SM and Marshall, CL (1986). Inhibition of rat neutrophil functional responses by azapropazone, an anti-gout drug. *Biochem Pharmacol*, **35**, 917–22
3. Tominaga, M (1969). Clinical results of azapropazone for post-operative pain. *Medic Treatment*, **2**
4. Oyamada, Y (1969). Examination of the effect of HK-70 used in operative cases. *J New Remedies & Clinic*, **18**
5. Vokner, J (1970). Klinische Erfahrung mit Azapropazon in der Chirurgie. *Praxis*, **50**, 1756–8
6. Schmökel, W (1971). Azapropazon in der Traumatologie. *Schweizer Rundschau Med (Praxis)*, **60**, 1114–6
7. Gabka, J and Foltin, E (1971). Objektivierung der Wirkung des neuen Antiphlogistikums Prolixan® 300 bei post-operativen Schwellungen. *Therapiewoche*, **21**, 2470–4
8. Perrini, F and Cocchi, G (1979). L'impiego di azapropazone in chirurgia odontostomatologica. *Dental Cadmos*, **11**, 56–60
9. Gabka, J (1983). The dose-dependent analgesic effect of intravenously administered azapropazone. *Clin Trials J*, **20**, 219–30
10. Christ, H and Frenkel, G (1985). Tolyprin® zur Behandlung von schmerzhaften Schwellungen und Entzündungen nach kieferorthopädischen Eingriffen. *ZWR*, **12**, 986–9
11. Gastpar, H (1988). Azapropazon in der Behandlung postoperativer Schwellungszustände nach maxillo-fazialen Eingriffen. *Med Welt*, **39**, 1383–5
12. Täger, KH and Brunner, E (1973). Therapeutische Erfahrungsberichte zur Anwendung von nicht-steroidalen Antiphlogistika bei postoperativen und posttraumatischen Schwellungen. *Med Welt*, **24**, 1752–3
13. Arquint, A (1987). Analgetisch-antiinflammatorische Therapie bei Operationen im Gelenkbereich. *Therapiewoche*, **3**
14. Köchermann, D and Holtfreter, K Ch (1987). Posttraumatische orthopädische Behandlung. *ZFA*, **63**, 156–8
15. Pfeil, J, Niethard, N and Kauth, J (1987). Azapropazon in der Traumatologie und Orthopädie. *Therapiewoche*, **37**, 895–8

16.   Esch, PM, Kapphan, J and Gerngross, H (1988). Objektive Schwellungsmessung am oberen Sprunggelenk im prä- und postoperativen Verlauf bei Aussenbandrupturen unter Prüfung der Wirksamkeit von Azapropazon. *Wehrmed Mschr*, **2**, 75–83

Summary

The findings from 20 years of experience with the clinical application of azapropazone in the area of ENT therapeutics, oral surgery (teeth and jaw), as well as orthopedics, traumatology and general surgery have been compiled.

The first studies, which in part do not meet the high methodical demands of today, already showed a good reduction in swelling using azapropazone, along with a relatively low number of adverse drug reactions.

The distinctive antiphlogistic potency of azapropazone was confirmed in further investigations, the area of ENT, surgery of the jaw and facial surgery, as well as in orthopedics and traumatology.

In addition, several scientific papers have also given a good analgesic efficacy.

Intravenous injection on the day of the injury, as well as operative intervention followed by continued oral treatment for more than 5 days (with a daily dose of 1200 mg of azapropazone), proved to be the most effective.

Zusammenfassung

Die Ergebnisse aus 20-jähriger Erfahrung mit der klinischen Anwendung von Azapropazon in den Bereichen HNO-Heilkunde und Zahn- und Kieferchirurgie sowie Orthopädie, Traumatologie und Allgemeinchirurgie werden zusammengefaßt.

Aus den ersten Studien, die teilweise den heutigen methodischen Anforderungen noch nicht genügten, zeichnete sich bereits die gute abschwellende Wirkung des Azapropazons ab, verbunden mit einer relativ geringen Nebenwirkungsrate.

Die ausgeprägte antiphlogistische Potenz von Azapropazon wurde in weiteren Untersuchungen sowohl im HNO-Bereich und der Kiefer- und Gesichtschirurgie als auch im Bereich von Orthopädie und Traumatologie bestätigt.

Darüberhinaus konnte in einigen Arbeiten eine zufriedenstellende analgetische Wirkung gezeigt werden.

Die intravenöse Gabe am Tag der Verletzung bzw. des operativen Eingriffs mit anschließender oraler Weiterbehandlung über 5 Tage (Tagesdosis 1200 mg Azapropazon) hat sich am besten bewährt.

Resumé

L'auteur passe en revue les résultats obtenus en 20 ans d'utilisation clinique de l'azapropazone dans le domaine de la médecine ORL, de la chirurgie dentaire et maxillaire, de l'orthopédie, de la traumatologie et de la chirurgie générale.

Les premières études, qui ne répondent pas totalement aux normes méthodologiques actuelles, montraient déjà l'efficacité antiphlogistique de l'azapropazone et son taux d'effets secondaires relativement bas.

L'action antiphlogistique puissante de l'azapropazone a été confirmée dans les études ultérieures, tant dans le domaine de la médecine ORL et de la chirurgie faciale et maxillaire que dans celui de l'orthopédie et de la traumatologie.

Certains travaux révèlent en outre une action analgésique satisfaisante.

Le schéma posologique qui s'est imposé comme le plus approprié est le suivant: administration intraveineuse le jour de la blessure ou de l'intervention chirurgicale, suivie d'un traitement oral pendant 5 jours (à raison d'une dose quotidienne de 1200 mg d'azapropazone).

16
Clinical trial methodology in rheumatoid arthritis: azapropazone studies

WW Buchanan and N Bellamy

'Millions o' wimmen bring forth in pain
Millions o' bairns that are no' worth ha'en!'

Hugh MacDiarmid (1892–1978)
A Drunk Man Looks at the Thistle

Some 21 years have elapsed since the first publication on azapropazone[1]. During this time, numerous clinical therapeutic trials have been published attesting the drug's efficacy as an anti-rheumatic non-steroidal anti-inflammatory analgesic (NSAID), and these have been the subject of several reviews[2-5]. In this communication, it is proposed to critically review the quality of the clinical therapeutic trials in rheumatoid arthritis (RA). This will be approached in terms of first reviewing the outcome measures employed and secondly, in terms of the trial design and interpretation. Finally, a codification of clinical trial methodology will be proposed which might segregate the quality of trials.

I. OUTCOME MEASURES

1. Pain

Currently, the most popular method of recording pain relief in clinical therapeutic trials is with the visual analogue scale[6]. Surprisingly, only one of the trials employed this method[7]. One of the problems encountered with the visual analogue scale is that patients may have difficulty in understanding the concept, at least initially[8,9]. This may have been the reason why the most popular choice was an adjectival scale, to which numerical values were given[10-13]. Only one study chose to employ a nine-point rating scale[14].

The visual analogue scale has been shown to have a good correlation with both adjectival and facial scales in RA[15,16] and osteoarthritis[17], and both of the former have proven sensitive to change[18]. Recently, Grossi *et al.*[19] have modified the standard 10 cm visual analogue scale with the addition of a chromatic component, which they have suggested might increase sensitivity. This remains, however, to be proven.

It is still a matter of contention whether patients should have access

Azapropazone – 20 years of clinical use. Rainsford, KD (ed)
© Kluwer Academic Publishers. Printed in Great Britain

to their previous scores when measuring such a subjective state as pain[20]. We agree with Scott and Huskisson[21], and Carlsson[22] that with progression of time, patients tend to overestimate their pain severity, but quickly correct this when shown their previous scores. There is clearly an important psychological component in long-term studies.

Pain varies at different times of the day and only a few of the studies[10-13] attempted to have assessments made at the same time of day. Weather also affects the patient's pain[23], which is important, particularly in long-term studies in countries with marked differences in climatic conditions such as England, Finland, Canada, and European countries. Pain is the major complaint of the patient with rheumatoid arthritis and is the most sensitive outcome measure in detecting change with NSAIDs[24]. It is surprising therefore, to find it not recorded in otherwise well-conducted trials with azapropazone[25] or only recorded in others on a four-point scale as 'state of the joints[26].

2. Patient and physician global assessments

Patient assessment of their progress[7,11,13,27] was more popular than investigator assessment[7]. Several studies with the title drug employed patient preference[12,28,29], and even one noted the patient's weight, which, not surprisingly, failed to change![27]. It is uncertain how global assessments are compiled by different authors, and to date there is no study to determine their reliability.

3. Joint counts

Scoring joint tenderness is second only to the patients' assessment of their pain relief as an index of change with NSAID therapy[24]. Since most of the trials of azapropazone were conducted by European workers, it is not surprising that the articular index of joint tenderness devised by Ritchie and her colleagues[30] was the most popular method of recording joint counts[10-13] (especially as this is the method recommended by the European League against Rheumatism Standing Committee on International Clinical Studies[31]. The Ritchie index correlates well with the articular index of the Co-operating Clinics Committee of the American Rheumatism Association[30]. Both show clear differences in short-term clinical therapeutic trials of NSAIDs[30]. The articular index of the Co-operating Clinics gives lower mean differences between active drugs and placebo, but this finding is offset by its smaller variability[30]. Both indices are equally satisfactory for clinical trial purposes. The finding that the American index was not used in any of the studies is merely due to the fact that none of the authors were American and the drug is not available in North America.

The obsolescent Lansbury index was used by two groups[14,25]. No articular index was used in one study[27] and in another, the method was neither described nor referenced[7]. The Ritchie index can be completed in 2–3 minutes with an amanuensis. Its reproducibility has been thoroughly studied both between the same observer, and different observers. The latter is too great to permit different observers to make the observations. It is essential that only one observer perform all the assessments; this also applies in general to other outcome measures.

4. Grip strength

Determination of grip strength using a Davis bag was a popular outcome measure[7,10–13,25–27]. Three studies failed to provide a description of the method which was employed[7,25,27]. Thus, no data were available to determine the intra- and inter-observer error. This aspect has been found by Lee et al.[32] to be up to 10 mmHg in the former and 20 mmHg in the latter. Grip strength index as determined by a Davis bag is not likely to change with anti-rheumatic drug therapy[24]. However, recently introduced automated hand grip procedures may prove of greater value[33].

5. Digital joint circumference

Digital joint circumference was measured by a plastic spring gauge[34] (unfortunately no longer available from Ciba–Geigy) in only three trials[11–13]. The method has a relatively small intra-observer error (2 mm), but a larger inter-observer error (10 mm)[34]. Reduction in joint circumference can only occur in patients with soft tissue inflammation and accompanying joint swelling.

Patients are selected for clinical trials on the basis of persistent pain rather than the ability of their finger joint circumference to respond to NSAIDs. The fact that three of the trials which used this outcome measure failed to show significant reduction in joint circumference does not invalidate the method and does not mean that azapropazone is without anti-inflammatory effect. If an anti-inflammatory effect of a drug is sought, then patients must be selected with soft tissue swelling of the proximal interphalangeal joints of the fingers and interphalangeal joints of the thumbs. It is a somewhat sobering thought that this relatively crude method is the only one available, other than determination of radionuclide joint uptake scans, and thermography, to study the anti-inflammatory effects of drugs in the joints in humans[35].

6. Morning stiffness, limbering-up time, and time of onset of fatigue

Morning stiffness was used in a number of trials[7,10–12,26], but none of the authors commented on the difficulty of measurement[36]. Two groups[11,13] preferred to record severity on a Likert scale, and this we find more acceptable than recording duration. Three groups who recorded morning stiffness failed to indicate whether this was in terms of severity or duration[14,25,27]. Lassitude was only recorded in one trial[27].

Morning stiffness is perhaps best measured from diurnal changes in grip[33]. Laboratory methods can only be applied to relatively few joints and have not to our knowledge ever been applied in clinical trials. Although morning stiffness probably arises from accumulation of fluid in and around joints during sleep[37], it is not relieved by diuretics[38]. Clearly, more attention needs to be placed upon how morning stiffness should be recorded, and some estimate in the error involved would be useful. At the very least a standardized procedure should be agreed upon.

7. Range of joint movement

Despite the fact that range of joint movement is highly reproducible[39], it is of limited value in assessing anti-rheumatic drug therapy in rheumatoid arthritis. Only one trial with azapropazone included measurement of the range of joint movement, but failed to specify which joint or joints were studied. Not surprisingly, no differences were found between azapropazone and placebo[27].

8. Functional indices

Functional impairment, or *functio laesa*, is a major feature of rheumatoid arthritis. The most popular method of assessing functional impairment is to record the time to walk a distance of 15 metres or some other specified distance. This is, however, not particularly sensitive to change[40]. None of the trials with azapropazone included any assessment of function, which is probably reasonable in view of the fact that the trials were of short duration, where this parameter would be less likely to change. Recently, a number of functional and quality-of-life indices have been evolved, some of which may prove useful in assessing outcome of trials with anti-rheumatic drugs such as azapropazone[41].

9. Radionuclide studies

Three trials[10,12,13] used ^{99m}Tc joint uptake measurements; none of these showed statistical improvement with azapropazone compared with placebo. ^{99m}Tc 04 has been found to be superior to radio-iodinated (^{125}I) human fibrinogen[42]. The technetium pyrophosphate and diphosphate compounds absorb to juxta-articular bone and consequently are less useful than ^{99m}Tc 04 itself[43]. It should be noted that an increased uptake of ^{99m}Tc pyrophosphate or diphosphonate compounds also occurs in bone in rheumatoid arthritis[44]. Although radionuclide joint uptakes have been shown to be reproducible and capable of being reduced by NSAID therapy, they are relatively insensitive[24] and so have not been widely accepted[45]. Nevertheless, radionuclide joint measurements are entirely objective and may give better resolution with improvements in technical performance.

10. Thermography

None of the studies with azapropazone utilized thermography despite the fact that it provides a non-invasive, sensitive, reproducible and quantifiable method of assessing improvement in joint inflammation. Nor is thermography subject to circadian variation. The initial cost of equipment is high and the method must be carried out with strict attention to ambient temperature[42].

11. Radiology

All of the trials were short term, and therefore did not include radiological assessment, which is appropriate only for long-term trials with second-line agents. Indeed, even in long-term trials of such agents there is controversy as to its usefulness[46].

II. OTHER STUDIES

So far, only double-blind cross-over trials of the title drug have been considered. However, other types of trials are also useful in assessing the therapeutic potential of drugs such as azapropazone. Thus, Brooks et al.[47], compared the analgesic effect of azapropazone 1200 mg/day with aspirin 3.9 g/day for effects on pain relief, number of days withdrawn from the trial, and patient satisfaction over a 2 week period. Although azapropazone was slightly better than aspirin in all three parameters, the differences did not reach statistical significance.

The method of assessing pain relief used in this trial was simple in that the patients kept a daily diary of their pain, which they recorded on an adjectival scale. At the end of the 2-week period, the subjects indicated their satisfaction with the drug on the same scale, and simply posted back the completed charts. Since it had been previously shown[48] that the initial pain rating provides the most useful measure in determining outcome of analgesic therapy, the average pain rating during treatment was statistically adjusted for differences in initial pain. The method used in this trial has been shown to be reproducible, as borne out by the fact that the average treated pain rating and mean satisfaction scores obtained for aspirin in this trial were similar to those obtained for aspirin in previous trials[49,50]. The results of studies using this method are summarized in Table 1. Prednisone 15 mg/day was statistically superior to all other treatments. All of the NSAIDs with the exception of phenylbutazone 50 mg daily, were statistically better than placebo. However, paracetamol, 4 g daily, was not. The important point is that no statistical differences could be found between any of the NSAIDs. This is consistent with the findings in other short-term trials of azapropazone[11,13,14,26,27] and NSAIDs in general[51].

Table 1 Pain ratings and satisfaction scores by the pain chart assessment method (mean ± SEM) (Lee et al[7-50,54,55])

Drug	Ref.	Daily dosage	Number of patients	Initial pain rating	Average treated pain rating	Number of withdrawals (%)	Mean days withdrawn	Average treated pain rating adjusted for initial pain rating	Mean satisfaction scores	Ranking
Azapropazone	47	1200 mg	49	3.0±0.16	3.0±0.1	16 (33%)	2.4±.062	3.0±0.2	2.7±0.2	5
Aspirin		3.9 g	36	3.2±0.14	3.2±0.12	17 (47%)	4.1±0.73	3.3±0.2	2.4±0.2	7
Placebo	49	-	41	3.0±0.2	3.5±0.1	28 (68%)	6.4±0.7	3.5±0.1	1.7±0.2	10
Prednisoline		15 mg	45	3.0±0.2	2.6±0.1	6 (13%)	1.3±0.7	2.6±0.1	3.7±0.2	1
Aspirin		3.9 g	42	2.9±0.2	3.0±0.1	14 (33%)	3.0±0.7	3.1±0.1	2.4±0.2	7
Aspirin	50	3.9 g	44	2.8±0.2	3.1±0.1	26 (59%)	4.9±0.7	3.3±0.1	2.4±0.2	7
Paracetamol*		4.0 g	38	2.7±0.2	3.4±0.1	20 (53%)	4.5±0.7	3.5±0.1	2.0±0.2	9
Indomethacin		100 mg	41	2.6±0.2	2.8±0.1	13 (32%)	2.0±0.7	2.9±0.1	2.8±0.2	4
Ketoprofen	54	100 mg	44	3.0±0.1	3.2±0.1	15 (34%)	2.8±0.7	3.2±0.1	2.3±0.2	8
Ketoprofen		200 mg	46	2.8±0.1	3.1±0.1	17 (37%)	2.7±0.7	3.2±0.1	2.5±0.2	6
Ibuprofen		1200 mg	45	2.9±0.1	3.1±0.1	16 (36%)	3.0±0.7	3.2±0.1	2.4±0.2	7
Indomethacin	48	100 mg	41	2.6±0.1	2.7±0.1	14 (34%)	2.2±0.6	2.9±0.1	2.9±0.2	3
Flurbiprofen		150 mg	45	2.8±0.1	2.7±0.1	13 (28%)	2.1±0.6	2.8±0.1	2.8±0.2	4
Mefanamic acid		1500 mg	46	2.8±0.1	2.6±0.1	12 (26%)	2.3±0.6	2.7±0.1	2.7±0.2	5
Alclofenac		3.0 g	45	2.7±0.1	3.1±0.1	17 (38%)	3.1±0.6	3.0±0.1	2.3±0.2	8
Benoylate		8.0 g	42	3.0±0.1	3.0±0.1	15 (36%)	3.6±0.6	3.0±0.1	2.5±0.2	8
Safapryn**	55	12 tabs	39	3.2±0.1	3.0±0.1	7 (18%)	1.7±0.6	3.1±0.2	2.9±0.2	3
Phenylbutazone		300 mg	43	2.8±0.1	2.7±0.1	3 (7%)	0.5±0.6	2.8±0.2	2.5±0.2	6
Phenylbutazone		50 mg	40	3.0±0.1	3.3±0.1	15 (38%)	3.5±0.6	3.3±0.2	3.6±0.2	2

*Acetaminophen.
**Safapryn® (Pfizer): each tablet contains 300 mg aspirin in an enteric coated core plus 250 mg paracetamol in an outer layer.

Capell and her colleagues[52,53] have employed a novel approach to assessing the acceptability and therapeutic efficacy of NSAIDs, using life-table analysis of lack of compliance, either due to side-effects or lack of effect. Unfortunately, they did not include azapropazone in these studies. An important finding by this group was that drop-out from all NSAIDs they tested occurred at the same rate for the first three months, and only after this time could differences be seen. This is presumably why short-term trials fail to show any differences between different NSAIDs.

The therapeutic effectiveness of a NSAID is a combination of its effectiveness as an analgesic and its overall toxicity. This was assessed in the studies of Lee et al.[47-50,54,55] and also by Capell and her colleagues[52,53]. The results of the Lee et al. studies[47-50,54,55] are summarized in Table 2, where it can be seen that the most common reason for withdrawal from

Table 2   Reasons for withdrawing from trials reported by Lee and his colleagues[47-50,54,55]

Drug	Reference	Reason for withdrawal			
		Pain	Side-effects	Pain and side-effects	Unknown
Azapropazone	47	6	10	0	0
Aspirin		1	12	0	4
Placebo		22	2	3	1
Prednisolone	49	2	3	1	0
Aspirin		7	3	4	0
Aspirin		6	13	4	3
Paracetamol	50	15	2	3	0
Indomethacin		4	5	2	2
Ketoprofen*		7	4	4	0
Ketoprofen**	54	10	1	5	1
Ibuprofen		9	3	2	2
Indomethacin		5	8	1	0
Flurbiprofen		6	3	4	0
Mefanamic acid	48	3	5	3	1
Alclofenac		9	2	5	1
Benonylate		4	10	1	0
Safapryn		1	6	0	0
Phenylbutazone***	55	2	1	0	0
Phenylbutazone****		15	0	0	0

* 100 mg daily.
** 200 mg daily.
*** 300 mg daily.
**** 50 mg daily.

placebo was pain. Azapropazone caused a significant number of side-effects, especially dyspepsia, and was second only to aspirin in this regard. Clearly, if the therapeutic effectiveness of azapropazone has to be established in relation to other NSAIDs, then studies of the type described by Capell et al.[52,53] will be required.

Isomäki et al.[29] compared the analgesic effect of azapropazone with placebo and nine other NSAIDs using a single-blind method in 90 patients with rheumatoid arthritis. The period of treatment, 3 days, was somewhat short, as was the wash-out period between each treatment, one day. Preference ranking revealed azapropazone (900 mg daily), along with ibuprofen (1200 mg daily), carprofen (450 mg daily), and aspirin (3 g daily), tolfenamic acid (600 mg daily), and diclofenac (100 mg daily).

Dieppe and his colleagues[28] also used patient preference to compare azapropazone (1200 mg daily) with soluble aspirin (2.4 g daily), naproxen (500 mg daily), fenoprofen (2.4 g daily) and ibuprofen (1200 mg daily) in a study which lasted one year. All of the patients had rheumatoid arthritis and were allowed to alter their treatment if they were dissatisfied with it. No patient was prescribed more than three drugs. The patients showed a significant preference for azapropazone over soluble aspirin, and a slight preference over naproxen. It should be noted, however, that the dose of soluble aspirin was relatively low, which might explain the apparent superiority of azapropazone. Nevertheless, it is from this type of study that one can best evaluate therapeutic effectiveness.

Two studies using adults with rheumatoid arthritis[56,57] have claimed corticosteroid sparing effects of azapropazone. Despite the fact that one of the studies was double-blind and cross-over in type, comparing azapropazone with phenylbutazone, no placebo was included. Without a placebo group all that can be demonstrated is that drug $A = $ drug $B = 0$.

III. DESIGN AND INTERPRETATION

Essentially, there are five types of trial design used to evaluate anti-rheumatic drugs: randomized parallel, randomized cross-over, sequential, non-randomized comparative groups, and one-group non-compartmental open designs[41]. Parallel designs are operationally more simple, but require larger sample sizes, and are unable to address issues of preference or within-patient response differences. Cross-over designs are more complex, especially as carry-over effects may occur with NSAIDs with a long half-life; this for azapropazone is estimated between 12[58] and 20 hours[59]. This aspect is especially important when the period of study is short, such as in the trial of Isomäki et al.[29].

Guyatt et al.[60] have recently suggested an 'n of 1' design, which is particularly useful in studying therapy in a single patient. In this type of study, the patient receives active medication and placebo sequentially, six or more times. This type of trial design requires clear-cut differences between active drug and placebo, which certainly does not occur with NSAIDs[24]. Non-randomized comparative group designs and one-group non-comparative open designs lack the rigour necessary to establish the pharmacological efficacy of NSAIDs. However, these designs are, as previously discussed, extremely useful in determining the therapeutic value of a new NSAID.

In the early stage trials it is essential to include a placebo control group to avoid the pitfall, discussed above, of drug A = drug B = 0. Some 50% of patients can be expected to respond over a 1–2 week period with placebo therapy[61]. No correlation has been found between placebo response and endomorphins[62]. In later trials, when the NSAID has been unequivocally proven to be superior to placebo, it is appropriate to compare the new compound with an established drug without using placebo, especially if the study is of long duration[63]. A placebo can be defined as any therapy or component of therapy that is deliberately or knowingly used for its non-specific psychological or psychophysical effect[64]. In most clinical trials, placebos are chosen to be not only pharmacologically inert, but also free from side-effects. This may not be entirely appropriate in assessing analgesic effects of drugs, since the recent studies of Max et al.[65] clearly show that side-effects produced by an analgesic drug augment its analgesic effects. Perhaps in the future design of NSAID trials it would be useful to include a placebo which gave side-effects, e.g. dyspepsia, similar to the drug being tested.

All clinical trials are highly biased, since patients are carefully selected for study. Patients at the extremes of age, those who are pregnant or with concurrent illnesses, and patients receiving other drugs are usually excluded. Great caution must therefore be exercised in generalizing the results to the population at large. However, in early trials, it is useful to study a homogeneous group of 'squeaky-clean' patients, especially when unexpected toxic effects may occur. Patients who volunteer for clinical trials differ prognostically from those who refuse to participate[66], a further reason for limiting generalizations of the results of such studies.

Most of the clinical trials reported for azapropazone, and indeed for all NSAIDs[51], are described by their authors as being randomized. Strictly speaking none of such trials was randomized, although most were stratified. With such a variable disease as rheumatoid arthritis, randomization would not necessarily guarantee group comparability: indeed, the reverse is more likely! Thus, since the major variable in determining the response to NSAID therapy is the amount of pain at baseline[49], it is quite justifiable to use the process of stratification followed by subsequent allocation to treatment groups as described by Lee and his colleagues[48]. It is of historical interest that Maclagan first noted, over a century ago in his paper on salicin in rheumatic fever, that the amount of pain and joint inflammation were the most important determinants of therapeutic response[67].

If it is important to include a placebo group in early stage therapeutic trials, then it is equally important to include a wash-out period. Essentially, this is restricted to trials of NSAIDs, since the sudden cessation of cortico-steroid therapy is not without its risks, and the suspension of disease-modifying drugs is impracticable, since the effects may not be apparent for weeks or months[41]. Because the withdrawal of NSAID medication is often poorly tolerated by patients with active rheumatoid arthritis, the provision of a 'trap-door' is useful. Only two trials of azapropazone included a wash-out, of one day[29], and the other of 3 days[12], although three other trials began with a 48 hour[11] or one week placebo period[10,26]. Washout periods are useful in minimizing sample size requirements by excluding those patients who are incapable of change, and in allowing baselines to be established in trials of cross-over design. In trials which last longer than 6 weeks or 2 months, a washout period at the end of the trial is useful in confirming persistence of patient responsiveness. A placebo washout period, or a washout period where simple analgesics are allowed *ad libitum*, are not as useful as a no-treatment period with a trap-door.

None of the clinical therapeutic trials of azapropazone commented on calculation of sample size. This is a function of several factors including trial design, the magnitude of the type I (α) and type II (β) errors, the size of the difference sought, and the variability of the outcome measures. Most of the trials were, however, conducted in the late 60s and early 70s, when the importance of calculation of sample size, although known, had not been widely publicized[68].

Most clinical trials use a variety of outcome measures, but this leads to the statistical problem that the more outcomes are assessed the more likely one will achieve a p value of <0.05 because of chance alone. Statistical adjustment for multiple comparisons is important, but currently seldom considered. In practice, it is useful to define *a priori* one or two major outcomes in calculation of sample size.

Co-intervention refers to the administration of another potentially efficacious treatment during the period of the trial. With NSAID trials, co-intervention is generally concomitant analgesic therapy. There is still controversy regarding the use of simple analgesics in rheumatoid arthritis[69, 70]; some authors declare them useless[70] while others[71–73] advocate their use. Some trials have reported no significant differences between simple analgesics and placebo in rheumatoid arthritis[48,50,74,75], whereas they have been found superior in others[76–79]. In view of the uncertainty of the effectiveness of simple analgesics in rheumatoid arthritis, we believe that their use should be avoided in clinical therapeutic trials of NSAIDs, even if return tablet counts are done. The possibility exists that simple analgesics, such as paracetamol, may be effective in mild disease, but not for patients with severe pain. Co-intervention is probably the most serious threat to the validity of any clinical therapeutic trial[80].

None of the clinical therapeutic trials of azapropazone attempted to test compliance, even with a tablet count, despite the fact that all the studies were performed on an out-patient basis. Compliance can be measured by patient report, either verbal or by diary, pill counting, and plasma drug monitoring. It should be noted, however, that even when the monitoring procedure is satisfactory, there is still no standard definition for any level of compliance below which the therapeutic response is significantly compromised. We believe that compliance with NSAID therapy is probably high in patients with rheumatoid arthritis who suffer continuous pain[81], and patient report by diary or pill counting are adequate for short-term NSAID trials. Such is not the case, however, with long-term trials with slow-acting drugs[82].

Essentially, there are two approaches to statistical analysis: explicative or per protocol, and management or intention-to-treat. In the former, all patients who do not complete the trial according to the protocol are excluded from the analysis. In the latter, all patients are included in the analysis[83]. The intention-to-treat strategy is now the preferred form of analysis. It is of interest that it was employed in one of the studies on azapropazone[47].

Finally, it is again worth emphasizing that caution is necessary in extrapolating the results of a trial and in generalizing them to other patient populations which may differ in their response potential and adverse effects. The results of a trial must be viewed in the appropriate clinical context, and interpreted with respect to data obtained from both open studies and clinical practice.

IV. CODIFICATION OF TRIALS

It is important, in reviewing publications of clinical trials, to know not only what was done, but how it was done. This, of course, should be described in 'Materials and Methods', but from what has been found in the present study of trials of azapropazone, it is quite clear that most of the publications are inadequate in this regard. Similar observations were made by Reiffenstein et al.[84], who found 20% of trials published in *The New England Journal of Medicine* and 42% in the *Canadian Medical Journal* failed to fulfill their methodoligical criteria of adequacy. Recommendations[85-87] and guidelines[88,89] have been suggested, and checklists for authors published[90-93], but without evidence of improvement[87]. Elsewhere, we[94] have proposed a codification system, an example of which is illustrated in Table 3, which we believe might greatly improve not only the quality of trials, but also facilitate their review. All that would be required is publication of the codes for design, measurement and analysis, as appears in the table. We have summarized the advantages of using such an international coding system for clinical trials of anti-rheumatic drugs as follows:

1. The provision of minimum requirements for detailed reporting design, measurement, and analytic components of clinical trials.

2. Standardization of the reporting procedure.

3. Enhancement in the speed and efficiency of the peer review process.

Table 3 Coding system for reporting clinical trials in the rheumatic diseases (92)

Design Stems	Characteristics	Analysis Stems	Characteristics
D = design	TB = triple-blind DB = double-blind SB = single blind U = unblinded (open) QE = quasi-experimental CO = cross-over P = parallel	*NR = number of patients responding to treatment (total) *NSE = number of patients with clinical side-effects *NW = Number of patients withdrawn from study (total)	(Indicate n) (Indicate n) (Indicate n)
NP = number of patients (total)	(Indicate n)	A = analysis (biostatistical tests)	T = Students T test CS = chi square test AV = analysis of variance AC = analysis of covariance SC = survival curve ST = sign test MW = Mann–Witney U W = Wilcoxen P = parametric (miscellaneous) NP = non-parametric (miscellaneous) ET = equivalence testing Subscripts 1 = one-tailed 2 = two-tailed
NG = number of (treatment) groups	(Indicate n)		
NT = number of treatments	(Indicate n)		
R = randomization	SR = simple randomization B = blocked randomization ST = stratified randomization BA = baseline adaptive randomization RA = response adaptive randomization M = minimization		
S = stratification	(Indicate number of strata)	E1 = type 1 error (α for principle variable (specify level)	
WP = washout period	DF = drug free P = placebo AGF = analgesia free AIF = anti-inflammatory free Subscripts 1 = preintervention 2 = inter-/intra-vention 3 = postintervention	E2 = type 2 error (β error for principle variable) (specify level)	
DU = duration of active treatment	(Indicate number in days)	P = power	(give power for specified Δ)

continued

Table 3 *continued*

Design Stems	Characteristics	Analysis Stems	Characteristics
Measurement		**Miscellaneous codes**	
NV = number of outcome variables measured	(Indicate n)	UNC = unclassified ? = unknown + = performed	
NO = number of individual observers	(Indicate n)	− = not performed (cf? = unknown)	
CP = compliance measures	PC = pill count DL = drug level monitoring PR = patient report	N/A = not applicable	
CV = co-intervention	AG + = analgesics (monitored) AG − = analgesics (not monitored) PT = physiotherapy AI = anti-inflammatory agents H = hospitalization S = surgery	*In cross-over designs n may exceed the total number of patients in the study and is an expression of the number of events (response, intolerance, withdrawal) which occurs across *all* treatment groups. The maximum value for n = NP × NT. (See stem codes.)	

Design: D = DB,P·NP = 83·NG = 2·NT = 2·
R = +,GC + ·S = ?·WP = P₁,SB·DU = 84.
Measurement: NV = 6 NO = ?·CP = DL·CV = ?·
Analysis: NR = 61·NSE = 38·NW = 21·A = W,MW·E1 = ?·E2 = ?·P = ?
(Reproduced by kind permission of the editor of the EULAR Bulletin.)

231

4.   Increased efficiency and clarity in interpersonal communication.

5.   Facilitation of computer-assisted data storage, retrieval, integration and analysis.

All of this may seem too much common sense, but as Voltaire remarked in his *Dictionnaire Philosophique*: 'Common sense is not so common!'

V. CONCLUSIONS

In spite of the apparent variability in quality of the clinical trials employed with azapropazone, this drug has clearly proven efficacious in the treatment of rheumatoid arthritis. The variable quality of clinical trials has also presented a major problem for assessing the effectiveness of other NSAIDs, and this is a difficulty in trying to assess the relative effectiveness and safety of azapropazone with other NSAIDs in RA. The problem is exacerbated by the variability which exists in long-term progress of RA. Attempts to overcome variability within RA subjects and with the natural course of the disease requires employing so-called n of 1 (sequential double-blind cross-over) study designs and it may be useful to employ these in future studies.

References

1.   Kiesewetter, E (1968). Klinische Ergebnisse mit der neuen antiphlogistisch wirksamen Substanz Azapropazon. *Wien Med Wschr*, **118**, 941–3

2.   Brooks, PM and Buchanan, WW (1976). Azapropazone—its place in the management of rheumatoid conditions. In *Recent Advances in Clinical Rheumatology: a Review and Clinical Assessment of Azapropazone. Curr Med Res Opin* (Special Issue), **4**, 94–100

3.   Eberl, RG and Bröll, RH (1977). *Langzeitbehandlung mit Azapropazon* In: Fenner, H and Eberl, RG (eds) *Erkrankungen des rheumatischen Formenkreises* (Karlsruhe: G Braun), pp. 7–10

4.   Hart, FD (1978). Azapropazone: a review of the literature. *Europ J Rheumatol and Inflamm*, **1**, 142–4

5.   Sondervost, M (1979). Azapropazone. *Clin Rheum Dis*, **5**, 465–80

6.   Huskisson, EC (1974). Measurement of pain. *Lancet*, **2**, 1127–31

7.   Templeton, JS (1981). Azapropazone—twice or four times daily? *Eur J Rheumatol Inflamm*, **4**, 401–7

8.   Maxwell, C (1978). Sensitivity and accuracy of the visual analogue scale: a psycho-physical classroom experiment. *Br J Clin Pharmacol*, **6**, 15–24

9.   Stubbs, DF (1979). Visual analogue scales. *Br J Clin Pharmacol*, **7**, 124

10.   Grennan, DM, Watkins, C and Kennedy, AC (1974). Preliminary clinical evaluation of azapropazone in rheumatoid arthritis. *Curr Med Res Opin*, **2**, 67–71

11.   Capell, HA, McLeod, MM, Hernandez, LA, Grennan, DM and Templeton, JS (1976). Comparison of azapropazone and naproxen in rheumatoid arthritis. *Curr Med Res Opin*, **4**, 285–9

12.   Grennan, DM, McLeod, M, Watkins, C and Dick, WC (1976). Clinical assessment of azapropazone in rheumatoid arthritis. *Curr Med Res Opin*, **4**,

44–9

13. Kean, WF, Kraag, GR, Rooney, PJ and Capell, HA (1981). Clinical therapeutic trial of aspirin and azapropazone in rheumatoid arthritis when prescribed singly and in combination. *Curr Med Res Opin*, **7**, 164–7

14. Pavelka, K, Vojtisek, O and Kankova, D (1975). Doppelblind-cross-over Versuch mit Azapropazon und Indomethacin in der Behandlung der pcP. In: Fenner, H and Eberl, R (eds), *Azapropazon bei Erkrankungen des rheumatischen Formenkreises*. (Karlsruhe: G Braun), pp. 31–5

15. Woodforde, JM and Merskey, H (1972). Some relationships between subjective measures of pain. *J Pshychosom Res*, **16**, 173–8

16. Revill, SI, Robinson, JO, Rosen, M and Hogg, MIJ (1976). The reliability of a linear analogue for evaluating pain. *Anaesthesia*, **31**, 1191–8

17. Frank, AJM, Moll, JMH and Hort, JF (1982). A comparison of three ways of measuring pain. *Rheumatol and Rehabil*, **21**, 211–7

18. Ohnhaus, EE and Adler, R (1975). Methodological problems in the measurement of pain: a comparison between the verbal rating scale and the visual analogue scale. *Pain*, **1**, 379–84

19. Grossi, E, Borghi, C, Cerchiari, EL, Puppa, TD and Francucci, B (1983). Analogue chromatic continuous scale (ACCS): a new method for pain assessment. *Clin Exp Rheumatol*, **1**, 337–40

20. Jacobsen, M (1965). The use of rating scales in clinical research. *Br J Psychiatry*, **111**, 545–6

21. Scott, J and Huskinsson, EC (1979). Accuracy of subjective measurements made with or without previous scores: an important source of error in serial measurement of subjective states. *Ann Rheum Dis*, **38**, 558–9

22. Carlsson, Am (1983). Assessment of chronic pain 7. Aspects of the reliability and validity of the visual analogue scale. *Pain*, **16**, 87–101

23. Dequeker, J and Wuestenraed, L (1986). The effect of biometerological factors on Ritchie articular index and pain in rheumatoid arthritis. *Scand J Rheumatol*, **15**, 280–4

24. Deodar, SD, Dick, WC, Hodgkinson, R and Buchanan, WW (1973). Measurement of clinical response to anti-inflammatory drugs in rheumatoid arthritis. *Quart J Med*, **42**, 387–401

25. Sigiyama, T, Okazaki, T and Onada, T (1969). A clinical trial of azapropazone in rheumatoid arthritis. *J Jap Rheum Assoc*, **9**, 16–7

26. Hicklin, JA, Hingorani, K, Lloyd, KN, Templeton, JS and Williamson, M (1976). Azapropazone compared with indomethacin in the treatment of rheumatoid arthritis. *Practitioner*, **217**, 799–803

27. Thune, S (1976). A comparative study of azapropazone and indomethacin in the treatment of rheumatoid arthritis. *Curr Med Res Opin*, **4**, 70–5

28. Dieppe, PA, Boyle, D and Jacoby, R (1981). Arthritis: anti-inflammatory drugs in practice. *Practitioner*, 225, 397–9

29. Isomäki, H, Martion, J, Kaarela, K *et al.* (1984). Comparison of the analgesic effect of ten nonsteroidal anti-inflammatory drugs. *Br J Rheumatol*, **23**, 61–5

30. Ritchie, DM, Boyle, JA, McInnes, JM *et al.* (1968). Clinical studies with an articular index for the assessment of joint tenderness in patients with rheumatoid arthritis. *Q J Med* (New Series), **37**, 393–406

31. Sequesne, M (1980). European guidelines for clinical trials of new anti-rheumatic drugs. *EULAR Bull*, **9**, (Suppl), 171–5

32. Lee, P, Baxter, A, Dick, WC and Webb, J (1974). An assessment of grip strength measurement in rheumatoid arthritis. *Scand J Rheumatol*, **3**, 17–23

33. Buchanan, WW, Gopa, DN, Ghista, DN, Grace, EM and Tugwell, P (1984). Rheumatoid hand weakness characterising indices and clinical data acquisition. *Eng Med*, **13**, 115–20

34. Webb, J, Downie, WW, Dick, WC and Lee, P (1973). Evaluation of digital joint circumference measurements in rheumatoid arthritis. *Scand J Rheumatol*, **2**, 127–31

35. Boardman, PL and Hart, FD (1967). Clinical measurement of the anti-inflammatory effects of salicylates in rheumatoid arthritis. *Br Med J*, **4**, 264–8

36. Steinberg, AD (1978). On morning stiffness. *J. Rheumatol*, **5**, 3–6

37. Scott, JT (1960). Morning stiffness in rheumatoid arthritis. *Ann Rheum Dis*, **19**, 361–8

38. Magder, R, Baxter, ML and Kassam, YB (1986). Does a diuretic improve morning stiffness? (Letter to the editor.) *Br J Rheumatol*, **25**, 318–9

39. Mitchell, WS, Miller, J and Sturrock, R (1975). An evaluation of goniometry as an objective parameter for measuring joint motion. *Scott Med J*, **20**, 57–9

40. Grace, EM, Gerecz, EM, Kassam, YB, Buchanan, HM, Buchanan, WW and Tugwell, PS (1988). 50-foot walking time: a critical assessment of an outcome measure in clinical trials of anti-rheumatic drugs. *Br J Rheumatol*, **27**, 372–4

41. Bellamy, N and Buchanan, WW (1989). Clinical evaluation in rheumatic diseases. In: McCarty, DJ (ed), *Arthritis and Allied Conditions*, 11th ed. (Philadelphia: Lea and Febiger), Chapter 9, pp. 158–86

42. Lee, P, Sturrock, RD, Buchanan, WW and Dick, WC (1974). The technetium (^{99}mTc) radioiodinated (^{125}I) human fibrinogen scan and clinical indices in the assessment of disease activity in rheumatoid arthritis. *J. Rheumatol*, **1**, 432–40

43. Hoffer, PB and Genant, HK (1976). Radionuclide joint imaging. *Semin Nucl Med*, **6**, 168–84

44. Rosenspire, KC, Kennedy, AC, Steinbach, J, Blau, M and Green, FA (1980). Investigation of the metabolic activity of bone in rheumatoid arthritis. *J Rheumatol*, **7**, 469–73

45. Lee, P (1982). Isotopes in the measurement of joint inflammation. *Rheumatol*, **9**, 767

46. Pullar, T, Hunter, JA, Capell, HA (1983). Does second-line therapy affect the radiological progression of rheumatoid arthritis? *Ann Rheum Dis*, **43**, 18–23

47. Brooks, PM, Mason, DIR, McNeil, R, Anderson, JA and Buchanan, WW (1976). An assessment of the therapeutic potential of azapropazone in rheumatoid arthritis. *Curr Med Res Opin*, **4**, 50–6

48. Lee, P, Anderson, JA, Miller, J, Webb, J and Buchanan, WW (1976). Evaluation of analgesic action and efficacy of anti rheumatic drugs. Study of 10 drugs in 684 patients with rheumatoid arthritis. *J Rheumatol*, **3**, 283–94

49. Lee, P, Webb, J, Anderson, JA and Buchanan, WW (1973). Method for assessing therapeutic potential of anti-inflammatory anti-rheumatic drugs in rheumatoid arthritis. *Br Med J*, **2**, 685–8

50. Lee, P, Watson, TL, Webb, J, Anderson, J and Buchanan, WW (1975). Therapeutic effectiveness of paracetamol in rheumatoid arthritis. *Int J Clin Pharmacol*, **11**, 68–75

51. Rosenbloom, D, Brooks, P, Bellamy, N and Buchanan, WW (1984). *Clinical Trials in the Rheumatic Diseases. A Selected Critical Review.* (New York: Praeger), pp. 70–187

52. Capell, HA, Rennie, JAN, Rooney, PJ et al. (1979). Patient compliance: a novel method of testing non-steroidal anti-inflammatory analgesics in rheumatoid arthritis. *J Rheumatol*, **6**, 586–93

53. Pullar, T, Zoma, AA, Madhok, R, Hunter, JA and Capell, HA (1985). Have the newer NSAIDs contributed to the management of rheumatoid arthritis? *Scott Med J*, **30**, 161–3

54. Anderson, JA, Lee, P, Webb, J and Buchanan, WW (1974). Evaluation of the therapeutic potential of ketoprofen in rheumatoid arthritis. *Curr Med Res Opin*, **2**, 189–97

55. Brooks, PM, Walker, JJ, Lee, P *et al.* (1975). Erprobung eines neuen Acetylsalicylsäure/Paracetamol-Präparates mit magensaftresistentem Überzug (Safapryn) und zweier verschiedenen Dosierungen von Phenylbutazon bei Patienten mit primär chronischer Polyarthritis anhand eines neuen Bewertungsverfahrens. *Z Rheumaforshc*, **34**, 350–65

56. Mathies, H and Kilani, S (1970). Untersuchungen zur Glukokortikoid— Einsparung durch Azapropazon bei chronischer Polyarthritis. *Fortschritte der Medizin*, **88**, 942–6

57. Mathies, H, Olbrich, E, Kilani, S and Sausgruber, H (1974). Glukokortikoid— Einsparung durch Azapropazon und Phenylbutazon im Doppelblind—cross-over Vergleich. *Therapiewoche*, **24**, 3646–52

58. Klatt, L and Koss, FW (1973),. Human pharmacokinetic studies with ^{14}C-tagged azapropazone dihydrate. *Arzneimittel-Forschung*, **23**, 920–1

59. Leach, H (1976). The determination of azapropazone in blood plasma. *Curr Med Res Opin*, **4**, 35–43

60. Guyatt, G, Sackett, D, Taylor, DW, Chong, J, Roberts, R and Pugsley, S (1986). Determining optimal therapy—randomized trials in individual patients. *N Engl J Med*, **314** (Suppl 14), 889–92

61. Langley, GB, Sheppeard, H and Wigley, RD (1983). Placebo therapy in rheumatoid arthritis. *Clin Exp Rheumatol*, **1**, 17–21

62. Mewa, A, Rosenbloom, D, Grace, EM *et al.* Effects of aspirin, naloxone, and placebo on serum beta endorphin concentration and joint pain in patients with rheumatoid arthritis. *Clin Rheumatol*, **6**, 526–31

63. Grace, EM, Mewa, A, Rooney, PJ and Buchanan, WW (1983). Clinical therapeutic trial of sodium meclofenamate and naproxen in rheumatoid arthritis, with comments on the use of placebos in clinical trials. *Curr Med Res Opin*, **8**, 417–24

64. Shapiro, AK, quoted by Bok, S (1974). The ethics of giving placebos. *Sci Am*, **231**, 17–23

65. Max, MB, Schafer, SC, Culnane, M, Dubner, R and Gracely, RH (1988). Association of pain relief with drug side effects in post herpetic neuralgia: a single dose study of clonidine, codeine, ibuprofen and placebo. *Clin Pharm Ther*, **43**, 363–71

66. Wilhelmsen, L, Ljungberg, S, Wedel, H and Werko, L (1976). A comparison between participants and non-participants in primary preventive trial. *J Chronic Dis*, **29**, 331–9

67. Maclagan, TJ (1876). The treatment of acute rheumatism by salicin. *Lancet*, **1**, 342–3

68. Frieman, JA, Chalmers, TC, Smith, H and Kuebler, RR (1978). The importance of beta, the type II error and sample size in the design and interpretation of the randomized control trial. *N Engl J Med*, **299**, 690–4

69. Rennie, JAM, Mason, DIR and Capell, HA (1977). Simple analgesics in rheumatoid arthritis. Editorial *Scott Med J*, **22**, 253–4

70. Nuki, G (1983). Non-steroidal analgesic and anti-inflammatory agents. *Br Med J*, **287**, 39–43

71. Huskisson, EC (1974). Simple analgesics for arthritis. *Br Med J*, **4**, 196–200

72. Kantor, TG (1980). Analgesics for arthritis. *Clin Rheum Dis*, **6**, 525–31

73. Hart, FD (1987). Rational use of analgesics in the treatment of rheumatic disorders. *Drugs*, **33**, 85–93

74. Fremont–Smith, P and Bayles, TB (1965). Salicylate therapy in rheumatoid arthritis. *J Amer Med Assoc*, **192**, 103–6

75. Nuki, G, Downie, WW, Dick, WC et al. (1973). Clinical trial of pentazocine in rheumatoid arthritis. Observations on the value of potent analgesics and placebos. *Ann Rheum Dis*, **32**, 436–43

76. Hardin, JG, Kirk, KA (1979). Comparative effectiveness of five analgesics for the pain of rheumatoid arthritis. *J Rheumatol*, **6**, 405–42

77. Brooks, PM, Dougan, MA, Mugford, A and Meffin, E (1982). Comparative effectiveness of five analgesics in patients with rheumatoid arthritis. *J Rheumatol*, **9**, 732–6

78. Emergy, P and Gibson, T (1986). A double-blind study of the simple analgesic nefopam in rheumatoid arthritis. *Br J Rheumatol*, **27**, 117–22

79. Seidman, P and Melander, A. (1986). Equianalgesic effects of peracetamol and indomethacin in rheumatoid arthritis. *Br J Rheumatol*, **27**, 72–6

80. Feinstein, AR (1970). Clinical biostatistics: III The architecture of clinical research. *Clin Pharm Ther*, **11**, 432–41

81. Lee, P and Tan, LJP (1979). Drug compliance in outpatients with rheumatoid arthritis. *Aust NZ J Med*, **9**, 274–7

82. Pullar, T, Peaker, S, Martin, MFR, Bird, HA and Feely, MP (1988). The use of a pharmacological indicator to investigate compliance in patients with a poor response to anti rheumatic therapy. *Br J Rheumatol*, **27**, 381–4

83. Sackett, DL and Gent, M (1979). Controversy in counting and attributing events in clinical trials. *N Engl J Med*, **301**, 1410–2

84. Reiffenstein, RJ, Schiltroth, AJ and Todd, DM (1968). Current standards in reported drug trials. *Canad Med Assoc J*, **99**, 1134–5

85. Mosteller, F, Gilbert, JP and McPeek, B (1980). Reporting standards in research strategies for controlled trials. *Controlled Clin Trials*, **1**, 37–58

86. Mosteller, F (1979). Problems of omission in communications. *Clin Pharm Ther*, **25**, 761–4

87. Dev Simonian, R, Charette, J, McPeek, P and Mosteller, F (1982). Reporting on methods in clinical trials. *N Engl J Med*, **306**, 1332–7

88. Chilton, NW and Barbano, JP (1974). Guidelines for reporting clinical trials. *J Periodontal Res*, **9**, (Suppl 14), 207–8

89. O'Fallon, JR, Dubey, SD, Salsburg, DS, Edmonson, JH, Soffer, A and Colton, T (1978). Should there be statistical guidelines for medical research papers? *Biometrics*, **34**, 687–95

90. Dev Simonian, R, Charette, J, McPeek, P and Mosteller, F (1978). Reporting on methods in clinical trials. *N Engl J Med*, **307**, 1220

91. Chalmers, TC, Smith, H, Blackburn, B et al. (1981). A method for assessing the quality of a randomized control trial. *Controlled Clin Trials*, **2**, 31–49

92. Colton, T (1982). Reporting on methods in clinical trials. *N Eng J Med*, **307**, 1219–20

93. Sackett, DL (1982). Reporting on methods in clinical trials. *N Engl J Med*, **307**, 1219

94. Bellamy, N and Buchanan, WW (1984). The codification of clinical trial methodology. *EULAR Bull*, **13**, 61–4

Summary

In spite of the apparent variability in quality of the clinical trials employed with azapropazone, this drug has clearly proven efficacious in the treatment of rheumatoid arthritis (RA). The variable quality of clinical trials has also presented a major problem for assessing the effectiveness of other NSAIDs, and this is a difficulty in trying to assess the relative effectiveness and safety of azapropazone with other NSAIDs in RA. The problem is exacerbated by the variability which exists in long-term progress of RA. Attempts to overcome variability within RA subjects and with the natural course of the disease requires employing so-called sequential double-blind crossover study designs and it may be useful to employ these in future studies.

Zusammenfassung

Trotz der offensichtlichen Qualitätsunterschiede bei klinischen Studien mit Azapropazon hat sich diese Substanz bei der Therapie der chronischen Polyarthritis (cP) eindeutig als wirksam erwiesen. Auch bei der Beurteilung der Wirksamkeit anderer nichtsteroidaler Antirheumatika (NSAID) stellt die unterschiedliche Qualität der klinischen Studien ein grosses Problem dar. Es ist deshalb schwierig, die relative Wirksamkeit und Sicherheit von Azapropazon bei cP im Vergleich zu anderen NSAIDs einzuschätzen. Diese Schwierigkeiten werden zudem durch den variablen Langzeitverlauf der cP potenziert. Um den Unterschieden innerhalb eines Kollektivs von cP-Patienten und dem unterschiedlichen Spontanverlauf der Krankheit Rechnung zu tragen, müsste ein sogenannter sequentieller, doppelblinder, gekreuzter Studienaufbau verwendet werden. Es wäre zweckmässig, künftige Studien auf diese Weise zu konzipieren.

Resumé

Malgré l'apparente variabilité de la qualité des essais cliniques effectués avec l'azapropazone, ce médicament s'est avéré nettement efficace dans le traitement de la polyarthrite rhumatoïde (PR). La qualité variable de ces essais cliniques fut également à origine d'un problème délicat posé dans l'évaluation de l'efficacité des autres AINS, et ceci représente une difficulté si l'on veut tenter d'apprécier l'efficacité relative et la sécurité de l'azapropazone et des autres AINS dans la PR. Le problème est encore plus difficile en raison de la variabilité inhérente à l'évolution à long terme de la PR. Si l'on veut tenter de maîtriser cette variabilité entre les sujets atteints de PR, et celle de l'évolution naturelle de cette affection, il faut recourir à des protocoles d'étude dits "cross-over double-insu séquentiel", et il serait utile de les suivre dans les études futures.

17
Comparative effects of azapropazone on the progression of joint pathology in osteoarthritis

FS Walker, P Revell, A Hemingway, F Low,
KD Rainsford and S Rashad

I. INTRODUCTION

If everyone over the age of 65 were to be X-rayed with sufficient diligence, there would be findings which are radiologically diagnostic of osteoarthritis (OA)[1]—but most people over the age of 65 are not deemed to have the condition[2]. The main reason for this apparent discrepancy is that the majority of these people do not have persistent episodes of pain, and in practice it is the presence of joint pain which causes a person who has the appropriate radiological findings to acquire the diagnostic label of 'osteoarthritis'.

Thus, the most important clinical feature of OA is pain. This is closely followed in importance by reduced mobility. At best, OA is an annoyance; at worst, the pain can substantially disrupt normal living. As Marcel Proust wrote, 'to kindness, to knowledge we make promises only: pain we obey'[3].

Being now a sufferer, the OA patient is usually—though by no means always—perceived to need treatment primarily for the relief of pain. If the pain is adequately treated, there may also be a beneficial effect on disability, since the relief of pain may be accompanied by increased ability to move and to perform the normal tasks of day-to-day living. Enthusiastic physicians with the means at their disposal may also add other measures to the therapeutic regimen aimed at improving mobility such as physiotherapy, counselling and the provision of aids for living, all of which may confer additional benefit to the patient.

Unfortunately, the management of OA over the years has not presented such a simple picture[4]. Physicians have generally felt that they had little to offer therapeutically; the measure of success in the treatment of OA has been rather low, and the condition has been regarded as having an inevitability as people age. This has resulted in a lack of enthusiasm among rheumatologists, and the genesis of somewhat negative terms for OA such as 'degenerative arthropathy' with its pejorative implication that little of real value can be done for these patients. The term 'osteoarthrosis' has also not been very helpful since, almost by definition it denies the existence of an inflammatory

Azapropazone – 20 years of clinical use. Rainsford, KD (ed)
© Kluwer Academic Publishers. Printed in Great Britain

component in OA. This inflammatory component undoubtedly exists in a proportion of OA patients[5], as judged by hot, tender joints and a pronounced therapeutic response to anti-inflammatory drugs[6], as opposed to centrally-acting analgesics such as dextropropoxyphene or a simple analgesic such as paracetamol.

The first milestone in the efforts to find an effective medicine for the pain and inflammation of arthritis was the discovery of aspirin in 1899. Since then, and with a growing understanding of the nature of both rheumatoid arthritis (RA) and OA, more scientifically logical work has been pursued since about 1930, leading to the proclamation by Hench et al.[7] in 1949 that cortisone and ACTH had dramatic pain-relieving effects in RA.

Within a year of this, semi-synthetic cortisone became available for clinical use. We must remember that in those days cortisone was used in what would now be regarded as very high dosage—and that it also had a brief vogue in the treatment of OA.

In 1952—two years after cortisone became available—Demartini et al.[8] reported that cortisone might be associated with pathological fractures in rheumatoid patients. Subsequently, Allen and Murray[9] described changes similar to those of neuropathic joints which they had observed in a review of 100 pre-1950 radiographs: these included steroid-treated OA patients.

The first of the modern non-steroidal anti-inflammatory drugs (NSAIDs) to be introduced was phenylbutazone in 1952, followed by indomethacin in 1965. Again, within 2 years, Allen and Murray[9] had observed that some arthritic patients being treated with indomethacin and who had never received steroids, developed a rapidly-progressing arthropathy (Figure 1) similar to that previously reported with steroids and they coined the expression 'analgesic hip'. Their retrospective radiological review also reported a similar arthropathy associated with phenylbutazone which they then realized that they had been seeing in 1964. Since then, there have been numerous reports describing accelerating OA associated primarily with indomethacin[10–14] and also with other drugs[9,15]. Almost all concern themselves with the hip joint and with the femoral head in particular. Newman and Ling[16], however, found a highly significant correlation between NSAID use and acetabular destruction in OA. There appears to be only one reference[17] to 'analgesic knee' and none to the condition in other joints; some investigators[18,19] doubt the existence of 'analgesic hip' at all.

Assuming that NSAIDs can actually accelerate the joint pathology of OA, what is the likely mechanism? A widely-held view is that these drugs produce an 'iatrogenic Charcot's arthropathy'[19], the analgesia encouraging the over-use of compromised joints. This may well be true in RA where the skeleton is weakened[20] and where the femoral head is in increased danger from trabecular microfractures, but there is little evidence for this in OA. There is also no evidence for the opposite view, namely that immobilization of an osteoarthritic joint promotes its healing: indeed, there is evidence that load-bearing and use are required for the integrity of articular cartilage to

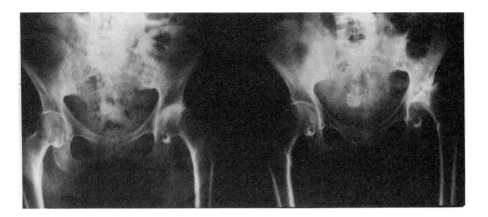

Figure 1 Radiographs before (left) and after (right) 18 weeks treatment with indomethacin 75 mg daily.

be maintained[21].

It is known, however, that perfusion of the osteoarthritic femoral head is increased[22] presumably due to inflammation; it is also known that NSAIDs attenuate the vasodilator response by inhibiting the synthesis of vasodilator prostaglandins (PG)[23]. It is possible that the osteoarthritic joint requires enhanced perfusion to maintain the increased biological demands of the repair processes, and that if perfusion is reduced by inhibition of PG synthesis, the already compromised joint will deteriorate more rapidly. If this is true, then it should be possible to demonstrate that, by comparison with a potent PG synthesis inhibitor, the progression of the osteoarthritic process will be slower if a weak inhibitor of PG synthesis is used to treat OA patients.

In order to test this hypothesis, patients were treated with either indomethacin, a potent inhibitor of PG synthesis[24] or with azapropazone, a weak inhibitor. The clinical progress of their OA was followed, together with radiological, biochemical and pathological investigations.

All of the studies so far reported on this question are retrospective or anecdotal: this is the first reported prospective clinical investigation of the subject.

II. PATIENTS AND METHODS

Between 1983 and 1988, 105 OA patients were recruited to the study and completed it. Details of the study population are shown in Table 1. The study inclusion and exclusion criteria are set out in Table 2. Basically, patients had to have primary uncomplicated OA of the hip so as to confine

Table 1 Study population

Treatment group:	Azapropazone	Indomethacin
n:	49 (19 M, 30 F)	56 (21 M, 35 F)
Mean age:	65.5 ± 11.75(SD)	67.1 ± 7.98(SD)
Mean initial joint space (sum in mm of 4 segments):		
Affected hip:	9.16 ± 0.54(SE)	9.89 ± 0.55(SE)
Contralateral hip:	13.56 ± 0.56(SE)	13.84 ± 0.51(SE)

Table 2 Study inclusion/exclusion criteria

Inclusion	Exclusion
1. Primary uncomplicated OA of the hip	1. IgM rheumatoid factor
2. Pain requiring treatment and admission to arthroplasty waiting list	2. Polyarticular disease
	3. Superior pole disease
3. Fit enough to be well at end of waiting period	4. Signs of avascular necrosis
	5. Destructive arthropathy
4. Fit enough to do well after arthroplasty	6. Crystals in joints
5. Able and willing to co-operate	7. Treatment with anticoagulant, steroid, immunosuppressant, lithium
	8. NSAID intolerance
	9. History of peptic ulcer
	10. Substantial obesity

the study as far as possible to one sub-set of OA. They had to be suffering pain or disability of sufficient intensity to justify admission to the waiting list for hip arthroplasty, but apart from this, they had to be fit and well. Patients were excluded from the study if they showed evidence of a rapidly destructive arthropathy or if they needed arthroplasty in less than 6 months.

During the pre-arthroplasty period, patients were randomly allocated either to azapropazone 600 mg or 900 mg daily, or to indomethacin 50 mg or 75 mg daily. Patients were assessed monthly, at which time their pain scores were recorded using a 5-point categorical pain scale. Patients were X-rayed 3-monthly using a standardized procedure: the same machine was used for each X-ray of a given patient, film stock dedicated to this particular study was used, and the same exposure was used each time on a given patient. For each patient, the hip which was associated with the most pain or restriction of movement—the 'affected' hip— and the contralateral hip were X-rayed, both antero-posterior and 45° oblique, with the patient supine. After preliminary exercises designed to ensure inter-observer concordance, the radiographs were examined by 2 independent radiologists: each radiological joint space was divided into 4 segments (Figure 2), the width of each segment in mm was measured and the 4 measurements added to give a combined joint space measurement (joint space).

Hip arthroplasty was performed when pain could no longer be adequately controlled, or when severe restriction of joint movement resulted in inability to perform normal tasks. This assessment was always made by

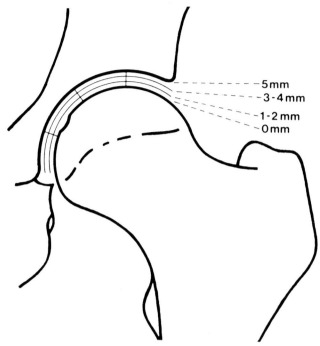

Figure 2 Radiological joint space measurement.

the same doctor. Each patient was given tetracycline 500 mg on days 16–18 and days 6–8 before arthroplasty in order to label appositional bone in the femoral head, so that the distance between the bands could be measured under UV microscopy and bone growth rate calculated. At arthroplasty, a sample of synovium for assay of eicosanoids was cut from that part of the joint capsule underlying the obturator internus and a small wedge was cut from the posterior rim of the femoral head to act as a marker, facilitating the subsequent coronal slicing of the femoral head.

The excised femoral head was cut into 8 or 9 slices. A part of the central slice was dehydrated, embedded in acrylic polymer sectioned to 10 μm and mounted in Fluormount mounting medium. Measurement of distance between bands of tetracycline fluorescence was carried out under UV microscopy using filters BG38 & UG1 (barrier) and 50 & 65 (excitor). Calculation of the appositional bone growth rate was performed using the method of Frost[26].

Femoral head slices were decalcified in 5% formic acid in 10% formol-saline, the process being monitored by periodic radiography. The decalcified slices were then processed in a Shandon Hypercentre II, embedded in paraffin wax, sectioned to 3μm and stained with haematoxylin and eosin (H & E, Figure 3). The image from each H & E section was computer-analyzed using a Quantimet 730 image analysis system to quantitate cysts, osteophytes,

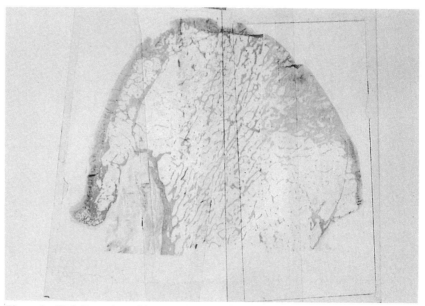

Figure 3   H & E section of femoral head: on the left can be seen a large osteophyte, with underlying cartilage remnant; on the right is an area of eburnated bone.

bone mass and cartilage, and using the data from these sections, the whole femoral head structure was calculated according to the Delesse principle[27].

Proteoglycan in cartilage samples taken from the cut wedge from the femoral head was extracted with GuHCl in the presence of protease inhibitors, precipitated with 2% CPC, and the concentration of GAGs in the precipitate after dialysis assayed using the method of Farndale et al.[28]. The eicosanoids present in synovial tissues were extracted with 0.2 M citric acid and ethanol, and fractions were purified on SepPak® reverse phase minicolums. The concentrations of prostaglandin E_2 (PGE_2), thromboxane B_2 (TXB_2) and 5-hydroxy-eicosatetraenoic acid (5-HETE) were assayed in the synovial samples using radioimmunoassay kits (Advanced Magnetics Inc.). Full details of the biochemical methods and validation will be reported elsewhere.

The time to arthroplasty data were processed using the product limit estimation method of Kaplan and Meier[29], the rate of change of joint space was determined by regression of the combined joint space measurements on time to arthroplasty and other data were analysed using χ^2 or Mann Whitney U as appropriate.

All measurements were done single-blind and the study was approved by the West Middlesex University Hospital ethics committee.

III. RESULTS

Both treatment groups were well matched for age and sex distribution (Table 1). As far as can be judged from the radiological joint space measurements, both groups were also well matched for the stage of primary OA of the hip at entry into the study.

Frequencies of individual pain scores at the beginning of the study and immediately before arthroplasty for each patient are shown in Table 3. Initial day pain scores for the azapropazone group tended to be higher (more pain) than for the indomethacin group, but this difference did not quite reach significance: the modal day pain score was 2 for both groups. The final modal day pain score was 3 for both groups, although the score for the azapropazone group was higher than for the indomethacin group ($p < 0.05$); both groups, however, changed their day pain scores to a similar extent. Night pain scores were lower than day pain scores for both groups and were similar; they also changed to a smaller extent than the day pain scores. A few patients (8 azapropazone, 5 indomethacin) reduced their pain scores during the day.

The time from entry into the study up to the end-point of arthroplasty was 50% longer ($p < 0.01$) in the azapropazone group than in the indomethacin group (Figure 4); a much greater proportion of the azapropazone group (30%) than of the indomethacin group (5%) took more than 18 months to reach the criteria for arthroplasty ($p < 0.001$).

Throughout the study there was an overall reduction in joint space (Figure 5) for both treatment groups; this reduction was slightly, though not significantly, slower in the azapropazone group. In those patients showing no change or a decrease in joint space, the rate of loss of joint space in the indomethacin group was greater in both hips ($p < 0.05$) than in the azapropazone group (Table 4). In indomethacin patients, the 'affected' hip lost joint space more rapidly ($p < 0.05$) than did the contralateral hip, a difference not seen in the azapropazone group.

The mean pre-arthroplasty joint spaces of the 'affected' hips (mm $\pm$ SE) were 8.87 ± 5.0 and 8.55 ± 4.0, and for the contralateral hips 13.14 ± 5.2 and 13.00 ± 5.4 in the indomethacin and azapropazone groups respectively.

There was little difference in the rates of appositional bone growth between the groups: the rate (mean μm/day $\pm$ SE) was 1.34 ± 0.07 (n = 38) for the azapropazone group and 1.22 ± 0.010 (n = 44) for the indomethacin group.

Histomorphometry of the excised femoral heads also varied little between groups (Table 5). Cartilage proteoglycan content (mean μg/mg $\pm$ SE) however, was greater ($p < 0.05$) at 13.42 ± 1.34 (n = 13) in the azapropazone group than in the indomethacin group 7.77 ± 1.34 (n = 18).

There was a significantly higher content of PGE_2, TXB_2 and 5-HETE in the synovium of azapropazone-treated patients than in indomethacin-treated patients (Table 6).

Side-effects in the study were those to be expected in patients taking NSAIDs. One indomethacin patient had an acute bleed (melaena).

IV. DISCUSSION

In this study the effects of a weak and of a strong inhibitor of prostaglandin synthesis on the progression of OA have been compared. Early in the study

Table 3 Frequencies of pain scores

	Day pain				Night pain			
	Azapropazone		Indomethacin		Azapropazone		Indomethacin	
	Initial	Final	Initial	Final	Initial	Final	Initial	Final
None	0	1	2	4	4	12	8	12	9
Slight	1	5	3	9	7	16	9	17	5
Moderate	2	29	19	37	12	13	19	24	22
Severe	3	11	20	6	33	4	12	3	20
Very severe	4	4	6	0	0	5	2	0	0

Day pain:
Aza vs. indo
Initial $\chi^2 = 9.07$ 4df $p = 0.06$
Final $\chi^2 = 12.74$ 4df $p < 0.05$

Night pain:
Aza vs. indo
Initial $\chi^2 = 8.13$ 4df $p = 0.09$
Final $\chi^2 = 2.15$ 3df $p = 0.30$

Aza = azapropazone; indo = indomethacin.

246

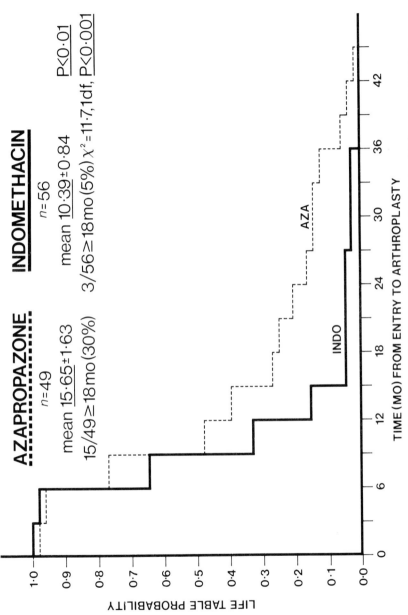

Figure 4 Kaplan–Meier plot of duration (months) from study entry to arthroplasty. AZA = azapropazone; INDO = indomethacin.

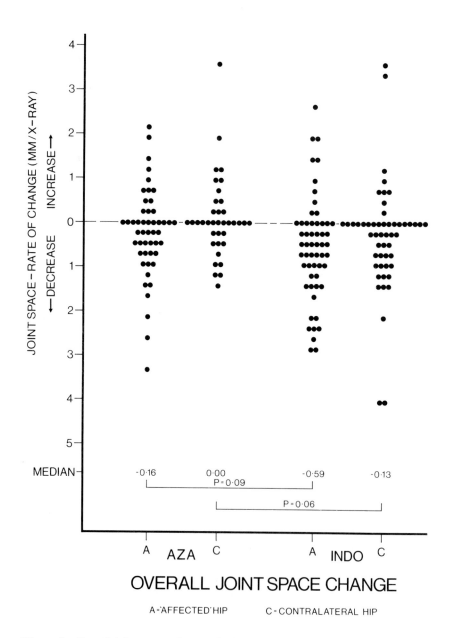

Figure 5 Overall joint space change. AZA = azapropazone; INDO = indomethacin.

Table 4   Patients showing no change or decrease in joint space

	Mean rate of joint space change, mm/X-ray $\pm$ SE		
	Azapropazone	*Indomethacin*	
'Affected' hip	0.66 ± 0.13 (n = 36)	0.97 ± 0.13 (n = 46)	$p < 0.05$
Contralateral	0.32 ± 0.09 (n = 25)	0.63 ± 0.14 (n = 43)	$p < 0.05$
	NS	$p < 0.05$	

Table 5   Cysts, osteophytes, cartilage and bone mass as mean % of femoral head $\pm$ SE

	Azapropazone n = 46	*Indomethacin* n = 55
Cysts	4.03 ± 0.94	5.11 ± 0.94
Osteophytes	8.21 ± 1.14	8.21 ± 0.80
Cartilage	46.05 ± 2.20	42.45 ± 2.52
Bone mass	28.51 ± 1.48	24.11 ± 3.09

Table 6   Eicosanoids in synovium

	Mean ng/mg $\pm$ SE		
	PGE_2	TXB_2	5-HETE
Azapropazone n = 16	10.10 ± 3.1	1.61 ± 0.32	7.35 ± 1.40
Indomethacin n = 28	3.17 ± 0.76	0.82 ± 0.30	4.18 ± 0.85
Azapropazone vs. indomethacin: PGE_2, $p < 0.05$			
TXB_2, $p < 0.001$			
5-HETE, $p < 0.01$			

attempts were made to include a control group of untreated patients, but this did not succeed: this is not surprising, since it is the pain of OA which makes the patient seek treatment and which seals the diagnosis of OA. Similarly, there were difficulties in recruiting a paracetamol-treated group, and this has also been the experience of others who have attempted to treat OA with simple analgesics[6].

Apart from being well matched for age and sex distribution, both treatment groups were comparable in their initial pain scores and in the stage of their OA as judged by their radiological joint space.

In this study, the end-point was arthroplasty, the timing of which was determined by failure to control pain, or severe restriction of joint movement, these assessments being made by the same doctor in all cases. Were the patients in the two treatment groups at a similar pathophysiological end-point when they eventually came to the end-point of arthroplasty? From the data presented, both treatment groups were very similar in this respect: there was little difference between the groups in the histomorphometric analysis of the femoral head or in bone growth rate, and there was also little difference between the groups in the final pre-arthroplasty joint space. The most substantial difference between the groups was the length of time which they took to reach this uniform end-point, the azapropazone group taking 50%

longer to do so and with slower radiological deterioration. This may be associated with the higher cartilage proteoglycan content in the azapropazone group; the suggestion also arises that cartilage 'quality' *per se* may be only a minor factor in the genesis of the end-point in this study.

Another important difference between the treatment groups is the relative behaviour of the 'affected' versus the contralateral hips. If one accepts that the contralateral hip serves as a similarly-treated control for the 'affected' hip, then the significant difference in rate of joint space loss between the 'affected' and the contralateral hips of the indomethacin patients—a difference not seen in the azapropazone patients—means that the more a hip is affected by OA, the faster it will deteriorate with indomethacin treatment. This view is further supported by work in animals[30].

Was there any effect of initial OA severity—as measured by joint space—in the time to arthroplasty? There was very little relationship between these two factors: correlations in both treatment groups were weak, with $r = 0.39$ for azapropazone and 0.29 for indomethacin.

Were there differences in pain relief between the groups which could have influenced the time to arthroplasty? The data suggest that any differences in this respect are really very small and unlikely to account in any way for the major difference between the groups in time to arthroplasty.

The differences in synovial eicosanoids between the treatment groups present no surprise, since azapropazone and indomethacin differ considerably in their capacity to inhibit cyclo-oxygenase products[24]. The concentration of PGE_2 and TXB_2 was reduced ($p < 0.05$ and 0.001 respectively) in the synovial tissues of the indomethacin treated patients and this was to be expected. The reduced synovial content of 5-HETE ($p < 0.01$) was, however, unexpected since NSAIDs have been shown not to inhibit the lipoxygenase pathway to eicosanoid synthesis[31]. A possible reason for this finding is that indomethacin may have a greater inhibiting effect on migration of eicosanoid-secreting leucocytes to sites of inflammation in OA.

The initial hypothesis has been tested: it has been shown that, in patients treated with a potent inhibitor of prostaglandin synthesis, OA of the hip progresses more rapidly as judged by clinical, radiological, biochemical and pathological criteria. In patients treated with a weak inhibitor of PG synthesis, the OA process is, by comparison, significantly slower according to all criteria measured.

Thus, evidence now exists that greater caution should be exercised in treating OA patients with the more powerful inhibitors of PG synthesis.

Acknowledgments

The authors would like to record their thanks to David Clayton for statistical advice, to Chris Pirie for preparation of the pathology specimens, to Linda Mundy and Candie Smellie for technical assistance, to Josephine Walker and Niki Woolven for data assembly and to Janet Wheeler for preparation of the typescript.

Part of the work reported here was published by *The Lancet* on 2nd September 1989.

References

1. Lawrence, JS, Bremner, JM and Bier, F (1966). Osteo-arthrosis: prevalence in the population and relation between symptoms and X-ray changes. *Ann Rheum Dis*, **25**, 1–24
2. Dieppe, PA (1984). Osteoarthritis: are we asking the wrong questions? *Br J Rheumatol*, **23**, 161–3
3. Proust, M (1871–1922). *Cities of the Plain* I, Part 2, Ch 1
4. Wood, PHN and Badley, EM (1986). Epidemiology of individual rheumatic disorders. In: Scott, JT (ed), *Copeman's Textbook of the Rheumatic Diseases*, Vol 1. (Edinburgh: Churchill Livingstone), p. 89
5. Peyron, J (1981). Inflammation in osteoarthritis (OA): review of its role in clinical picture, disease progress, subsets and pathophysiology. *Arthritis Rheum*, **11**, 115–6
6. Doyle, DV, Dieppe, PA, Scott, J, Huskisson, EC (1981). An articular index for the assessment of osteoarthritis. *Ann Rheum Dis*, **40**, 75–8
7. Hench, PS, Kendall, EC, Slocumb, CH and Polley, HF (1949). The effect of a hormone of the adrenal cortex (17-hydroxy-11-dehydrocorticosterone: compound E) and of pituitary adrenocorticotropic hormone on rheumatoid arthritis. *Proc Staff Meet Mayo Clin*, **24**, 181–97
8. Demartini, F, Grokoest, AW and Ragan, C (1952). Pathological fractures in patients with rheumatoid arthritis treated with cortisone. *JAMA*, **149**, 750
9. Allen, EH and Murray, RO (1971). Iatrogenic arthropathies. *Europ Assoc Radiol Proc*, **249**, 204–10
10. Coke, H (1967). Long-term indomethacin therapy of coxarthrosis. *Ann Rheum Dis*, **26**, 346–7
11. Rubens-Duval, A, Villiaumey, J, Kaplan, G and Bailly, D (1970). Surmenage et détérioration rapide de coxo-fémorales arthrosiques au cours de thérapeutiques anti-inflammatoires non corticoïdes. *Revue de Rheumatisme*, **37**(8–9), 535–41
12. Foss Hauge, M (1975). Hofteleddsartrose—indometacin. *Tidsskrift Norske Laegeforen*, **95**(28), 1594–6
13. Milner, JC (1973). Osteoarthritis of the hip and indomethacin. *J Bone Jt Surg*, **54B**, 752
14. Desproges–Gotteron, G, Loubet, R, Dunoyer, J and Laures J–C (1971). Enquête anatamopathologique sur les têtes fémorales prélevées lors des arthroplasties de hanches. *Revue de Rheumatisme*, **38**(10), 623–30
15. Watson, M (1976). Femoral head height loss: a study of the relative significance of some of its determinance in hip degeneration. *Rheumatol Rehab*, **15**, 264–9
16. Newman, NM, Ling, RSM (1985). Acetabular bone destruction related to non-steroidal anti-inflammatory drugs. *Lancet*, **2**, 11–3
17. Murray, RO and Jacobson, HG (1977). *The Radiology of Skeletal Disorders*, 2nd ed, Vol. II. (Edinburgh: Churchill Livingstone)
18. Solomon, L (1973). Drug induced arthropathy and necrosis of the femoral head. *J Bone Jt Surg*, **55B**, 246–61
19. Doherty, M, Holt, M, MacMillan, P, Watt, I and Dieppe, P (1986). A reappraisal of 'analgesic hip'. *Ann Rheum Dis*, **45**, 272–6
20. Mueller, MN and Jurist, JM (1973). Skeletal status in rheumatoid arthritis: a preliminary report. *Arthritis Rheum*, **16**, 66–70
21. Gay, RE, Palmoski, MJ, Brandt, KD and Gay, S (1983). Aspirin causes *in vivo* synthesis of type I collagen by atrophic articular cartilage. *Arthritis Rheum*,

26(10), 1231–6

22. Harrison, MHM, Schajowitz, F and Trueta, J (1953). Osteoarthritis of the hip: a study of the nature and evolution of the disease. *J Bone Jt Surg*, **35B** 598–626

23. Vane, JR (1971). Inhibition of prostaglandin synthesis as a mechanism of action for aspirin-like drugs. *Nature New Biol*, **231**, 232–5

24. Walker, FS (1985). Azapropazone and related benzotriazines. In: Rainsford, KD (ed), *Anti-Inflammatory and Anti-Rheumatic Drugs*, Vol II: *Newer Anti-Inflammatory Drugs*. (Boca Raton: CRC Press), pp. 1–32

25. Revell, PA (1986). Quantitative methods in bone biopsy examination. In: *Pathology of Bone*. (Berlin: Springer–Verlag), pp. 87–111

26. Frost, HM (1976). Histomorphometry of trabecular bone. I. Theoretical correction of appositional rate measurements. In: Meunier PJ (ed), *Bone Histomorphometry*, 2nd International Workshop, (Paris: Armour-Montagu), pp. 361–78

27. Delesse, MA (1848). Procédé mechanique pour determiner la composition des roches. *Ann Mines*, **13**, 379–88

28. Farndale, RW, Buttle, DJ and Barrett, AJ (1986). Improved quantitation and discrimination of sulphated glycosaminoglycans by use of dimethylmethylene blue. *Biochim Biophys Acta*, **883**, 173–7

29. Kaplan, EL and Meier, P (1958). Nonparametric estimation from incomplete observations. *J Am Statist Ass*, **53**, 457–81

30. Pettipher, ER, Henderson, B, Edwards, JCW and Higgs, GA (1986). Indomethacin enhances proteoglycan loss from articular cartilage in antigen-induced arthritis. *Br J Pharmacol*, **94**, 341P

31. Moncada, S, Flower, RJ and Vane, JR (1985). Prostaglandins, prostacyclin, thromboxane A and leukotrienes. In: Gilman, AG, Goodman, LS, Rall, TW and Murad, F (eds) *The Pharmacological Basis of Therapeutics*, 7th ed. (New York: Macmillan), pp. 660–673

Summary

Since the introduction of indomethacin there have been reports that the use of NSAIDs in osteoarthritis (OA) can be associated with rapidly-developing arthropathy. It is suggested that this effect is mediated by NSAID-induced reduction of the synthesis of vasodilator prostaglandins (PG), thereby diminishing joint perfusion. To test this hypothesis 105 OA patients awaiting hip arthroplasty were treated prospectively wtih a strong or with a weak PG synthesis inhibitor, indomethacin or azapropazone respectively. Pain and radiological joint space were monitored during the period up to arthroplasty and the condition of the excised femoral head was determined. From radiological and histopathological data, both treatment groups were at a similar pathophysiological end-point when they came to arthroplasty. In the indomethacin group the 'affected' hips lost joint space more rapidly than the contralateral hips, a difference not seen in the azapropazone group. The azapropazone group took longer than the indomethacin group to reach the arthroplasty end-point with a substantially greater proportion of these patients taking more than 18 months to do so. These differences were associated with higher concentration to synovial vasodilator PG in the azapropazone group. It is suggested that the more potent inhibitors of PG synthesis may be inappropriate in the management of OA of the hip, and that weaker inhibitors such as azapropazone may be suitable.

Zusammenfassung

Seit der Einführung des Indomethacins wurde immer wieder darüber berichtet, daß die Anwendung von NSAR bei Osteoarthritis von einer sich schnell entwickelnden Arthropathie begleitet ist. Man vermutet, daß die von den NSAR verursachte Herabsetzung der Synthese der vasodilatatorisch wirksamen Prostaglandine (PG) für diese Wirkung verantwortlich ist und zu einer Minderdurchblutung der Gelenke führt. Zur Untersuchung dieser Hypothese wurden 105 Patienten mit Osteoarthritis, die einer Hüftgelenksoperation unterzogen werden sollten, prospektiv mit einem starken oder mit einem schwachen PG-Synthese-Hemmer, d.h. entweder Indomethacin oder Azapropazon, behandelt. Bis zum Zeitpunkt der Hüftgelenksoperation wurde die Schmerzstärke gemessen und der Gelenkraum radiologisch überwacht. Außerdem wurde der Zustand des entfernten Femurkopfes bestimmt. Die radiologischen und histopathologischen Daten zeigten, daß beide Behandlungsgruppen vor Durchführung der Hüftgelenksoperation einen ähnlichen pathophysiologischen Endpunkt erreicht hatten. Bei den Patienten in der mit Indomethacin behandelten Gruppe zeigte sich bei der erkrankten Hüfte ein schnellerer Gelenkraumverlust als bei der gegenüberliegenden Hüfte. Bei der mit Azapropazon behandelten Gruppe konnte dieser Unterschied nicht festgestellt werden. Die mit Azapropazon behandelte Gruppe brauchte länger, um den Endpunkt, d.h. die Hüftgelenksoperation, zu erreichen, als die mit Indomethacin behandelte Gruppe, und ein viel größerer Anteil der Patienten in der Azapropazon-Gruppe brauchte dazu über 18 Monate. Der Unterschied war auf höhere PG-Konzentrationen in der Synovia in der Azapropazon-Gruppe zurückzuführen. Daraus läßt sich die Schlußfolgerung ziehen, daß die stärkeren Hemmer der PG-Synthese zur Behandlung der Hüftgelenksarthritis ungeeignet sind und schwächere Hemmer, wie z.B. Azapropazon, für diesen Zweck besser geeignet sind.

Resumé

Depuis l'introduction de l'indométacine, on a signalé que l'emploi des anti-inflammatoires non stéroïdiens dans le traitement de l'ostéoarthrite (OA) pourrait être associé à une arthropathie à évolution rapide. Il est suggéré que cet effet a pour médiateur la réduction de la synthèse des prostaglandines (PG) vasodilatatrices, provoquée par les anti-inflammatoires non stéroïdiens, ce qui diminue l'irrigation des articulations. Pour vérifier cette hypothèse, 105 patient atteints d'ostéoarthrite, qui attendaient une arthroplastie de la hanche, ont été soumis à un traitement prospectif par un inhibiteur fort ou un inhibiteur faible de la synthèse des PG – indométacine ou azapropazone respectivement. La douleur et l'interligne articulaire radiologique ont été surveillées jusqu'au moment de l'arthroplastie, et l'on a examiné l'état de la tête fémorale excisée. Au point de vue des données radiologiques et histopathologiques, les deux groupes traités avaient atteint un point de virage physio-pathologique analogue au moment de leur arthroplastie. Chez le groupe traité à l'indométacine, les hanches "affectées" présentaient une interligne articulaire qui avait diminué plus rapidement que celle des hanches contro-latérales, différence qui n'avait pas été constatée chez le groupe traité par l'azapropazone. Le groupe traité par l'azapropazone a été plus long à atteindre le point de virage de l'arthroplastie, une proportion assez importante de ces patients ayant mis plus de 18 mois à l'atteindre. Ces différences étaient associées à de plus fortes concentrations de PG vasodilatatrices synoviales chez le groupe traité à l'azapropazone. Ceci laisse présager que les inhibiteurs plus puissants de la synthèse des PG sont peut-être mal adaptés au traitement de l'OA de la hanche, mais que des inhibiteurs plus faibles, tels que l'azapropazone, pourraient mieux convenir.

18

Serious gastrointestinal reactions to azapropazone: an estimate of the risk

B Simon and JF Hort

'Science is the father of knowledge but opinion breeds ignorance'

Aristotle

I. INTRODUCTION

It would be ideal if physicians could be told precisely what the chance was of a serious gastrointestinal reaction a particular patient would experience from taking any particular non-steroidal anti-inflammatory drug (NSAID). At present this is not possible but enough data do exist to provide at least some estimate for azapropazone. These data derive from three sources: National Regulatory Authorities, large post-marketing surveillance studies and from clinical trials.

II. NATIONAL REGULATORY AUTHORITIES

1. Committee on Safety of Medicines (CSM)

The yellow card scheme for reporting suspected adverse drug reactions to the CSM has produced data which show that NSAIDs are responsible for a substantial segment of all reports of adverse drug reactions. A thorough review of these reports[1] resulted in the following conclusions, among others:

1. As a group NSAIDs are an important cause of serious reactions.
2. The toxicity of marketed NSAIDs varies between products and the CSM considers that these drugs fall into three categories.
   (a) A group of five drugs which have been withdrawn as substantially more toxic than the others;
   (b) One drug which, at least at low dosage, appears to be less toxic;
   (c) The remainder.

Of this remainder, which includes azapropazone, the CSM considers that 'in terms of overall safety, the drugs cannot be clearly distinguished from each other on the basis of yellow card reports'.

Azapropazone – 20 years of clinical use. Rainsford, KD (ed)
© Kluwer Academic Publishers. Printed in Great Britain

This difficulty arises both from confounding factors and from reporting bias. These conclusions were based on the numbers of yellow card reports of serious ADRs received in the first five years of the marketing of each of the drugs. For each drug, this number was then related to the number of prescriptions written in that first five years.

Apart from the confounding factors (reports seldom prove causation; effects of publicity; incomplete reporting; number of prescriptions overestimates the number of patients, due to repeat prescriptions; serious gastrointestinal events frequently occur in elderly person in the absence of drug therapy) acknowledged by the CSM, there is a further factor peculiar to azapropazone. For this drug in the first five years of marketing, the recommended daily dose for all patients was 1200 mg. Almost precisely at the end of that five years, the reduced dosage of 600 mg daily was introduced for patients over the age of 65.

The yellow card data for azapropazone is therefore not pertinent to the present day and the dosage factor must be added to the other factors affecting the data for all NSAIDs.

III. OTHER REGULATORY AUTHORITIES

1. Bundesgesundheitsamt (BGA)

Although the BGA have received some reports of gastrointestinal reactions associated with azapropazone, the number of these is too small for use in this present context.

2. Swedish Adverse Drug Reaction Advisory Committee (SADRAC)

In the period 1978–1984, SADRAC received a total of seven reports of gastrointestinal ulcers and bleedings associated with azapropazone[2]. During this period, reporting of serious reactions was compulsory and for about half of the period, there was no recommendation for a reduced dosage of azapropazone in elderly patients. SADRAC use the technical term "defined daily doses" (DDD) which equals the estimated average daily dose for adults when a drug is used in its main indication. The incidence of serious gastrointestinal reactions associated with azapropazone is given by SADRAC as 42 per 100 000 DDD years. Expressed in the same way, the incidence for piroxicam was 151, for indomethacin 5 and for diclofenac 3. SADRAC state "that the ranking of the NSAIDs in Sweden in almost every instance agrees with that reported from the United Kingdom..."

IV. POST-MARKETING SURVEILLANCE (PMS)

There have been no formal PMS studies of azapropazone. Studies which are to some extent equivalent have been carried out in the United Kingdom and are discussed under Clinical Trials. One study, performed in the Federal Republic of Germany, although not strictly a PMS exercise, incorporated close monitoring of patients and is therefore of value in this context[3]. This study is unique among the larger studies in that dosage for all patients did not exceed 900 mg. 1025 patients took part and the time period was from 1 to 5 years. Table 1 gives the number of gastric and duodenal ulcers encountered during this study, revealed either by symptoms and subsequent endoscopy or by loss of blood.

Table 1 Gastrointestinal reactions occurring among 1025 patients during from 1 to 5 years therapy with from 600 mg to 900 mg azapropazone daily

Reaction	Time of event (years)				
	1	2	3	4	5
Gastric ulcer	0	0	0	0	0
Duodenal ulcer	0	0	0	4	1

Although other gastrointestinal reaction may have occurred without being recognized, and although dosage was low for the younger patients, this study provides perhaps the best available data for the present purpose.

V. CLINICAL TRIALS, UNITED KINGDOM

1. Short term studies

Studies in which azapropazone was given for 28 days or less have in the main involved patients in the age range 18 to 70 with a preponderance of these being aged less than 65. The majority of these studies were conducted at an early stage after introduction of the drug and so dosages of 1200 mg azapropazone daily were used for all patients. The relevant details of these studies are summarized in Table 2. (For the purpose of this review, a 'serious gastrointestinal ADR' is defined as any firm evidence of ulceration or bleeding.)

Few elderly patients were admitted to these trials.

In five short term studies the dosage of azapropazone was less than 1200 mg daily. Berry and colleagues used 900 mg daily for 1 week in 60 subjects and encountered no serious adverse reactions[15]. Kamal, in a study in 40 patients all of whom were older than 65 years (range 67–90) employed 600 mg daily for 4 weeks and 1200 mg daily for 4 weeks in crossover fashion[16]. One patient suffered a haemetemesis on the higher dosage. Fernandez used 600 mg daily for patients older than 65 and 1200 mg daily for the younger patients, 40 patients in all taking these dosages for 21 days[17]. There were no serious gastrointestinal reactions. Rooney employed this same dosage schedule in 30 patients over a 14 day period and also encountered no serious gastrointestinal reactions[18].

Table 2 Studies of 28 days duration or less employing 1200 mg azapropazone daily for all patients

Ref:	No. of patients	Age range	Duration (days)	Serious GI ADRs
4	59	>18	14	0
5	15	18–69	14	0
6	58	>18	14	0
7	50	20–70	7	0
8	24	>18	7	0
9	24	>60	14	0
10	20	>18	28	0
11	23	>18	7	0
12	58	>18	28	0
13	50	33–76	21	0
14	2538	>18	28	1
Total	2919			1 (0.034%)

Calcraft and colleagues used 900 mg daily for 2 weeks in 22 patients encountering no serious adverse reaction[19].

A study employing the currently recommended dosage was conducted to discover if there was any difference between two capsule formulations of azapropazone for their respective gastrointestinal tolerance[20]. No difference was shown. Since the patients were given the drug for 4 weeks in two periods of two weeks on each formulation, the results provide information on gastrointestinal tolerance to azapropazone over the entire period. A total of 635 patients took part in this study. Those aged 65 and over were given 600 mg azapropazone daily and those under 65, 1200 mg daily.

One patient left the study having vomited and exhibited melaena; endoscopy on this subject showed gastritis only. All the above results are summarized in Table 3.

Table 3 Studies using less than 1200 mg azapropazone daily for some or all patients

Reference	No. of patients	Duration (days)	Serious GI ADRs
15	60	7	0
16	40	28	1 (1200 mg)
17	40	21	0
18	30	14	0
19	22	14	0
20	635	28	0
Total	827		1 (0.12%)

2. Long-term studies

There have been 4 long-term studies in which azapropazone was given at a dosage of 1200 mg for all patients. These are summarized in Table 4.

Table 4   Long-term studies employing 1200 mg azapropazone daily for all patients

Ref.	No. of patients	Duration (days)	Serious GI ADRs
21	839	< 180 (n = 418)	4
		180–600 (n = 421)	
22	51	365	0
23	40	180	0
24	46	225	1
Total	976		5 (0.5%)

3. Studies organized outside the United Kingdom

Clinical trials of azapropazone have been conducted in a number of other countries and tabulations of all these would occupy many pages. The main details are summarized in Table 5 which omits all figures derived from studies already discussed. The incidence of reactions occurring in French and Italian studies was considerably greater than in studies in other countries.

Taking all of these studies together, 8771 patients have been involved and 38 serious gastrointestinal reactions were reported (0.43%). During the course of some of these studies, patients reported gastrointestinal symptoms, some of them leaving a study because of this. It is not known whether ulceration was the cause of those symptoms, nor is it known whether the reactions which did occur were due to the drug. Therefore these data provide only an approximate incidence of actual gastrointestinal mucosal damage.

Rainsford made calculations on a similar basis for a number of NSAIDs[25]. Table 6 reproduces the figures presented in that paper with the addition of the above figure for azapropazone, providing a comparison with other NSAIDs.

Although providing some estimate of the risk of serious gastrointestinal reactions, regardless of dosage, these data do not provide information on

Table 5   Serious gastrointestinal side-effects encountered among patients in studies in mainland Europe and in Japan (Adapted from *Rheuma Forum*, special issue 2, p. 37, ed. Eberl, R and Fellman, N (G Braun Verlag, Karlsruhe))

Country	No. of patients	Serious GI side-effects (%)
Switzerland	409	0
German F.R.	1226	0.7
France	297	3.0
Austria	257	1.6
Italy	37	2.7
Yugoslavia	65	0
Hungary	87	0
Japan	329	1.2
Others	317	0
Total	3024	0.79%

Table 6 Percentage of patients with symptomatic ulcers in the upper gastrointestinal tract in patients with rheumatoid arthritis. The percentage for azapropazone is that of serious gastrointestinal reactions in patients with a variety of disorders

Substance	% with ulcers	Number of patients
Acetylsalicylic acid	2.9	447
Diclofenac	0.3	268
Fenclofenac	0	159
Fenoprofen	0.9	107
Ibuprofen	0.8	377
Indomethacin	2.1	2487
Piroxicam	1.4	771
Sulindac	0.4	1865
Tolmetin	2.0	1359
Azapropazone	0.43	8771 (All diagnoses)

the risk if azapropazone is prescribed exactly as currently recommended. That inappropriate dosage in older patients is accompanied by an increased risk is at least suggested by data derived from adverse reaction reports.

Since the launch of azapropazone in the United Kingdom in 1976, A.H. Robins (UK) Ltd. has received 49 reports of serious gastrointestinal reactions. Since all of these reports were followed up, full details of the reactions and the events preceding them are known; in this respect they are better documented than are reports to the CSM of which the company was not aware at that time.

Table 7 Serious gastrointestinal reactions reported to A.H. Robins (UK) Ltd since 1976

Age	Sex		Total
	Male	Female	
65 and older	12	25	37 (8)
64 and younger	3	6	9
Not known	1	2	3
Total	16	33	49

Table 7 shows in parentheses the proportion of these in which the dosage used was in accordance with current recommendations. The unreliability of these data can be illustrated by two case reports:

A female patient age 78 suffered a gastrointestinal bleed following a single 300 mg dose of azapropazone, having up until then been receiving another NSAID.

Another female patient, aged 79, taking 1200 mg azapropazone daily, was admitted to a small nursing home because of intractable vomiting. Azapropazone was continued throughout the following week, during which the vomiting also continued. At the end of the week, the patient suffered perforation of a duodenal ulcer, and this proved fatal.

Those who deal directly with drug reaction reports are aware of histories such as these and become concerned when these reports are treated as one would treat validated scientific data. However, in spite of these and other shortcomings, Table 7 contains interesting information. That elderly female patients are more likely to suffer serious reactions than are male patients has been pointed out by the Committee on Safety of Medicines. This difference, also shown in Table 7, cannot be entirely explained by the greater use of NSAIDs by female patients since, for azapropazone, prescription data shows that, for patients over 65, the proportion of prescriptions for females is 53%.

Although of course using the correct dose in older patients would not eliminate serious gastrointestinal reactions, it is probable that their incidence would be reduced. Omitting the reports in which azapropazone was used concurrently with warfarin, of the remaining 45, four were of suspected reactions in patients under the age of 65 and, of these four, one was known to have a duodenal ulcer when commencing azapropazone therapy and another suffered the reaction four days after changing from diclofenac to azapropazone. This suggests that serious gastrointestinal reactions are relatively uncommon in younger patients.

These data should be treated as providing guidance and not as showing actual incidence since little detail is available about individual cases and the 'reactions' must be regarded as 'associated' with azapropazone and not necessarily as caused by the drug.

VI. CONCLUSION

The three sources previously listed yield all available data and an estimate of the risk of serious gastrointestinal reactions to azapropazone therapy must therefore be drawn from these.

There is a contrast between the estimates from Regulatory Authorities and from clinical studies. The confounding factors of co-prescription of warfarin and of inclusion of cases in which the drug was very unlikely to have been causative are peculiar to the data from Regulatory Authorities. These factors account for a part of the discrepancy but probably not for all of it. The remaining discrepancy must be left unexplained.

Without giving emphasis to data from one source rather than another, the following conclusions appear to be justified.

1. Azapropazone, like all NSAIDs, is capable of producing severe gastro-intestinal reactions.
2. These reactions are more likely to occur in elderly female patients.
3. These reactions are more likely to occur if dosages in excess of those recommended are used, especially so again in elderly females.
4. In a population of both sexes and of all ages (over 18), using dosages which in some cases would now be considered excessive, the risk of

such a reaction can be estimated as about 0.43%.

Finally, to quote again from the CSM, 'NSAIDs should not be given to patients with active peptic ulceration. In patients with such a history and in the elderly they should be given only after other forms of treatment have been carefully considered. In all patients it is prudent to start at the bottom end of the dosage range.'

References

1. Mann, RD (ed.) (1987). *Adverse Drug Reactions* (Parthenon: Carnforth (UK) and Park Ridge (USA)) pp. 36–46
2. Rainsford, KD and Velo, GP (eds.) (1987). *New Developments in Antirheumatic Drugs.* (Lancaster: MTP Press) pp. 55–70
3. Faust-Tinnefeldt, G (1977). Wirkung von Azapropazon auf den Gastrointestinaltrakt und die Leber. *Therapiewoche*, **28**, 8567–8574
4. Brooks, PM and Buchanan, WW (1976). Azapropazone, its place in the management of rheumatoid conditions. *Curr Med Res Opin*, **4**, 94–100
5. Capell, HA, McLeod, MM, Hernandez, LA, Grennan, DM and Templeton, JS (1976). Comparison of azapropazone and naproxen in rheumatoid arthritis. *Curr Med Res Opin*, **4**, 285–289
6. Hicklin, JA, Hingorani, K, Lloyd, KN, Templeton, JS and Wilkinson, M (1976). Azapropazone compared with indomethacin in the treatment of rheumatoid arthritis. *Practitioner*, **217**, 3–7
7. Hingorani, K and Templeton, JS (1975). A comparative trial of azapropazone and ketoprofen in the treatment of acute backache. *Curr Med Res Opin*, **3**, 407–412
8. Kean, WF, Kraag, GR, Rooney, PJ and Capell, HA (1981). Clinical therapeutic trial of aspirin and azapropazone in rheumatoid arthritis when prescribed singly and in combination. *Curr Med Res Opin*, **7**, 164–167
9. Panayi, XIth European Congress of Rheumatology, Athens, 1987
10. Frank, AJM, Moll, JMN and Hort, JF (1982). A comparison of three ways of measuring pain. *Rheumatol Rehab*, **21**, 211–217
11. Grennan, DM, McLeod, M, Watkins, C and Dick, WC (1976). Clincial assessment of azapropazone in rheumatoid arthritis. *Curr Med Res Opin*, **4**, 44–49
12. Lassus, A. (1976). A comparative pilot study of azapropazone and indomethacin in the treatment of psoriatic arthritis and Reiter's disease. *Curr Med Res Opin*, **4**, 65–69
13. Thune, SA (1976). A comparative study of azapropazone and indomethacin in the treatment of rheumatoid arthritis. *Curr Med Res Opin*, **4**, 70–75
14. Robins, AH. Data on file (1984)
15. Berry, H, Bloom, B, Mace, BEW, Hamilton, EBD, Fernandes, L, Molloy, M and Williams, IA (1980). Expectation and patient preference – does it matter? *J Roy Soc Med*, **73**, 34–38
16. Kamal, A (1983). Azapropazone in elderly patients. *Br J Rheumatol* (letter)
17. Robins, AH. Data on file (1988)
18. Rooney, M. XIth European Congress of Rheumatology, Athens, 1987
19. Calcraft, B, Tildesley, G, Evans, KT, Gravelle, H, Hole, D and Lloyd, KN (1974). Azapropazone in the treatment of ankylosing spondylitis: A controlled clinical trial. *Rheumatol Rehab*, **13**, 23–29
20. Robins, AH. Data on file (1987)

21. Robins, AH. Data on file (1978)
22. Wheatley, D (1984). Azapropazone in arthritis: a long-term treatment. *Curr Med Res Opin*, **9**, 86–92
23. Eberl, R (1976). Prolonged treatment with azapropazone. *Curr Med Res Opin*, **4**, 76–79
24. Fraser, RC, Davis, RH and Walker, FS (1987). Comparative trial of azapropazone and indomethacin plus allopurinol in acute gout and hyperuricaemia. *J Roy Coll Gen Practit*, September 1987, 409–411
25. Rainsford, KD (1982). An analysis of the gastro-intestinal side effects of non-steroidal anti-inflammatory drugs, with particular reference to comparative studies in man and laboratory species. *Rheumatol Int*, **2**, 1–10

Summary

The gastro-intestinal tolerance of azapropazone can be assessed by examining data on serious reactions from three sources: National Regulatory Authorities, post-marketing surveillance studies and clinical trials.

The data from the first of these are subject to more unquantifiable variables than are data from clinical studies but have the advantage of being derived from much larger populations and of reflecting use of the drug in actual practice.

From these data, an estimate of the risk of a serious gastro-intestinal reaction to azapropazone may be estimated.

Zusammenfassung

Die Magen-Darm-Verträglichkeit von Azapropazon läßt sich anhand von Daten über schwere Nebenwirkungen aus drei verschiedenen Quellen beurteilen: Registrierungsbehörden, Post-Marketing-Studien und klinische Versuche.

Die Daten aus der ersten Quelle basieren zwar auf mehr unquantifizierbaren Variablen als die Daten aus klinischen Studien, bieten dafür aber den Vorteil, daß sie aus viel größeren Populationen stammen und die Anwendung des Arzneimittels in der Praxis widerspiegeln.

Aus diesen Daten läßt sich das Risiko schwerer Nebenwirkungen auf den Magen-Darm-Trakt abschätzen.

Resumé

On peut évaluer la tolérance gastro-intestinale de l'azapropazone en examinant les données sur les réactions graves provenant des trois sources suivantes: Autorités Nationales de Réglementation, surveillance des études de post-marketing et essais cliniques.

Les données provenant de la première source sont sujettes à davantage de variables, dont on ne peut déterminer la quantité, que ne le sont les données provenant des essais cliniques mais elles présentent l'avantage d'être dérivées de populations bien plus grandes et de refléter l'usage du médicament dans la practique réelle.

A partir de ces données, on peut évaluer le risque d'une sérieuse réaction gastro-intestinale avec l'administration d'azapropazone.

19
Tolerance of azapropazone: allergic and pseudo-allergic reactions and comparison with other NSAIDs

A Szczeklik, E Nizankowska and G Czerniawska-Mysik

I. INTRODUCTION

Pyrazolone drugs can precipitate adverse symptoms ranging from urticaria and angio-oedema to asthma and anaphylactic shock. Patients with these symptoms do not form a homogeneous population, but can be clearly divided into two groups with different pathogenesis.

In the first group, the mechanism responsible for the reactions appears to be allergic. In these patients: (i) noramidopyrine and aminophenazone induce anaphylactic shock and/or urticaria; (ii) skin tests with these drugs are highly positive; (iii) phenylbutazone, sulphinpyrazone and several other cyclo-oxygenase inhibitors, including aspirin, can be taken with impunity; (iv) chronic bronchial asthma is present only in about one fourth of the subjects.

In the second group, the reactions precipitated do not depend on the allergic mechanism (antigen-antibody reaction) but are due to inhibition of cyclo-oxygenase. Thus, in these patients; (i) noramidopyrine, aminophenazone, sulfinpyrazone and phenylbutazone, as well as several other inhibitors of cyclo-oxygenase, including aspirin, lead to open asthmatic attacks; (ii) skin tests with pyrazolone drugs are negative; (iii) all patients have chronic asthma.

The existence of these two groups, first noticed in 1977[1], and described in detail in later years[2-4] has been confirmed by several authors[4-7].

Azapropazone, a non-steroidal anti-rheumatic drug, is a tricyclic compound that has a pyrazolidine moiety in its molecule. There are large differences between azapropazone and other phenylpyrazolone drugs in acidity, basicity characteristics, solubilities, shapes and internal chemistry such that azapropazone should be classed separately. We, therefore, studied the tolerance of azapropazone in patients responding with allergic or pseudo-allergic reactions to pyrazolone drugs. Any results indicating good tolerance of azapropazone would obviously be of clinical interest and importance, since intolerance to mild analgesics constitutes a significant medical problem.

Azapropazone – 20 years of clinical use. Rainsford, KD (ed)
© Kluwer Academic Publishers. Printed in Great Britain

II. PATIENTS AND METHODS

1. Patients

We studied the tolerance of azapropazone in two groups of patients. The first consisted of 12 patients with aspirin-induced asthma (AIA). The second group was formed by 15 patients with hypersensitivity to noramidopyrine and/or aminophenazone with good tolerance of aspirin.

In the first group, there were 9 women and 3 men aged 27–52 years (average 40 years). The intolerance to aspirin manifested itself by dyspnoea and in the majority of cases also by profound rhinorrhoea; it was confirmed by oral challenge tests[1], performed at least two months prior to the study. The first symptoms of aspirin intolerance appeared from 2–22 years before, when the patients were on average 30 years old. The mean duration of aspirin intolerance was 10 years (Table 1).

Nine of these patients also had episodes of adverse drug reactions to noramidopyrine and/or aminophenazone, which manifested as typical attacks of bronchospasm, accompanied in all cases by severe rhinorrhoea. The patients found these symptoms comparable to those precipitated by aspirin, though their intensity was less pronounced.

The second group consisted of subjects hypersensitive to noramidopyrine and/or aminophenazone. There were 12 women and 3 men aged 18–55 years (average 36 years). Only one patient from this group had mild bronchial asthma; another one had hay fever. Adverse drug reactions varied in their intensity: six of the subjects had typical symptoms of anaphylactic shock with hypotension and loss of consciousness, usually within 5–15 minutes after the administration of the drugs. In the majority of the subjects, generalized urticaria, and oedema of the skin were observed. Anaphylactic shock developed 3 months to 6 years before the study. In all cases, anaphylactic shock was preceded by pruritus, urticaria or oedema (Table 2).

In the remaining 9 patients, symptoms of hypersensitivity were of moderate intensity, and consisted of generalized urticaria, laryngeal and skin oedema with intense pruritus. Most patients had several reactions to either of the pyrazolones. The first symptoms appeared 1–24 years and the last ones from 3 months to 6 years before the study. All gave a history of good tolerance to aspirin. This was confirmed by oral challenge tests in 12 of them.

Seven of those 15 patients had also hypersensitivity to other drugs, not related structurally to pyrazolones, i.e. antibiotics, sulphonamides, vitamins, etc.

2. Methods

Skin tests with azapropazone. Increasing concentrations of azapropazone (w/v) in Sörensen phosphate buffer (pH 7.2) were employed in skin tests. We used 0.1% solution of the drug for prick tests and 0.01 and 0.1% solutions

Table 1 Aspirin-induced asthma: characteristics of the patients

Initials	Age	Sex	First reaction to aspirin	Reactions to noramidopyrine/ aminophenazone		Skin tests with noramidopyrine i.d. (0.001% or 0.01% solutions)	Skin tests with azapropazone i.d.	Oral azapropazone challenges
				Dyspnoea	Rhinorrhoea			
B.B.	46	M	1945	−	−	−	−	−
I.S.	37	F	1981	+	+	−	−	−
S.J.	40	F	1987	−	−	−	−	−
N.W.	33	M	1970	+	−	−	−	−
P.D.	35	F	1985	+	+	−	+	−
K.M.	27	M	1987	−	−	−	−	−
G.J.	52	F	1981	+	−	−	−	−
W.H.	41	F	1968	+	−	−	−	−
B.S.	39	F	1982	+	+	−	−	−
J.E.	39	F	1982	+	+	−	−	−
T.H.	48	F	1967	+	+	−	−	−
S.Z.	40	F	1986	+	−	−	−	−

Table 2 Intolerance to noramidopyrine and/or aminophenazone. Characteristics of the patients. Skin tests with azapropazone were negative in all patients. Oral challenge tests with azapropazone were negative in all subjects except for one (Z.E.)

Initials	Age	Sex	First reaction to pyrazolones	Last reaction to pyrazolones	Type of reaction*				Skin tests with noramidopyrine and/or aminophenazone			Adverse reactions to antibiotics, sulphonamides
					S	U	E	D	Year	Results	Results in June '98	
G.M.	18	F	1988	1988	–	+	+	+	1988	–	–	+
G.D.	54	F	1981	1983	–	+	+	+	1988	–	–	+
G.B.	30	F	1987	1988	+	+	+	+	1988	++	–	+
K.S.	42	M	1984	–	–	+	–	+	not done		+	–
K.H.	31	F	1971	1988	+	+	+	+	not done		++	+
L.D.	39	F	1979	1983	+	+	+	+	1983	++++	++++	+
M.J.	20	F	1984	1984	–	+	+	+	1985	++	++	–
P.Z.	42	F	1980	–	–	+	+	–	1980	++	–	–
R.W.	55	F	1955	1989	+	+	+	+	1979	++	+++	+
W.H.	36	M	1977	1987	+	+	+	+	not done		+	–
W.J.	36	F	1987	1989	++	+	+	–	not done		+++	–
Z.H.	44	F	1972	1983	–	+	+	+	1983	+++	+++	–
Z.H.	33	M	1985	1986	–	+	–	+	1987	–	–	–
Z.E.	30	F	1988	1989	–	+	+	–	not done		++	–
Z.I.	33	F	1984	1986	–	+	+	+	1986	++	–	+

*S = shock; U = urticaria; E = skin oedema; D = dyspnoea (laryngeal oedema).

for intradermal tests. Histamine (1 mg/ml), Sörensen phosphate buffer alone and saline served as positive and negative two controls. Skin tests with noramidopyrine were also done in all the patients. First a prick test with a 0.1% solution of noramidopyrine in saline was done. Than an intradermal test with 0.001% and 0.01% solutions of noramidopyrine were done. In patients with a strongly positive prick test and/or with a history of anaphylactic shock the intradermal testing was started with a 0.0001% solution of noramidopyrine[3,4].

A. Oral challenges with increasing doses of azapropazone

These were done single-blind for 5 days according to the following scheme:

1st day: placebo, twice in 2-hour interval
2nd day: 1 mg followed by 5 mg of azapropazone (if no adverse reaction appeared during the two hours following the first dose)
3rd day: 10, 25 and 50 mg, each dose separated by 2-hour intervals
4th day: 100 and 100 mg separated by 2 hours
5th day: 300 and 300 mg separated by 2 hours

The first four challenges were performed on four consecutive days, while the last one (fifth day) was separated from the preceding one by 3–5 days.

3. Clinical and laboratory measurements

Prior to entry, each patient had a standard medical history taken and a general physical examination performed. Physical examination was repeated at the end of the study or at termination of test drug treatment. Patients were observed by both physician and a nurse for the 5-hour study period.

Pulmonary function tests (FVC, FEV_1, PEF, $MEF_{25,50,75}$) were measured on a flow-integrating computerized pneumotachograph (Jaeger, FRG),. The measurements were made 30, 60, 120, 180, 240 and 300 minutes following ingestion of drug or placebo.

III. DESIGN OF THE STUDY

The study consisted of two phases and was carried out in two distinct groups of patients, i.e. pyrazolone allergy, and aspirin-induced asthma. The aim of the first phase was to give to the investigator the rough estimate of the drug's tolerance. First, skin tests were performed (see above). The drug was then administered in an open trial, as described above, starting with very low doses, to be increased gradually until the dose equivalent to one tablet (600 mg) was reached.

The second phase was to be carried out if the results of the first phase indicated that the patients could tolerate a dose equivalent to one tablet without any major risks. The second phase was a double-blind randomized cross-over trial on the effects of azapropazone vs. placebo in patients with pyrazolone intolerance. The patients received, in a random manner, either placebo or azapropazone 600 mg. Clinical observations and pulmonary function tests were monitored for 5 hours following this challenge. A week or two later each went through the same procedure; if placebo was administered first, then the drug was given at the second session and vice versa. The trial was double-blind.

IV. RESULTS

1. Open study

A. Skin testing

All 12 patients with AIA had negative both prick and intradermal tests with the solvent of azapropazone. Prick tests with 0.1% solution of azapropazone were negative in all 12 patients. Intradermal skin tests with 0.01% solution were negative in all patients. Only one of them had weakly positive skin tests with 0.1% solution of azapropazone. Noramidopyrine tests, both prick and intradermal, were negative in all patients.

In all 15 subjects with hypersensitivity to noramidopyrine and/or aminophenazone, skin tests with azapropazone were negative. In the same subjects, noramidopyrine gave moderately positive skin tests in 5 patients, strongly positive in 4, and negative in the remaining 6.

B. Oral challenges

Twelve patients with aspirin-induced asthma tolerated increasing doses of azapropazone well. None of them developed any adverse symptoms, and the pulmonary function tests remained unaltered.

Similarly, 14 of 15 patients with hypersensitivity to noramidopyrine and/or aminophenazone tolerated azapropazone very well up to the dose of 600 mg. However, in one subject we did observe evident symptoms of adverse reaction. This was a 30 year-old female nurse who for the first time had experienced an attack of urticaria following administration of noramidopyrine i.m. a year before the study. She then suffered from sporadic urticarial eruptions – without any known offending factors. She was accidentally given noramidopyrine after cholecystectomy performed in another hospital 4 months before the study, which resulted in an attack of generalized urticaria. For at least one month preceding the study she was without any urticarial eruptions. Following ingestion of 100 mg of azapropazone, she developed sporadic wheals and mild erythema of the face. When challenged on another occasion with 300 mg azapropazone, she experienced urticaria of the face and trunk with minor oedema of the lips. No hypotension, dyspnoea or changes in spirometric values were observed.

2. Double-blind cross-over study

The patients were the same as in the open study, except for the 30 year-old woman who showed skin eruptions following azapropazone. All 12 patients with AIA and all 14 subjects with intolerance to noramidopyrine/aminophenazone showed very good tolerance of azapropazone. In none of them did we observe any adverse symptoms, and the pulmonary function tests remained unchanged throughout the observation period.

V. DISCUSSION AND CONCLUSIONS

In this study, we have focused our attention on two common types of intolerance to NSAID. Their clinical presentation is reminiscent of allergic reactions. They can be extremely dangerous, leading rapidly to death[4]. The patient is often unaware of his intolerance and there are no biochemical tests to make a diagnosis[4,8]. The problem is further complicated by existence of several distinct types of adverse reactions to NSAIDs[1]. Moreover, in some of these types, the spectrum of intolerance is wide and encompasses various groups of minor analgesics and antiphlogistics.

AIA is the best example of the latter type. It is a common clinical syndrome, which affects about 10% of adult asthmatics[4,9]. In the sensitive patients, the attacks can be precipitated by a large variety of NSAIDs, including such pyrazolones as noramidopyrine, aminophenazone, sulfinpyrazone and phenylbutazone. Those drugs have different chemical structures, but they all share the ability to block cyclo-oxygenase. Azapropazone is a very weak inhibitor of cyclo-oxygenase in $vitro$[10,11]. On a molar basis, indomethacin was found to be 139 times more active than azapropazone and 44 times more active than aspirin in inhibiting the biosynthesis of prostaglandin $F_{2\alpha}$ from arachidonic acid in guinea pig lung homogenates. Similarly, in cultured macrophages, azapropazone was able to diminish prostaglandin production only at high concentrations as compared to other NSAIDs. Our results indicate that, in man, this very weak, if any, inhibitory effect must be negligible, since the tolerance of azapropazone by aspirin-intolerant asthmatics was excellent. It seems, therefore, that azapropazone can be added to a short list of a few NSAIDs prescribed safely to patients with AIA. Before such a conclusion is reached, a study on long-term tolerance of azapropazone in AIA should be performed to evaluate cumulative effects of the drug. Such study is now being carried out in our department.

Patients in the second group studied by us were sensitive to noramidopyrine/aminophenazone. Clinical symptoms produced by those drugs varied from urticaria to shock. The clinical evidence of these reactions was well documented in the medical records. Because of these reactions, most of the patients had already been examined and followed up by us in the past. At the time of the study, skin tests with noramidopyrine were positive in 2/3 of patients. On the contrary, not a single positive reaction was observed with

271

azapropazone. The drug was very well tolerated by 14 of the 15 subjects studied. The mechanism of mild urticaria evoked twice by 100 and 300 mg azapropazone in the same patient is unclear. Perhaps, it had no relation to intolerance to noramidopyrine/aminophenazone since patients with this type of intolerance, as evidenced also in our group, are known to develop adverse reactions to drugs from widely different groups such as antibiotics, sulphonamides and vitamins.

In conclusion, both in an open study and in a double-blind cross-over trial, patients with aspirin-induced asthma showed very good tolerance to azapropazone. Under similar conditions, the drug was also well tolerated by 14 of 15 patients with idiosyncrasy to noramidopyrine/aminophenazone. In only one patient of the latter group, ingestion of azapropazone produced mild urticaria without symptoms of dyspnoea, hypotension or shock.

References

1. Szczeklik, A, Gryglewski, RJ and Czerniawska-Mysik, G (1977). Clinical patterns of hypersensitivity to nonsteroidal anti-inflammatory drugs and their pathogenesis. *J Allergy Clin Immunol*, **60**, 276–84
2. Czerniawska–Mysik, G and Szczeklik, A (1981). Idiosyncrasy to pyrazolone drugs. *Allergy*, **36**, 381–4
3. Szczeklik, A, Czerniawska–Mysik, G and Nizankowska, E (1985). Allergische und pseudoallergische Reaktionen auf Pyrazolonpräparate. In: Brune, K and Lanz, R (eds), 100 *Jahre Pyrazolone—eine Bestandsaufnahme*. (München-Wien-Baltimore: Urban & Schwarzenberg), pp. 247–52
4. Szczeklik, A (1986). Analgesics, allergy and asthma. *Drugs*, **32**, (Suppl. 4), 148–63
5. Voigtländer, V (1985). Dermatologische Nebenwirkungen von Pyrazolonen. In: Brune, K and Lanz, R (eds), 100 *Jahre Pyrazolone—eine Bestandsaufnahme*. (München-Wien–Baltimore, Urban & Schwarzenberg), pp. 261–6
6. Virchow, Chr, Schmitz–Schumann, M and Juhl–Schaub, E (1985). Pyrazolone und Analgetika–Asthma Syndrome. Ibidem, pp. 253–260
7. Fabro, L, Wuetrich, B and Walti, M (1987). Acetylsalicylic acid allergy and pyrazone allergy and pseudoallergy? Results of the skin tests and antibody determinations in a multicenter study. (In German). *Z Hautkr*, **62**, 470–8
8. Schneider, CH, Kasper, MF, De Weck, AL, Rolli, H and Angst, BD (1987). Diagnosis of antibody-mediated drug allergy. Pyrazolinone and pyrazolidine-dione cross-reactivity relationship. *Allergy*, **42**, 597–603
9. Szczeklik, A (1988). Aspirin-induced asthma as a viral disease. *Clin Allergy*, **18**, 15–20
10. Bray, MA and Gordon, D (1978). Prostaglandin production by macrophages and the effect of anti-inflammatory drugs. *Br J Pharmacol*, **63**, 635–42
11. Brune, K, Rainsford, KD, Wagner, K and Peskar, BA (1981). Inhibition by anti-inflammatory drugs of prostaglandin production in cultured macrophages. *Naunyn-Schiedeberg's Arch Pharmacol*, **315**, 269–78

Summary

Both in an open study and in a double-blind cross-over trial patients with aspirin-induced asthma showed very good tolerance to azapropazone. Under similar conditions the drug was also perfectly well tolerated by 14 of 15 patients with idiosyncrasy to noramidopyrine/aminophenazone. In only one patient of the latter group ingestion of azapropazone produced mild urticaria without symptoms of dyspnea, hypotension or shock.

Zusammenfassung

Sowohl in einer offenen als auch in einer doppelblinden, gekreuzten (cross-over) Studie zeigten Patienten mit Aspirin-induzierten Asthma bronchiale eine sehr gute Azapropazon-Toleranz. Unter ähnlichen Bedingungen tolerierten auch 14 von 15 Patienten mit Idiosynkrasie gegenüber Noramidopyrin/Aminophenazon die Substanz ausgezeichnet. Lediglich bei einem Patienten der letzteren Gruppe stellte sich nach Einnahme von Azapropazon eine milde urtikarielle Reaktion ein, wobei Symptome wie Dyspnoe, Hypotonie oder Schock fehlten.

Resumé

Aussi bien dans une étude ouverte que dans un essai en double-insu et cross-over, des patients présentant un asthme induit par l'aspirine, se sont révélés très bien tolérer l'azapropazone. Dans les mêmes conditions, le médicament fut également parfaitement toléré par 14 patients sur 15 qui présentaient une idiosyncrasie à la noramidopyrine/aminophénazone. Chez un seul des patients de ce dernier groupe, l'administration d'azapropazone provoqua un urticaire discrèt, sans symptômes de dyspnée, d'hypotension ou état de choc.

20
Haematological reactions

JF Hort

I. INTRODUCTION

Blood dyscrasias have been associated with virtually all currently available non-steroidal anti-inflammatory drugs (NSAIDs), but the deficiencies in the information available are such that the role of a particular drug in a particular reported dyscrasia has seldom been certain, except in the case of pyrazolones.

In the United Kingdom, the main source of information consists of 'yellow card' reports to the Committee on the Safety of Medicines (CSM). Log–linear trend analysis has been applied by Weber to the number of these reports associated with the occurrence of haematological and other side-effects by different drugs[1]. This author has, however, stressed that the method is 'essentially only a monitoring and signalling system which does not give any indication of the incidence or prevalence of adverse drug reactions (ADR)'. Without describing the reactions further than as 'serious blood dyscrasias', the author gave the estimated number of such reports for azapropazone as 5 per million prescriptions.

Clinically, the conclusions from this mathematical manipulation must depend on the content of the reports which are the raw data, before the value of the figures as a signal can be decided.

Details of these reports are described in this chapter.

II. HAEMOLYTIC ANAEMIA

Although azapropazone is known to have been associated with a positive direct antiglobulin test (DAT), how often this occurs is not known. A total of 22 cases of haemolytic anaemia were reported to the CSM as associated with azapropazone therapy between April 1976 and December 1988. Two patients with strongly positive DATs have been investigated serologically[2]. Two different antibodies were demonstrated in both of these patients, one of the penicillin type and the other of the alpha-methyldopa type.

Azapropazone – 20 years of clinical use. Rainsford, KD (ed)
© Kluwer Academic Publishers. Printed in Great Britain

III. OTHER HAEMATOLOGICAL EFFECTS

Other haematological disorders have been reported as associated with azapropazone therapy, but in no specific case have these been definitely attributed to the drug. Since rechallenge in these situations is unacceptable ethically, absolute certainty as to causation or its absence is impossible. The available evidence can provide only the basis for suggestive implication until an accumulation of sufficient numbers of cases means that some degree of certainty can at least be approached.

IV. CASE REPORTS

Table 1 presents the chief details of all reports to the CSM and Bundesgesundheitsamt (BGA) of blood dyscrasia associated with azapropazone. The type of dyscrasia may be assumed to be the type under which the reporting physician classified a case, but the exact definitions used are not known. For instance, the platelet count which was used in a particular instance to lead the reporter to diagnose thrombocytopenia is not known, nor in one of the cases of pancytopenia are the criteria for this diagnosis known.

The case reports are listed in Table 1 and the known details are given below.

Thrombocytopenia has been reported in two patients who were taking only azapropazone but in neither case was any information on dosage, duration of therapy or temporal relationship between drug and appearance of symptoms provided. In two further cases, thrombocytopenia was the only finding. Both patients were also taking indomethacin and receiving gold salts in the preceding period. In one case, hydrochlorothiazide was also being taken, an agent known to be associated with haematological disorders.

Pancytopenia has been reported twice. In one case, the patient had been on mianserin (which has been associated with bone-marrow depression) for some time and on azapropazone for 3 days. In the second case, the patient had a long history of anaemia associated with a bleeding tendency which culminated in a pancytopenia. During this period he had received phenylbutazone, isopyrin and azapropazone.

Hypoplastic anaemia was reported in a patient who initially developed an influenza-like illness and was given azapropazone for the accompanying aches and pains, taking the drug for 3 days and then stopping because of a rash. One week later, staphylococcal septicaemic shock developed and proved fatal. At post-mortem, the bone marrow was found to be hypoplastic with only scanty haemopoietic activity. Extramedullary haemopoiesis was found in the spleen, suggesting the marrow damage may have been long standing. The inference is that the drug may not have been the cause of the marrow depression.

A further case of hypoplastic anaemia occurred in an elderly man who

276

Table 1 Blood dyscrasias associated with azapropazone reported to CSM and BGA

Type	Drug	Duration of drug use	Additional information
Thrombocytopenia	Azapropazone	Not known	
	Azapropazone	Not known	
	Azapropazone Indomethacin Gold salts	Not known Not known Not known	
	Azapropazone Hydrochlorothiazide Indomethacin Gold salts	Not known Not known Not known Not known	
Pancytopenia	Azapropazone Mianserin	3 days Not known	
	Azapropazone Phenylbutazone Isopyrin	Not known Not known Not known	Long history of anaemia 'Bleeding tendency'
Hypoplastic anaemia	Azapropazone	3 days	
	Azapropazone	10 months at excessive dosage	
Aplastic anaemia	Azapropazone	After discovery of aplasia and during the episode	
	Azapropazone	3 days	
	Azapropazone Another NSAID	Not known 2 months	
	Azapropazone	No information	
Granulocytopenia	Azapropazone	2 months	
	Azapropazone Carbamazepine	14 days Not known	
	Azapropazone Cotrimoxazole	1 month 3 days	Azapropazone continued throughout recovery
	Azapropazone Phenylbutazone	5 days 5 weeks	Dyscrasia discovered 2 months after both drugs stopped
	Azapropazone Gold salts D-penicillamine	Not known Not known } Not known }	Stopped 2 years before dyscrasia During the 2 years before dyscrasia
	Azapropazone Indomethacin Diclofenac Piroxicam	Not known Not known Not known Not known	Intermittently over the 2 years preceding dyscrasia
Marrow depression	Azapropazone Cotrimoxazole	Not known Not known	

had been taking an excessive dose of azapropazone for 10 months. No other details were provided.

Aplastic anaemia has been reported 4 times in association with azapropazone. In one case, the patient started the drug after aplasia was discovered and recovered without azapropazone being withdrawn. In a second case, the only information provided was that the patient had been on azapropazone for 3 days. In a third case, the patient had been taking another NSAID for 2 months and no information was given as to the duration of azapropazone therapy. For the fourth case, there are no details of any kind available.

There have been 6 reports of *granulocytopenia*. In one, the patients had been taking azapropazone for 2 months and no other drug had apparently been taken. In a second case, the patient had been taking carbamazepine for an unknown period and azapropazone for 14 days. Agranulocytosis and aplastic anaemia have been associated with carbamazepine.

In a third case, the patient had been taking cotrimoxazole for 3 days and azapropazone for one month. Cotrimoxazole has been associated with blood dyscrasias. Azapropazone continued to be taken during the period of the patient's recovery. In a fourth case, azapropazone was taken for 5 days and phenylbutazone was taken for 5 weeks, the dyscrasia being discovered 2 months later. The fifth case concerned a patient who developed the dyscrasia some 2 years after ceasing to take azapropazone, during which time she was given both gold salts and D-penicillamine.

A sixth patient had been taking azapropazone, indomethacin, diclofenac and piroxicam at various times and intermittently over the 2 years preceding admission for a fractured femur.

Marrow depression has been reported once in association with cotrimoxazole plus azapropazone.

V. COMMENTS

The 'yellow card' reports of positive DATs and of haemolytic anaemia provided a clear signal that azapropazone could have been causative, since the 22 cases of haemolytic anaemia accumulated in the records at a steady rate over the years and in the great majority of these cases there were no other drugs involved which might have been responsible.

In contrast, reports of other haematological abnormalities associated with azapropazone give a confused picture. Marrow depression or damage from any NSAID is a rare event, but after 20 years of use of this drug, a definite propensity for it to produce a blood dyscrasia has not been signalled. Very rare events would not, however, have produced such a signal; from the cases described above, the possibility of azapropazone being capable of potentiating such effects from other drugs could perhaps be inferred. However, this is unlikely as there is no pattern of co-prescription with any one such drug, and because the low lipophilic activity of azapropazone to a great extent prevents entry of the drug into the bone marrow substance.

References

1. Weber, JCP (1987). Epidemiology in the United Kingdom of adverse drug reaction from non-steroidal anti-inflammatory drugs. In: Rainsford KD and Velo GP (eds), *Side-effects of Anti-Inflammatory Drugs*, Pt.1. Lancaster: MTP Press), pp. 27–35
2. Bird, GWG, Wingham, J, Babb, RG, Bacon, P and Wood, D (1984). Azapropazone association antibodies. *Vox Sang*, **46**, 336–7

Summary

Azapropazone is known to have induced haemolytic anaemia. Other haematological disorders have been associated with azapropazone but the case reports do not provide clear evidence that any of the dyscrasias were caused by the drug.

Zusammenfassung

Es ist bekannt, dass Azapropazon eine hämolytische Anämie auslösen kann. Auch andere hämatologische Störungen wurden mit Azapropazon in Verbindung gebracht, doch die vorliegenden Fallberichte liefern keine eindeutigen Anhaltspunkte dafür, dass zwischen Azapropazon und einer dieser Dyskrasien ein kausaler Zusammenhang besteht.

Resumé

Il est connu que l'azapropazone a induit des anémies hémolytiques. D'autres anomalies hématologiques ont été mises sur le compte de l'azapropazone, mais les dossiers n'apportent pas la preuve définitive que l'une ou l'autre de ces dyscrasies soient dûes au médicament.

21
Epilogue, with some thoughts for research on azapropazone

KD Rainsford

"If it be true that 'good wine needs no bush', 'tis true that a good play needs no epilogue: Yet to a good wine they do use good bushes; and good plays prove the better by the help of good epilogues".

William Shakespeare

Is this the justification for an Epilogue? The first half of this quotation (i.e. to ". . . needs no epilogue") is much quoted (see *The Oxford Dictionary of Quotations*, 2nd Edn. Oxford University Press), but clearly gives the wrong impression without the latter! So by analogy we trust the reader will see the goodness of the content. For the sake of unity or unification of thought an Epilogue is helpful to summarize salient features about azapropazone. This logically serves as a basis to bring forth some reflections and thoughts for future research which the author has taken the liberty of detailing.

We have seen that azapropazone is chemically and pharmacologically somewhat unique among the NSAIDs. We are told the drug is a benzotriazine oxide and in this respect the aromatic moiety of this drug is not evident in any other NSAID. The casual observer may say that the drug is simply a keto-enolic acid and that the aromatic moiety may, by contribution of lipophilicity, simply influence the pharmacokinetics and metabolism of the drug. This is, in fact, true, but ignores the role of the N-dimethylamino group at the 5 position. As Dean and McCormack have elegantly shown the latter group may impose important properties, for the internal molecular association of this group with the 3-carbon enolate group may lead to alterations in ionizability and solubility. This may have profound importance for understanding the low intrinsic ulcerogenicity of the drug in the gastrointestinal (GI) tract. It might also be important in the ways the drug exerts its anti-inflammatory actions by way of its effects on leucocyte emigration, oxyradical production, and lysosomal stabilization, though there is unfortunately no evidence for this suggestion. Likewise, too, it might be asked whether the intramolecular association suggested by McCormack and Dean has any significance in the weak inhibitory effects of azapropazone on the prostaglandin cyclo-oxygenase system. Thus many lines of evidence

Azapropazone – 20 years of clinical use. Rainsford, KD (ed)
© Kluwer Academic Publishers. Printed in Great Britain

suggest that the acidic group of NSAIDs serves as one of the main points of interaction with the active site of the prostaglandin cyclo-oxygenase. The inhibitory effects of these drugs are thought to result from this interaction combined with that from aromatic groups at a "flat site" on the enzyme. If intra-molecular interactions occur between the 3-enolate and the nitrogen of the dimethamino moiety as proposed by Dean and McCormack, then it is possible that this could restrict the potential of the former group to participate in interactions at the active site of the cyclo-oxygenase. This would result in weaker inhibitory actions than would otherwise be possible in a drug without the dimethylamino- moiety. Clearly, this aspect deserves consideration as well as the other structural features of azapropazone which could account for its specific pharmacological properties.

The low GI ulcerogenicity of azapropazone seen in experimental investigations in laboratory animals and in human clinical studies could result from a combination of (a) the weak inhibitory actions on prostaglandin cyclo-oxygenase, (b) its propensity to stabilize the lysosomal membrane at high drug concentrations (in contrast to that of phenylbutazone and other NSAIDs which labilize the membrane of this organelle), and (c) its weak liposolubility which may influence the pattern of GI absorption. It is conceivable that the membrane-stabilizing effect of this drug seen in respect of lysosomal membranes may also be evident with the surface mucosal cell membrane. Could it be that this also accounts for the low ulcerogenicity of the drug, perhaps from the unique intramolecular interaction postulated by McCormack and Dean?

While on the matter of GI ulcerogenicity, there is, paradoxically, a somewhat higher incidence in population studies of adverse drug reaction (ADR) reports. Thus, the low intrinsic GI ulcerogenicity observed in controlled experiments in man and laboratory animals is not vindicated by the ADR reports. What are the reasons for this striking difference? We know that ADR reporting is influenced by a number of non-drug-related effects, e.g. prescribing and usage patterns, various denominator factors etc. What is not known is whether the elderly have a particularly higher incidence of GI, or indeed other, side-effects with azapropazone and whether this is related to the presence of concomitant diseases (other that the arthritic conditions for which these patients receive the medication), or whether the treatment for the non-arthritic conditions affects the efficacy or safety of azapropazone. These are all questions still unresolved. These points could, however, be of considerable significance in explaining the relatively high incidence of ADR reports from azapropazone.

In the comprehensive reviews on the published clinical trials of azapropazone for the treatment of various arthropathies we have seen that this drug gives comparable effectiveness to that of conventional standard drugs. Yet as noted by Buchanan and Bellamy we have seen the need for continuous refinement of clinical trial methodologies (especially the need for placebo controls) for all NSAIDs, not only for azapropazone. This is especially important if we are going to understand:

(a)   Which NSAIDs are best suited for particular arthritic conditions, to enable quantification of benefits of drug therapy for the patient.

(b)   How the drug dosage may need to be adjusted at different phases of the arthritic disease process to improve efficacy and safety.

(c)   Which combinations of NSAIDs such as azapropazone with DMARDs are going to be most efficacious.

One of the successful applications of azapropazone has been in the therapy of gout. A number of studies including previously unpublished work by researchers at duPont (USA) attest to it having urate-lowering properties equal to that of allopurinol. Azapropazone has additional pain-relieving properties which may arise from its other actions as an anti-inflammatory agent and possibly even direct analgesic actions from effects on components of peripheral nerve transmission. In the context of the latter the studies by Wright, Davies, Walker and their co-workers on the analgesic actions at joints of azapropazone were investigated by a novel non-invasive ultrasound–EEG technique. This has given important information on the potential of the drug to inhibit or modulate pain transmission at the level of peripheral or higher nervous centres. While it may be still difficult to eliminate localized anti-inflammatory activity of the drug (i.e. in respect of effects on production of prostaglandins and other inflammatory mediators) it may be possible in the future to modify this model system to include assays of inflammatory mediators, so as to discriminate the anti-inflammatory effects of the drug from its potential influences on pain transmission.

The potential life-threatening side-effects of NSAIDs, though of low frequency, present a major problem for the practising clinician. We have seen from the paper by Hort that in the UK and FRG the overall incidence of haematological reactions with azapropazone is well below that of phenylbutazone. The UK 'Yellow card' reports of positive direct antiglobulin tests and of haemolytic anaemia provide a clear signal that azapropazone could have been causative in a total of 22 cases. No definite cases of bone marrow depression have been identified and no signal for it having the propensity of causing blood dyscrasias has been obtained. In this respect the drug is totally different from the pyrazolones, phenylbutazone and oxyphenbutazone, which are classically regarded as exhibiting such side-effects. As suggested by Hort the physicochemical properties of azapropazone may, with the shorter plasma half-life of the drug, reduce its propensity to accumulate in the bone marrow.

The allergic reactions to NSAIDs are thought to be related, in part, to their actions as cyclo-oxygenase inhibitors. The preliminary studies of Szczeklik and his co-workers suggest that the aspirin sensitivity may not be shared by azapropazone. We await further more detailed investigations of these initial observations with much interest, together with information on the mechanisms of the relative actions of these two drugs.

Some NSAIDs have been implicated in accelerating cartilage and bone destruction in osteoarthritis, while others have been claimed to be 'cartilage-sparing', 'cartilage-protective' or 'chondro-protective'. No agent has, in the opinion of the author, been strictly shown to have the latter two properties in osteoarthritic joints. The effects of NSAIDs on cartilage and bone metabolism and function are potentially very important. The results reported by Walker and co-workers suggest that azapropazone may be less likely to accelerate cartilage and bone destruction in osteoarthritis compared with that of indomethacin. These effects may be related to differences in the effects of the two drugs on cartilage proteoglycan and prostaglandin metabolism. Further comparative studies are underway and, with the inclusion of some placebo-treated subjects (which are difficult to recruit in such a study), will help elucidate the clinically-important features of these various NSAIDs on the progress of joint destruction in osteoarthritis.

We should not forget that the pattern of bone and cartilage destruction in osteoarthritis and the factors that control it may be quite different in this condition from that evident in rheumatoid and other arthropathies. Thus NSAIDs may have quite different effects in different arthritic diseases in the prevention or control of joint destruction. The complex interactions between NSAID effects on prostaglandin synthesis with their resultant actions on production of those cytokines controlling the resorption and turnover of macromolecules in cartilage and bone are also deserving of further detailed investigation.

In conclusion the 'state of the art' of investigations into the mode of action and use of azapropazone give this drug some exciting and interesting prospects for the future.

"Ist es wahr, daß 'der gute Wein keines Kranzes bedarf', so ist es auch wahr, daß ein gutes Stück keinen Epilog nötig hat; jedoch braucht man beim guten Wein gute Kränze, und gute Stücke werden durch gute Epiloge nur um so besser." (*William Shakespeare*)

Ist das die Rechtfertigung für einen Epilog? Die erste Hälfte dieses Zitats (d.h.: bis... "keinen Epilog nötig hat") wird häufig gebraucht, aber vermittelt ohne den Rest natürlich ein völlig falsches Bild! Wir wollen also hoffen, daß der Leser den Inhalt zu schätzen weiß. Zum Zwecke der Geschlossenheit oder der gedanklichen Klärung ist ein Epilog hier durchaus hilfreich, weil er die wichtigsten Merkmale von Azapropazon noch einmal zusammenfaßt. Logischerweise dient er damit als Basis für Überlegungen und Gedanken hinsichtlich zukünftiger Forschungen und der Autor nimmt sich hier die Freiheit, diese Gedanken etwas ausführlicher darzustellen.

Wir haben gesehen, daß Azapropazon aufgrund seiner chemischen und pharmakologischen Eigenschaften eine gewisse Sonderstellung unter den NSAR einnimmt. Wir haben erfahren, daß es sich bei dieser Substanz um ein Benzotriazin-Oxid handelt und der aromatische Teil dieser Substanz wurde bei keinem anderen NSAR gefunden. Der oberflächliche Betrachter wird vielleicht sagen, daß es sich bei dieser Substanz ganz einfach um eine Keto-Enol-Säure handelt und daß der aromatische Teil aufgrund der Lipophilität die Pharmakokinetik und den Metabolismus der Substanz beeinflußt. Das ist in der Tat richtig, aber man läßt dabei die Rolle der N-Dimethylamino-Gruppe in der 5er Stellung außer Acht. Dean und McCormack haben gezeigt, daß diese Gruppe wichtige Eigenschaften für die intramolekulare Assoziation dieser Gruppe mit der 3-Kohlenstoff-Enolat-Gruppe beisteuert, die möglicherweise die Ionisierbarkeit und die Löslichkeit verändern. Das könnte eventuell für das Verstehen der geringen gastrointestinalen Ulzerogenität der Substanz von großer Wichtigkeit sein. Möglicherweise ist das auch wichtig für die Art und Weise, in der die Substanz ihre entzündungshemmende Wirkung entfaltet, nämlich durch ihre Einwirkung auf den Leukozytenaustritt, die Bildung von Sauerstoffradikalen und die Stabilisierung der Lysosomen. Leider gibt es für diese Vermutung keinerlei Beweise. Man fragt sich vielleicht auch, ob der intramolekularen Assoziation, die McCormack und Dean vermuten, irgendeine Bedeutung bei der schwachen Hemmwirkung des Azapropazon auf das Prostaglandin-Cyclooxygenase System zukommt. Verschiedenes Beweismaterial deutet darauf hin, daß die säurebildende Gruppe der NSAR als eine der Hauptinteraktionsstellen mit der aktiven Stelle der Cyclooxygenase fungiert. Man nimmt an, daß die Hemmwirkungen dieser Arzneimittel aus dieser Interaktion in Verbindung mit einer Interaktion der aromatischen Gruppen an einer "flachen Stelle" des Enzyms resultieren. Wenn zwischen dem 3-Enolat und dem Stickstoff des Dimethylamino-Teils intramolekulare Interaktionen auftreten, wie Dean und McCormack vermuten, dann ist es möglich, daß diese Interaktionen das Potential der erstgenannten Gruppe, an den Interaktionen an der aktiven Stelle der Cyclooxygenase teilzunehmen, verringern. Das führt zu einer Schwächung der Hemmwirkung, die sonst bei einer Substanz ohne Dimethylamino-Teil stärker wäre. Diese Möglichkeit ist auf alle Fälle in Betracht zu ziehen, und außerdem sind die anderen strukturellen Merkmale des Azapropazon zu berücksichtigen, die ebenfalls für die spezifischen pharmakologischen Eigenschaften mitverantwortlich sein könnten.

Die in Experimenten mit Versuchstieren und in klinischen Humanstudien festgestellte, geringe gastrointestinale Ulzerogenität des Azapropazons könnte auf eine Kombination aus (a) der schwachen Hemmwirkung auf die Cyclooxygenase, (b) der Neigung zur Stabilisierung der Lysosomenmembran nach Gabe hoher Dosen (diese Wirkung unterscheidet sich von der des Phenylbutazon und anderer NSAR, die die Membran der Organellen destabilisieren) und (c) der schwachen UO-Löslichkeit der Substanz zurückzuführen sein, die das Absorptionsverhalten im Magen-Darm-Trakt beeinflußt. Es ist denkbar, daß die Substanz ihre stabilisierende Wirkung nicht nur auf die Lysosomenmembran ausübt, sondern auch auf die Membranen der obersten Schleimhautzellen. Wäre es dann möglich, daß die geringe Ulzerogenität der Substanz vielleicht auch von der einzigartigen intramolekularen Interaktion herrührt, die McCormack und Dean vermuten?

Da wir uns gerade mit der gastrointestinalen Ulzerogenität befassen, möchte ich dazu noch anmerken, daß paradoxerweise die Anzahl der berichteten Nebenwirkungen bei Populationsstudien höher lag. Das heißt also, daß die in kontrollierten Versuchen am Menschen und an Versuchstieren festgestellte geringe gastrointestinale Ulzerogenität der Substanz nicht durch diese Berichte über unerwünschte Nebenwirkungen bestätigt werden kann.

Was sind die Gründe für diese Diskrepanz? Wir wissen, daß die Erfassung von Nebenwirkungen von einer Reihe von Faktoren beeinflußt wird, bei denen es sich nicht um arzneimittelbedingte Faktoren handelt, wie z.B. bestimmte Verschreibungs- oder Gebrauchs-Gewohnheiten. Dazu kommen noch verschiedene Unterschiede in der Bezeichnung usw. Nicht bekannt ist, ob bei älteren Patienten nach der Azapropazon-Behandlung besonders häufig gastrointestinale Nebenwirkungen oder insgesamt überhaupt mehr Nebenwirkungen auftreten, oder ob das mit den bestehenden Begleiterkrankungen (außer der Arthritis, für die die Patienten eine Begleitmedikation erhalten) zusammenhängt oder ob die Behandlung der nicht-arthritischen Erkrankung die Wirksamkeit und Sicherheit von Azapropazon beeinträchtigt. Alle diese Fragen sind bisher noch ungeklärt. Sie können jedoch sehr wichtig sein, wenn sie dazu beitragen, die relativ hohe Nebenwirkungsrate bei der Azapropazon-Behandlung zu erklären.

Wir haben in den umfassenden Stellungnahmen zu den veröffentlichten klinischen Studien zur Anwendung von Azapropazon bei der Behandlung verschiedener Arthropathien gesehen, daß diese Substanz in ihrer Wirksamkeit mit den herkömmlichen Standardarzneimitteln vergleichbar ist. Schon Buchanan und Bellamy haben auf die Notwendigkeit zur ständigen Verbesserung der Methodologie klinischer Studien hingewiesen, und das gilt für alle NSAR und nicht nur für Azapropazon. Das ist besonders wichtig, wenn wir folgendes verstehen wollen:

(a) Welche NSAR für bestimmte Arthritis-Formen am besten geeignet sind und eine Quantifizierung der Vorteile dieser Behandlung für den Patienten ermöglichen.

(b) Wie die Dosis in unterschiedlichen Stadien der Arthritis anzupassen ist, damit die Wirksamkeit und Sicherheit des Arzneimittels verbessert werden kann.

(c) Welche Kombinationen von NSAR, wie z.B. Azapropazon, mit einem anderen Rheumamittel am wirkungsvollsten sein werden.

Eine der erfolgreichsten Anwendungen von Azapropazon gelang bei der Gichtbehandlung. Eine Reihe von Studien sowie unveröffentlichte Arbeiten von Wissenschaftlern bei duPont (USA) bestätigen, daß die Substanz eine uratsenkende Wirkung hat, die der des Allopurinol vergleichbar ist. Azapropazon hat darüberhinaus auch schmerzlindernde Eigenschaften, die wahrscheinlich von seinen anderen Wirkungen als entzündungshemmende Substanz herrühren, und möglicherweise sogar eine direkte analgetische Wirkung infolge des Einflusses auf die an der Reizübertragung im periphären Nervensystem beteiligten Komponenten. Im Hinblick auf die zuletztgenannte Wirkung untersuchten Wright, Davies, Walker und Mitarbeiter in ihren Studien die analgetische Wirkung von Azapropazon auf die Gelenke mit Hilfe eines neuartigen nichtinvasiven Ultraschall-EEGs. Diese Untersuchungen ergaben wertvolle Informationen über das Potential der Substanz zur Hemmung oder Modulation der Schmerzübertragung auf der Ebene periphärer oder höherer Nervenzentren. Es wird immer noch schwierig sein, die lokale entzündungshemmende Wirkung der Substanz auszuschalten (d.h. angesichts der Wirkung auf die Bildung von Prostaglandinen und anderer Entzündungsvermittler), aber vielleicht wird es in Zukunft eine Möglichkeit geben, dieses Modell zu modifizieren, so daß damit auch die Entzündungsvermittler analysiert werden können, damit man zwischen den entzündungshemmenden Wirkungen der Substanz und seinem potentiellen Einfluß auf die Schmerzübertragung trennen kann.

Die potentiell lebensbedrohenden Nebenwirkungen der NSAR sind zwar selten, stellen aber trotzdem für den praktizierenden Kliniker ein großes Problem dar. Wir haben in der Arbeit von Hort gesehen, daß die Häufigkeit hämatologischer Reaktionen auf Azapropazon in Großbritannien und der BRD insgesamt weit unter der von Phenylbutazon liegt. In Großbritannien sind die "Gelbe Karte"-Berichte über positive, direkte Antiglobulin-Tests und hämolytische Anämie ein deutliches Anzeichen dafür, daß Azapropazon in insgesamt 22 Fällen der auslösende Faktor hätte sein können. Es wurden keine definitiven Fälle von Knochenmarkhemmung festgestellt, und es gibt keine Anhaltspunkte dafür, daß die Substanz zu Dyskrasie führt. In dieser Beziehung unterscheidet sich die Substanz völlig von den Pyrazolonen, Phenylbutazon und Oxyphenbutazon, die bekanntermaßen diese Nebenwirkungen verursachen. Wie Hort vermutete, können die physikalischen und chemischen Eigenschaften des Azapropazon zusammen mit der kürzeren Halbwertszeit der Substanz im Plasma die Tendenz der Substanz, sich im Knochenmark anzureichern, verringern.

Man glaubt, daß die allergischen Reaktionen auf NSAR teilweise mit deren Hemmwirkung auf die Cyclooxygenase zusammenhängen. Die ersten Untersuchungen von Szczeklik und Mitarbeitern deuten darauf hin, daß Azapropazon nicht die Sensitivität des Aspirin besitzt. Gegenwärtig stehen ausführlichere Untersuchungen dieser anfänglichen Beobachtungen noch aus, und wir warten mit Interesse auf weitere Informationen über die Mechanismen der relativen Wirkungen dieser beiden Substanzen.

Bei der Osteoarthritis wurden einige NSAR für die Beschleunigung der Zerstörung von Knorpel und Knochen verantwortlich gemacht, wohingegen von anderen NSAR behauptet wurde, sie seien "knorpelschonend" oder "knorpelschützend". Nach Meinung des Autors konnte streng genommen bei keiner Substanz nachgewiesen werden, daß sie bei Gelenken, die von Osteoarthritis betroffen waren, diese Eigenschaften tatsächlich entwickelt hat. Die Wirkungen der NSAR auf den Metabolismus und die Funktion von Knorpel und Knochen sind sehr wichtig. Die Ergebnisse, über die Walker und Mitarbeiter berichteten, deuten darauf hin, daß Azapropazon im Gegensatz zu Indomethacin dazu neigt, die bei der Osteoarthritis auftretende Knorpel- und Knochenzerstörung zu beschleunigen. Das könnte eventuell mit den unterschiedlichen Wirkungen der beiden Substanzen auf die Knorpel-Proteoglykane und den Prostaglandin-Metabolismus zusammenhängen. Weitere noch laufende Vergleichsstudien, die auch Patienten mit Placebo-Behandlung einschließen (solche Patienten sind für eine derartige Studie schwer zu finden), werden neue Aufschlüsse über die klinisch wichtigen Merkmale der verschiedenen NSAR und deren Einfluß auf den Verlauf der Gelenkzerstörung bei der Osteoarthritis bringen.

Wir sollten dabei aber nicht vergessen, daß das Muster der bei der Osteoarthritis auftretenden Knochen- und Knorpelzerstörung und die Faktoren, die diese Zerstörung steuern, bei diesem Krankheitsbild ganz anders sein können als bei rheumatischen Erkrankungen oder anderen Arthropathien. Deshalb haben NSAR bei verschiedenen Arthritis-Typen ganz unterschiedliche Wirkungen im Hinblick auf die Vorbeugung vor Gelenkzerstörung oder deren Einschränkung. Die komplexen Interaktionen zwischen den Wirkungen der NSAR auf die Prostaglandin-Synthese und die daraus resultierenden Wirkungen auf die Bildung der Zytokine, die die Absorption und den Metabolismus der Makromoleküle im Knorpel und im Knochen steuern, bedürfen ebenfalls noch detaillierterer Untersuchungen.

Abschließend sei gesagt, daß der gegenwärtige Stand der Untersuchungen der Wirkungsweise und Anwendung von Azapropazon diesem Arzneimittel einige vielversprechende Zukunftsaussichten bietet.

> "S'il est vrai qu' 'un bon vin n'a pas besoin de bouchon', il est tout aussi vrai qu'une bonne pièce de théâtre n'a pas besoin d'épilogue: pourtant, pour un bon vin, on utilise un bon bouchon; et les bonnes pièces n'en sont que meilleures grâce aux bons épilogues."
>
> *William Shakespeare*

Est-ce là la justification d'un épilogue? La première partie de cette citation (c'est-à-dire jusqu'à ... "n'a pas besoin d'épilogue") est souvent rapportée (voir *The Oxford Dictionary of Quotations – Dictionnaire des Citations d'Oxford –*, 2ème édition, Oxford University Press), mais donne en réalité une fausse impression si la deuxième partie n'est pas citée! Par analogie, nous espérons que le lecteur réalisera la valeur du texte. Pour respecter l'unité ou la coordination des pensées, un épilogue résumant les caractéristiques principales de l'azapropazone semble approprié. Il doit logiquement servir de base à toute réflexion ou considération portant sur des recherches futures, que l'auteur a pris la liberté de détailler.

Nous avons vu que l'azapropazone a un caractère chimique et pharmacologique quelque peu unique parmi les AINS. On nous dit que ce produit est un oxyde de benzotriazine et, à cet égard, la fraction aromatique de cette substance n'est apparente dans aucun autre AINS. L'observateur occasionnel dira peut-être que le produit est simplement un acide céto-énolique et que la fraction aromatique peut, grâce à la lipophilicité, simplement influencer la pharmacocinétique et le métabolisme du médicament. En réalité, ce fait est correct mais ne tient pas compte du rôle joué par le groupe N-diméthylamine en position 5. Comme Dean et McCormack l'ont parfaitement démontré, ce dernier groupe peut imposer d'importantes propriétés pour l'association moléculaire interne de ce groupe avec le groupe 3-carbone-énolate, conduisant éventuellement à des modifications de l'ionisabilité et de la solubilité. Ce fait peut être d'une importance considérable pour comprendre la faible ulcérogénicité intrinsèque du produit dans le tube gastro-intestinal (GI). Egalement, il peut être important dans la manière dont le produit exerce son action anti-inflammatoire en causant un effet sur la diapédèse leucocytaire, la production d'oxyradicaux, la stabilisation lysosomiale, bien qu'il n'y ait malheureusement aucune preuve corroborant cette hypothèse. De même on pourrait se demander si l'association intramoléculaire suggérée par McCormack et Dean a une signification quelconque relativement au faible effet inhibiteur de l'azapropazone sur le système cyclo-oxygénase des prostaglandines. Donc, d'après différents témoignages, il semblerait que le groupe acide des AINS agisse en tant que l'un des points principaux d'interaction avec le lieu actif de la cyclo-oxygénase des prostaglandines. On pense que les effets inhibiteurs de ces produits sont dus à cette interaction combinée avec celle de groupes aromatiques sur un "lieu plat" de l'enzyme. Si des interactions moléculaires se produisent entre le 3-enolate et l'azote de la fraction diméthylamine, comme le suggèrent Dean et McCormack, il est alors possible que ce fait restreigne le potentiel du groupe antérieur dans sa participation aux interactions du lieu actif de la cyclo-oxygénase, ce qui pourrait causer une action inhibitrice plus faible que celle généralement attendue d'un produit sans fraction diméthylamine. Il est clair que cet aspect mérite d'être étudié ainsi que les caractéristiques structurelles de l'azapropazone qui peuvent expliquer ses propriétés pharmacologiques spécifiques.

Le faible taux d'ulcérogénicité GI de l'azapropazone, relevé lors d'expérimentations sur des animaux de laboratoire et d'études cliniques sur des êtres humains, peut résultater d'une combinaison a) de sa faible action inhibitrice sur la cyclo-oxygénase des prostaglandines, b) de sa tendance à stabiliser la membrane lysosomiale à hautes concentrations (contrairement à la tendance de la phénylbutazone et des autres AINS qui déstabilisent la membrane de cet organite), et c) sa faible solubilité-UO qui peut influencer l'évolution de l'absorption GI. Il est possible que l'effet stabilisateur de ce produit sur la membrane, observé sur les membranes lysosomiales, soit aussi apparent avec la membrane de la cellule muqueuse superficielle. Est-il possible que ce fait soit aussi responsable de la faible ulcérogénicité du produit, peut-être en raison de l'unique interaction intramoléculaire postulée par McCormack et Dean?

Et, à propos d'ulcérogénicité, on note paradoxalement une incidence un peu plus élevée de rapports de réactions indésirables au produit (RIP) lors d'études sur la population. Ainsi, la faible ulcérogénicité GI intrinsèque, observée lors d'essais contrôlés chez l'homme et chez des animaux de laboratoire, n'est pas corroborée par les rapports RIP.

Quelles sont les raisons de cette différence flagrante? Nous savons que les rapports de RIP sont influencés par un nombre d'effets non associés au produit, par exemple les méthodes de prescription et d'utilisation, différents facteurs dénominateurs, etc ... Ce que l'on ne sait pas c'est si les personnes âgées ont une incidence plus élevée d'effets secondaires GI, ou même d'autres effets dus à l'azapropazone, et si ce fait est associé à la présence de maladies concomitantes, (indépendantes de la condition arthritique pour laquelle le malade est soigné), ou si le traitement des symptômes non-arthritiques affecte l'efficacité ou la sécurité de l'azapropazone. Ces questions sont toutes sans réponse. Elles pourraient cependant avoir une signification considérable sur les raisons de la fréquence relativement élevée des rapports de RIP l'azapropazone.

Dans l'étude complète des essais cliniques publiés sur l'azapropazone pour le traitement de différentes arthropathies, nous avons observé que le produit présentait une efficacité comparable à celle des produits classiques standard. Pourtant, comme le remarquent Buchanan et Bellamy, nous avons noté la nécessité d'une amélioration continue des méthodologies cliniques des essais pour tous les AINS, pas seulement pour l'azapropazone. Ce fait est particulièrement important pour que nous arrivions à comprendre:

a) quels sont les AINS les plus appropriés dans le traitement des affections arthritiques spécifiques pour permettre d'accroître les bénéfices thérapeutiques du produit chez le malade;

b) comment la posologie du produit peut être ajustée aux différentes phases de l'évolution de la maladie arthritique pour améliorer l'efficacité et la sécurité du produit;

c) quelles sont les combinaisons les plus efficaces d'AINS comme l'azapropazone, et de PARMA (Produits anti-rhumatismaux modificateurs d'affections – Disease Modifying Anti-rheumatic Drugs – DMARDs).

L'une des applications les plus efficaces de l'azapropazone est son utilisation dans le traitement antigoutteux. Une série d'études, y compris les travaux non publiés de chercheurs de chez duPont (Etats-Unis), rapportent qu'elle présente des propriétés de diminution de l'acide urique égales à celles de l'allopurinol. L'azapropazone a d'autres propriétés anti-douleur découlant sans doute de ses autres actions en tant qu'agent anti-inflammatoire et peut-être même d'actions analgésiques directes provenant d'effets sur les composés de la transmission périphérique nerveuse. Dans le contexte de cette dernière interprétation, au cours d'études réalisées par Wright, Davies, Walker et leurs collègues, l'action analgésique de l'azapropazone sur les articulations fut recherchée au moyen d'une nouvelle technique EEG ultrasonique non sanglante. Ce procédé a fourni d'importantes données sur le potentiel du produit à inhiber ou à moduler la transmission de la douleur au niveau des centres nerveux périphériques ou supérieurs. Même s'il est toujours difficile d'éliminer l'activité anti-inflammatoire localisée du produit (c'est-à-dire en ce qui concerne les effets sur la production des prostaglandines et autres médiateurs inflammatoires) il se peut qu' à l'avenir on puisse modifier ce système-modèle et inclure des essais de médiateurs inflammatoires pour pouvoir distinguer les effets anti-inflammatoires du produit de ses influences éventuelles sur la transmission de la douleur.

Les effets secondaires des AINS pouvant mettre en jeu la vie du malade, bien que rares, présentent cependant un problème crucial pour le clinicien exerçant. Nous avons noté dans le rapport de Hort qu'au Royaume-Uni et en RFA l'incidence générale de réactions hématologiques dues à l'azapropazone est de loin inférieure à celle de la phénylbutazone. Les rapports de "Cartes Jaunes" du Royaume-Uni, relatifs à des tests positifs directs d'antiglobuline et des tests d'anémie hémolytique sont une claire indication du fait que l'azapropazone aurait pu être l'agent pathogène dans un total de 22 cas. Aucun cas certain de dépression médullaire osseuse n'a été observé et aucun signal indiquant une tendance à causer des troubles de la crase sanguine n'a été relevé. Sous ce rapport, le médicament est totalement différent des pyrazolés phénylbutazone et oxyphenbutazone, qui sont connues pour être la cause de tels effets secondaires. Comme le suggère Hort, les propriétés physico-chimiques de l'azapropazone peuvent, avec la demi-vie plasmatique réduite du produit, diminuer sa tendance à s'accumuler dans la moelle osseuse.

Les réactions allergiques aux AINS sont considérées comme étant en partie associées à leur action inhibitrice de la cyclo-oxygénase. Les études préliminaires de Szczeklik et de ses collègues indiquent que la sensibilité à l'aspirine peut ne pas être partagée par l'azapropazone. Nous attendons d'autres investigations plus détaillées de ces premières observations avec grand intérêt, ainsi que des informations sur le mécanisme des actions relatives de ces deux médicaments.

288

Certains AINS ont été impliqués dans l'accélération de la destruction du cartilage et des os dans des cas d'arthrose tandis que d'autres ont été décrits comme "ménageant le cartilage", "protégeant le cartilage" ou tout simplement comme "chondro-protecteurs". Selon l'auteur, aucun agent n'a jamais réellement démontré les deux dernières propriétés dans le cas d'arthrose des articulations. Les effets des AINS sur le métabolisme et la fonction du cartilage et des os sont potentiellement très importants. Les résultats rapportés par Walker et ses collègues indiquent que l'azapropazone est probablement moins susceptible d'accélérer la destruction du cartilage et des os en cas d'arthrose que l'indométacine. Ces effets peuvent être liés à des différences dans les effets des deux médicaments sur le protéoglycane du cartilage et le métabolisme des prostaglandines. D'autres études de comparaison sont en cours, et la collaboration de sujets soumis à des placébos (recrutement difficile pour ce genre d'étude), permettra d'éclairer les caractéristiques cliniquement importantes de ces différents AINS sur l'évolution de la destruction des articulations dans les cas d'arthrose.

Nous ne devons pas oublier que l'évolution de la destruction du cartilage et des os dans les cas d'arthrose ainsi que les facteurs qui la contrôlent peuvent être très différents dans ces cas-ci comparativement aux facteurs rhumatoïdes et autres arthropathies. Donc, selon le genre de maladie arthritique, les AINS peuvent avoir des effets très différents sur la prévention ou le contrôle de la destruction articulaire. D'autres recherches détaillées devraient aussi couvrir les interactions complexes entre les effets des AINS sur la synthèse des prostaglandines, avec les actions qu'ils causent sur la production des cytocines contrôlant la résorption et le renouvellement des macromolécules dans le cartilage et les os.

Pour conclure, les investigations les plus récentes relatives au fonctionnement et à l'utilisation de l'azapropazone offrent à ce produit des perspectives d'avenir captivantes et fort intéressantes.

Index